Medical Herbalism: Principles and Practices of Herbal Medicine

Medical Herbalism: Principles and Practices of Herbal Medicine

Editor: Jonathan Cook

MURPHY & MOORE
www.murphy-moorepublishing.com

www.murphy-moorepublishing.com

MURPHY & MOORE

Cataloging-in-Publication Data

Medical herbalism : principles and practices of herbal medicine / edited by Jonathan Cook.
p. cm.
Includes bibliographical references and index.
ISBN 978-1-63987-360-9
1. Herbs--Therapeutic use. 2. Materia medica, Vegetable. 3. Medicinal plants. 4. Botany, Medical. I. Cook, Jonathan.
RM666.H33 M43 2022
615.321--dc23

Murphy & Moore Publishing,
1 Rockefeller Plaza,
New York City, NY 10020, USA

ISBN 978-1-63987-360-9 (Hardback)

Contents

Preface

It is often said that books are a boon to mankind. They document every progress and pass on the knowledge from one generation to the other. They play a crucial role in our lives. Thus I was both excited and nervous while editing this book. I was pleased by the thought of being able to make a mark but I was also nervous to do it right because the future of students depends upon it. Hence, I took a few months to research further into the discipline, revise my knowledge and also explore some more aspects. Post this process, I begun with the editing of this book.

The use of medicinal plants for the management of diseases and promoting health is termed as medical herbalism. One of the fundamental principles of herbal medicine is that the effect of the whole plant is more potent than its parts. Therefore, the active ingredients are not derived and isolated in herbal medicine. The major focus of herbal medicine is to return the body to a state of balance wherein the body can naturally recover from ailments. Ginger, garlic, Echinacea and dong quai are some of the herbs which are commonly used within this field. Herbal medicine is produced in a variety of forms such as tablets, powders, capsules, teas and extracts. This book discusses the fundamentals as well as modern approaches of medical herbalism. Also included herein is a detailed explanation of the various concepts and applications of herbal medicine. The extensive content of this book provides the readers with a thorough understanding of the subject.

I thank my publisher with all my heart for considering me worthy of this unparalleled opportunity and for showing unwavering faith in my skills. I would also like to thank the editorial team who worked closely with me at every step and contributed immensely towards the successful completion of this book. Last but not the least, I wish to thank my friends and colleagues for their support.

Editor

1

Powerful Properties of Ozonated Extra Virgin Olive Oil

Elisabetta Carata, Bernardetta Anna Tenuzzo and Luciana Dini

Abstract

Extra virgin olive oil has been mainly produced and consumed in Mediterranean countries since ancient times; olive oil is one of the principal ingredients in the Mediterranean diet, and it constitutes the main source of nutritional fat. Aside from the high nutritional content of olive oil, it is also known for its cosmetic and therapeutic properties. In 1956, Thiers obtained satisfactory results in the treatment of scleroderma, stating that olive oil and its derivatives could be considered "a new group of therapeutic agents." Hincky reported the beneficial properties of olive oil in the treatment of dry, senescent and sensitive skins. This has opened a new perspective for the use of the olive fruit, thus contributing to the increase in research about new applications. One such application is ozonized olive oil, which combines the properties of ozone with those of olive oil, to obtain a peerless compound. The composition of olive oil makes it a suitable vehicle for cutaneous absorption, as it is able to stabilize ozone, which is a highly reactive molecule. The oxidant power of ozone has interesting effects on microorganism and on wound healing.

Keywords: extra virgin olive oil, ozone, herbal medicine, antimicrobial activity, wound healing

1. Introduction

Herbal medicine is commonly used to treat skin disorders, and the ethnobotanical remedies are developed in different regions, based on local plants. In particular, two different systems, Ayurvedic herbs, estabilished in India, and the traditional Chinese medicine, which uses the combination of different herbs, are known. In the occidental world, the use of herbal medicine is relative to purified extracts, often substituted for synthetic chemical drugs. In the last years, we assisted an intense return, in the occidental world, to herbal medicine, probably because we are living in the green revolution [1]. The use of vegetable raw materials in the preparation of products for local application on the skin dates back to ancient times. The term phytocosmetics, from Greek *kosmesis,* which means adorn, and *phytos,* which means plant, is used to indicate the predominant and preferential use of botanical derivatives in cosmetic products. The vegetable field is an inexhaustible source of raw materials that, transformed by various processes, find many applications, both as functional substances and as excipients of the products. Contrary to some 50 years ago, when the cosmetic use of medicinal herbs was largely based on the mere observation of the traditional use, today, numerous scientific studies on the properties of plant-based drugs, as well as advanced knowledge on technical-scientific ones that allow to extract the active principles contained in the plants, are available. The herbal phytonutrient offers an enormous amount and heterogeneity of substances, which, by means of various extracellular processes, give rise to extracts with various functional applications. The active constituents of plants are in fact represented by a complex mixture of substances of different chemical nature (tannins, pectins, saponins, flavonoids, essences, fixed oils, etc.) whose concentration in the extract is essentially linked to the particular extraction process. The most widely used vegetable extracts are glycolic extracts, hydroalcoholic extracts, distilled water, dried extracts, oily extracts, essential oils, and vegetable oils. Vegetable oils are obtained by cold squeezing of plant drugs whose active ingredients are characterized by oily texture. The oil is predominantly made up of polyunsaturated fatty acids rich in triglycerides and also contains antioxidant substances, liposoluble vitamins, and the so-called insaponifiable fraction, a complex mixture of substances of extreme interest both from the dermatological and cosmetic field. Olive oil, coconut oil, wheat germ oil, borage oil, and almond oil are the main types of vegetable oils used in cosmetics. Compared to other types of oily ingredients, the advantage of using vegetable oils in cosmetics and cosmeceuticals lies primarily in their particular lipid composition, which is very close to the structure and function of that of the physiologic sebum present in the interstices and the surface of the corneal layer of the epidermis. The very high affinity to the skin sebum gives them an excellent ability to restore the physiological skin barrier by means of a protective, filmogenic, and emollient action. In this chapter, we describe the advantageous effects of ozonated olive oil in the treatment of skin disorders; in fact, olive oil is considered one of the most excellent foods for diet, but it has anti-inflammatory action, so it is used for skin disease. In the chapter, we report information about the safety and mechanism of action on microorganism and on wound healing.

1.1. Olive oil

Olive oil consists of glycerides, such as oleic, arachidic, palmitic, linoleic, and stearic acids, and of phenolic compounds. It is very important in the culinary use, but it has important applications in cosmetic and pharmaceutical fields. The olive tree *Olea europaea* is a common feature of the Mediterranean landscape, with the olive fruit and olive oil being the basic elements in the nutrition of civilizations around the Mediterranean basin for millennia. The principal reason is due to the tree's climatic requirements, which are found in limited areas of the earth's surface [2]. This longevous tree integrates and identifies economically, socially, and culturally with the inhabitants of this land and determines its rural landscape [3]. Even olive leaves have been used in popular medicine. The therapeutic and health properties of olive oil have been known for millennia so much that Hippocrates advised the juice of fresh olives to cure mental illness and wraps to heal ulcers. During the Middle Ages and during the Renaissance, olive oil was used to cure gynecological infections and was considered useful in the treatment of heart disease, fever, and hypertension.

1.1.1. Beneficial effects of olive oil: health properties

Virgin olive oil has been and still is the subject of numerous studies that have attributed great properties to it, both in the field of health and in cosmetology. Various epidemiological studies have shown that the incidence of inflammatory, cardiovascular, and tumor illnesses is generally lower in Mediterranean European countries (such as Greece, Italy, and Spain) than in other western and northern countries [4]. This can be attributed to the high consumption of olive oil in the Mediterranean diet, which contributes to the daily requirement of vitamin E, essential fatty acids, and specific antioxidants, particularly represented by phenolic compounds and tocopherols. In addition, antioxidants have a primary role in resistance to oxidation and hence in the stability of olive oil and have been shown to exert numerous beneficial effects on the human body. The antioxidants' protective effect is mainly due to their ability to inhibit the action of oxygen free radicals, indicated by the acronym ROSs [5]. ROSs are highly reactive species represented by atoms or molecules with one or more electrons being dissipated, capable of generating the so-called oxidative stress. When the organism is subject to an increase in oxidative stress, an increase of F2-isoprostanes (IsoPs) in plasma levels and of urinary excretion is observed. IsoPs are a type of novel compound, structurally similar to prostaglandins, biosynthesized *in vivo* from the free radical–catalyzed peroxidation of arachidonate independent of the cyclooxygenases (COX) [6]. Oxidative stress seems to be the main reason for many chronic and degenerative diseases and skin aging. More specifically, ROSs induce (i) DNA mutations and protein alterations that are the basis of carcinogenesis [7]; (ii) oxidation of low density lipoproteins (LDL) involved in the formation of atherosclerotic plaques [8]; (iii) the onset of chronic intestinal inflammatory diseases, such as Crohn's disease [9]; (iv) probable onset of neurodegenerative diseases, such as Parkinson's disease [10]; and (v) cellular aging, by lipid peroxidation of the membranes, which become more permeable and less effective. All this evidence allows us to understand the importance of antioxidants, even from exogenous sources such as diet. The beneficial effects, and in particular the antitumor activity, of olive oil on human health are attributed to the high content of phenolic substances with high antioxidant power [11]. Phenolic compounds, in synergy with α-tocopherol and coenzyme Q, protect cells from oxidative damage by contrasting the toxic effects of ROS [12]. Through various epidemiological studies, the correlation between the consumption of virgin olive oil and the risk of onset of certain types of cancer has been demonstrated, such as breast [13], lung [14], colon [15], ovary [16], pancreas [17], and prostate cancer [18]. It has been shown that among the phenolic compounds, one of the most biologically active is hydroxytyrosol (3,4-DHPEA) that is able to inhibit the 5-lipoxygenase enzyme, by reducing the production of leukotriene B4 in the leukocytes, originating from the metabolism of the eicosanoids [19]. In addition, hydroxytyrosol is able to inhibit *in vitro* the oxidation of LDL [20] and *in vivo* [21] the aggregation of platelets [22]. Some experimental studies have also shown that the phenolic extract of virgin olive oil and two isolated compounds, the dialdehyde form of hydroxytyrosol (3,4-DHPEA-EDA) and thiol (p-HPEA-EDA), are able to inhibit uncontrolled cellular proliferation by blocking the cell cycle at G0/G1 and to induce apoptosis in some lines of cancer cells, as demonstrated for HL60 cells of promyelocytic human leukemia [23, 24]. However, compounds with greater biological activity are those containing the ortho-diphenol residues; it has been shown that 3,4-DHPEA and 3,4-DHPEA-EDA are more effective than p-HPEA and p-HPEA-EDA in protecting DNA from damage caused by oxidation [25]. In an *in vitro* study, by examining different virgin olive oil extracts, a chemoprotective effect was demonstrated on HL60 cell lines in relation to their composition but not to the total content of phenolic substances [26]. ROS production is also closely related to inflammatory processes in which the cyclooxygenase enzymes (COX-1 and COX-2), belonging to the oxidoreductase class, catalyze the conversion of arachidonic acid into prostaglandins. The p-HPEA-EDA, also called oleocanthal, has the ability to inhibit the activity of such enzymes and has a pharmacological effect similar to that of ibuprofen, which belongs to the class of nonsteroidal anti-inflammatory drugs [27]. It has also been shown that the consumption of olive oil may improve blood pressure regulation and cholesterol content in the blood; these events, together with the inhibition of platelet aggregation and the reduction of LDL oxidation, are important to prevent the onset of atherosclerotic plaques and, in general, cardiovascular pathologies [28, 29]. Olive oil also contains many monounsaturated fatty acids, including oleic acid, which is a key component of cellular membranes and can progressively replace polyunsaturated fatty acids. Membranes rich in monounsaturated fatty acids are more fluid and less subject to lipid peroxidation [30]. Some studies have also shown that regular intake of this food may result in a reduction in the risk of developing diabetes [31]. The therapeutic properties of olive oil include a laxative effect and stimulation of biliary function [32]. Finally, some studies on animal models have shown that the intake of olive oil can help to counteract the damage caused by epidermal ultraviolet radiation [33].

1.1.2. Dermatological and cosmetic properties

In recent years, in a number of fields, including cosmetics, there has been a renewed interest in materials of natural origin, particularly those of vegetable origin. Since ancient times, olive oil has been known not only for its high nutritional power but also for its cosmetic and therapeutic properties [34]. In 1971, Thiers was still pointing to its potential use in the cosmetic sector. To date, olive oil is certainly the most appreciated natural ingredient, alongside jojoba and avocado oils. The topical application of olive oil may be advised for its soothing action and its beneficial effects on eczema, surface wounds, and burns [35, 36]. In particular, the presence of phytosterols and triterpenoid compounds offers revitalizing and soothing properties for the skin. Vitamins E and A have an intense antioxidant action and have the ability to prevent irritation and aging of the skin, to help maintain its softness, smoothness, stability, and elasticity. As a result, in the cosmetic field, olive oil can be used to prevent signs of aging as a soothing emollient for dry skin and to strengthen hair [37]. Indeed, it is very often a component of lotions, lip balms, shampoos, bath oils, and massage oils. From a dermatologic point of view, olive oil has also proven to have antimicrobial activity, *in vitro*, against some positive and negative Gram and various types of fungi, including *Candida* spp. [38]. Some components of olive oil, especially certain aliphatic aldehydes, inhibit elastase activity; this enzyme is involved in the virulence process [39]. Olive oil is an important component of some topical formulations used in the treatment of inflammatory and mycotic skin diseases [40]. The unsaponifiable fraction is rich in numerous active ingredients with sebum-regulating and moisturizing properties, as well as emollients; it can be a component of cosmetic products (in the form of creams, balms, gels, etc.) for the treatment of delicate, dry, and cracked skin. In fact, the unsaponifiable fraction is very useful in the case of particularly vulnerable skin, such as that of infants and children, or in the case of xerotic skin, such as that of the elderly. Skin hydration is above all important in the neonatal period and especially in premature infants: some clinical trials have been conducted to highlight the beneficial effects of emollient topical treatment [41, 42]. Furthermore, the unsaponifiable fraction exerts a good photoprotective effect on ultraviolet exposed skin: various studies have shown that the application of olive oil may reduce the incidence of skin epithelial tumors on UV-B–exposed mice compared to a control group [43, 44]. The unsaponifiable fraction can also be an additive in makeup products with the purpose of making them easier to apply, softer, and smoother. Butter contains high quantities of squalene (which is the most important constituent of sebum), waxes, and esters that guarantee high penetration of the skin. Butter is ideal for massages or as a vehicle for other active ingredients used in skin care. It acts also as an emollient and moisturizing agent, promoting skin elasticity and preventing the onset of wrinkles. Finally, it can be used as an additive in photoprotective products or in skin hygiene products due to its ability to neutralize aggressive detergent action.

An interesting and powerful way to use extra virgin olive oil is with ozone. The process of ozonization allows the properties of ozone gas to be combined with those of olive oil; the result is a peerless compound. Since ancient times, ozone has also been used in a large number of medical indications [45–49].

2. Ozone

Ozone is an oxygen derivative and is known primarily for its ecological role in the Earth's balance, absorbing most of the ultraviolet radiation from the sun and preventing it from reaching humans in a harmful way. It is an unstable gas that cannot be stored; in fact, it dissolves in very short time. Ozone is totally neutral to the human body, and in fact, it does not (i) modify pH, (ii) irritate skin or mucous membranes, (iii) damage hair or clothing, (iv) interact with drugs, and (v) cause allergic reactions. This molecule has been subjected to countless studies, and in particular, its strong oxidation capacity has been tested in order to underline its disinfectant and sanitizing properties principally applied as a disinfectant of drinking and waste water [45–47]. To this purpose, the dedicated design and construction of equipment for the production of gaseous ozone for air and water purification are increasing. But research into the properties of ozone has yielded promising results in biological applications, thus confirming the ozone activity in stimulating natural cell defenses and increasing their energy availability. Indeed, since ancient times, ozone has also been used in a large number of medical indications [48, 49]. Scientific studies have shown that ozone, while being highly unstable, can be trapped inside vegetable oils. These are composed of triglycerides in which saturated and unsaturated fatty acids are present, which have the ability to retain ozone, thus allowing them to prolong their use. In addition, the greater the amount of unsaturated fats present, the greater the amount of ozone that will be retained [50]. Therefore, when extra virgin olive oil is ozonated, the produced product combines the beneficial properties of extra virgin olive oil with those of ozone. There are countless ozone-based products on the market, and in particular, in our laboratory, we have developed Bioxoil™, an ozonated extra virgin olive oil available in pharmacies. This product is exclusively made from olive cultivars from Puglia and Salento and the oil is ozonated by an innovative patented method (number: M2011A001045 titled: "Process for the ozonization of a vegetable oil") that confers quality and efficiency in various fields of application; in particular, Bioxoil™ is indicated for the treatment of acne, herpes, psoriasis, fungal infections, bed sores, and wounds in general, due to its healing and disinfectant properties (**Figure 1**).

Bioxoil™ is produced from extra virgin olive oils from two local *cultivars*, *Ogliarola* and *Cellina*, in Salento (Apulia, Italy). The ozone reacts with unsaturated compounds through the known Criegee mechanism. The quality of extra virgin oil is very important to obtain a higher grade of ozonization; for this reason, during the process, it is necessary to control different physical and chemical parameters. Of these parameters, the most important is the temperature, and in fact, during the reaction, the temperature increases provoking an alteration of antioxidant content. The oils' peroxide content and acidity value that indicate the level of hydrolytic modification and primary and secondary oxidation of oil are analyzed and reported in **Table 1**. Peroxide index (PI) and acidity index (AI) after ozonization of oils increase with respect to relative controls. In particular, *Cellina*'s oil sample has an acidity index of 0.2% and a peroxide index of 12 mmol O_2 kg^{-1}, while related ozonated oil has an AI of 1.8% and a PI of 533 mmol O_2 kg^{-1}. *Ogliarola*'s oil sample presents an acidity index of 0.3% and a peroxide index of 13 mmoli O_2 kg^{-1}, while respective ozonated oil has an AI of 1.3% and the PI increases to 677 mmoli O_2 kg^{-1}.

In our experiments, the ability of ozone to react with olive oil and in particular with the carbon-carbon double bonds present in unsaturated fatty acids was demonstrated by gas liquid

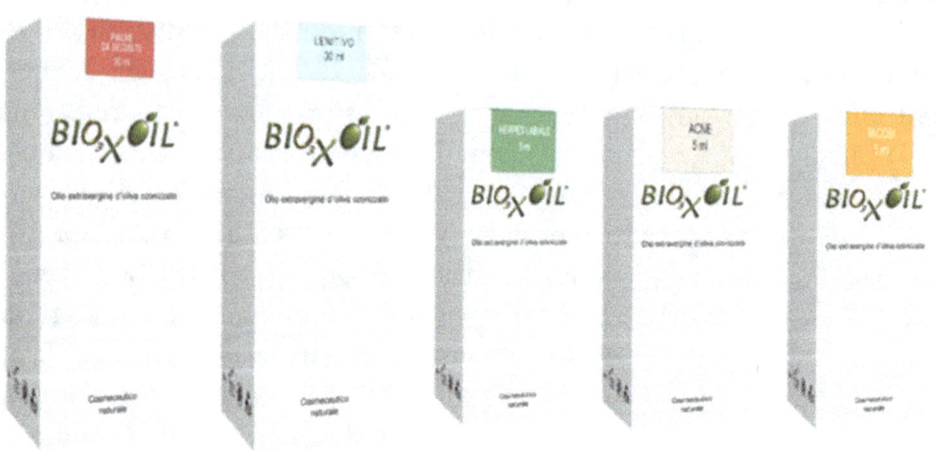

Figure 1. Bioxoil™ products. The Bioxoil products have different applications. Bioxoil with a red label is indicated for bed sores; the sky blue label is indicated as soothing medication; the green label is indicated for herpes labialis; the pink label is indicated for acne; and the orange tag is indicated for mycosis.

Sample	Acidity index (AI), % (means ± SD)	Peroxide index (PI), mmol O_2 kg^{-1}, (means ± SD)
Ogliarola olive oil	0.2 ± 0.03	12 ± 1.2
Ozonated Ogliarola olive oil	1.8 ± 0.02	533 ± 1.5
Cellina olive oil	0.3 ± 0.02	13 ± 1.5
Ozonated Cellina olive oil	1.3 ± 0.01	677 ± 1.6

Table 1. Physicochemical parameters of *Ogliarola* olive oil and *Cellina* olive oil after ozonization procedure.

Composition of fatty acids (%)	*Cellina*	*Cellina*	*Ogliarola*	*Ogliarola*
	Control	Ozonated oil	Control	Ozonated oil
Palmitic acid	12.45	11.91	11.89	11.30
Linolenic acid	5.57	2.19	4.96	2.06
Cis-oleic acid	**70.27**	**39.82**	**67.00**	**41.25**
Trans-oleic acid	8.22	6.68	7.88	7.2
Stearic acid	3.48	1.29	3.32	3.22
Nonanal	0	11.69	0	10.07
Nonanoic acid	0	1.36	0	1.98

Table 2. Composition of fatty acids in olive oil samples *Cellina* and *Ogliarola*.

chromatography (GLC). The composition of fatty acids of each olive oil and respective ozonated oil are analyzed by GLC. Data demonstrate that the amount of oleic acid decreases in both ozonized oil samples: in *Cellina*'s ozonated oil, we observed a 30% reduction, while in *Ogliarola*'s ozonized oil, the reduction was about 26% (**Table 2**). During the ozonization reaction, ozone etches mainly the double bond of acid oleic, the most abundant fatty acid in olive oil (about 80%). This explains the decrease in oleic acid and the contemporary appearance of new compounds, which are the reaction's products, among which are nonanal aldehyde and nonanoic acid, both compounds with nine carbon atoms (**Table 2**). In both cultivar ozonized oils, the composition of fatty acids changes, showing a gradual decrease in unsaturated fatty acids (C 18:1, C 18:2), with a gradual increase in ozone doses.

3. Biocompatibility of ozonated olive oil with skin

The skin is the largest organ of the body and is the major barrier between the inside and outside of our body. It is formed of two main layers: the epidermis, a thin outer portion, and the dermis, the connective tissue layer of skin. This portion is involved in the thermoregulation process, and the resident dermal fibroblasts secrete collagen, elastin, and substances that offer support and elasticity of the skin. The epidermis is subdivided into four layers: (i) the stratum germinativum (SG) that provides the germinal cells necessary for the regeneration of epidermidis; (ii) the stratum spinosum (SS), in which the cells divided in the SG start to accumulate many desmosomes on their surface; (iii) the stratum granulosum (SGR), in which the keratinocytes accumulate dense basophilic keratohyalin granules that contain lipids, which help to form a waterproof barrier; and (iv) the stratum corneum (SC), the outermost layer, in which the cells are dead. The skin is constantly exposed to the environmental stress of pollutants or cigarette smoke, for example, so it is necessary for the wellness of the skin to preserve it from oxidative stress. To this purpose, there are a variety of antioxidants that include glutathione peroxidase, superoxide dismutase, catalases, and nonenzymatic low-molecular weight antioxidants such as vitamin E isoforms, vitamin C, glutathione (GSH), uric acid, and ubiquinol. Interestingly, the distribution of antioxidants in the SC follows a gradient with higher concentrations in deeper layers [51].

The biocompatibility of Bioxoil™ was investigated by MTT assay on fibroblast 3T3 and on keratinocytes HaCaT and compared with ozonated *dulcis* almond oils and nonozonated olive oil as controls. The MTT test values the cell metabolic activity and, in particular, measures the activity of oxidoreductase by reduction of the tetrazolium bromide dye in formazan. The *dulcis* almond oil was chosen because it is largely used in cosmetics, and as it is an oil, it is a possible vector of ozone. Data reported in **Figure 2** demonstrate the Bioxoil™ biocompatibility for both cell types. The viability of cells never significantly decreased in relation to the control and was the same as the nonozonated oil. Conversely, once ozonated, 10% of *dulcis* almond oil had a very significant negative effect on the viability of fibroblasts and keratinocytes but not when *dulcis* almond oil was nonozonated. Interestingly, the vitality test demonstrated that when these cells are exposed to a mixture of ozonated olive oil and 10% of ozonated *dulcis* almond oil (3:1), the adverse event induced by the ozonated almond oil alone was partially prevented (**Figure 2**).

3.1. Biological action of ozonides

By combining the beneficial properties of extra virgin olive oil with that of ozone, the ozonated extra virgin olive oil becomes very powerful for the topical treatment of acute and chronic skin lesions. The ozonides generated during the ozonization procedure possess many properties including a high germicidal activity on fungi, yeasts, viruses, and bacteria; activation of local microcirculation; stimulation of granulation and tissue growth; and revitalization of epithelial tissues.

3.1.1. Germicidal activity

The excessive consumption of antibiotics for the treatment of infectious diseases has fuelled the drug resistance phenomenon, *i.e.*, the microorganisms are resistant to antibiotics. Therefore, it is necessary to develop new molecules with antibiotic properties, preferably natural and nonsynthetic. In fact, this research is divided into the field of synthetic molecules produced by the chemical/pharmaceutical industry and the field of natural active compounds, in which plant extracts are studied also by the use of green chemistry. The plants are able to withstand fungal and bacterial infections and therefore their secondary metabolites can be applied in the field

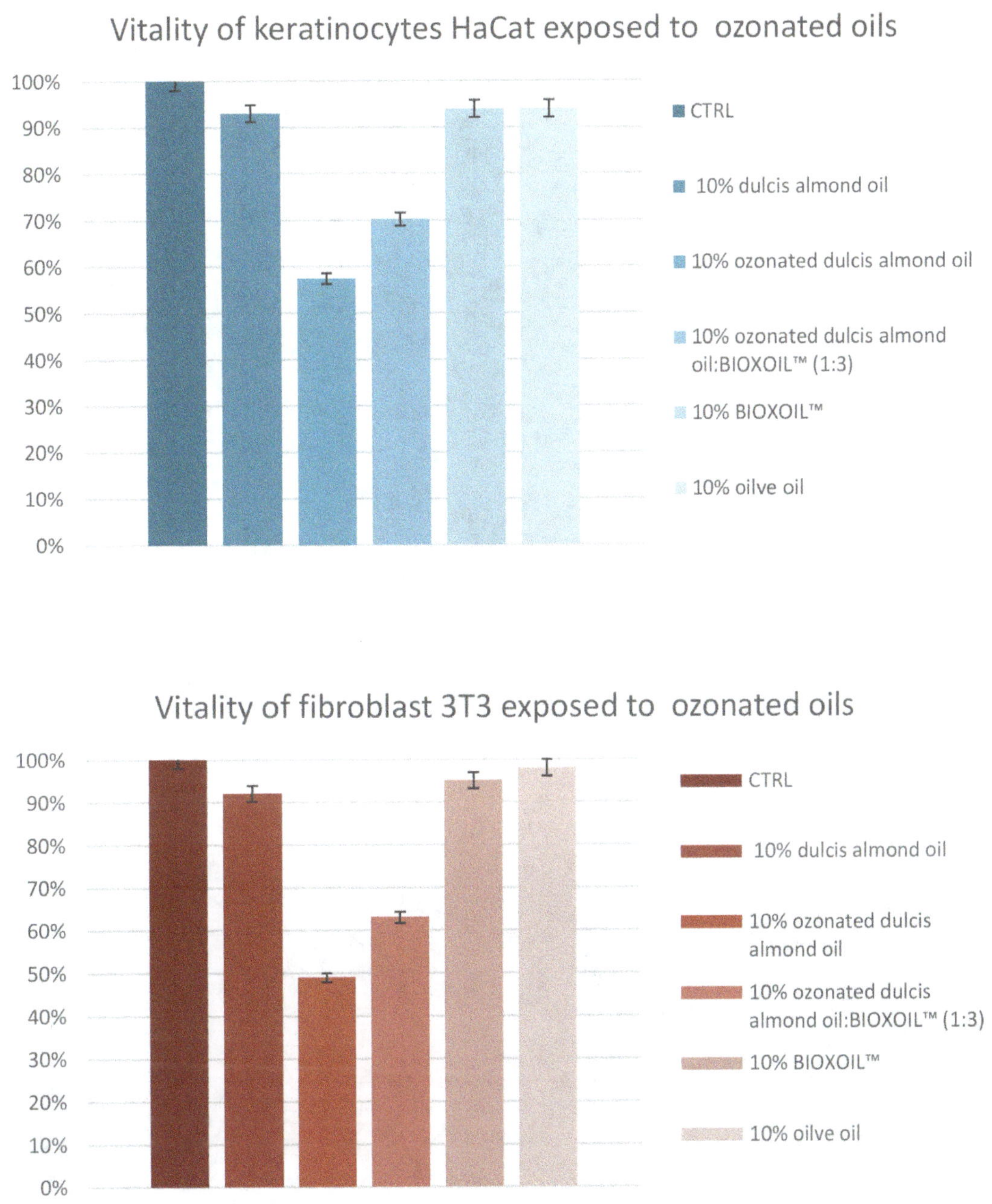

Figure 2. MTT assay on fibroblasts and keratinocytes.

of medicinal herbs. Maoz and Neeman in their research reported an antifungal action of olive oil due to the high content of oleic acid [52]. The ozonated oil increases this natural capacity, because ozone acts on microorganisms, thanks to its greater oxidizing power; in fact, it is able to break down the macromolecules that are the basis of the vital integrity of bacterial cells, fungus, protozoa, and viruses. The ozone in contact with the microorganism's lipoproteins forms H_2O_2 and the final products of lipid oxidation (LOP); H_2O_2 assures bacteriostatic and bactericidal activity, while final lipid oxidation products have induction activity and reactivate metabolic functions (**Figure 3**). Nagayoshi et al. [53] reported the capability of ozone to destroy Gram-positive and -negative microorganisms, and in particular, Gram-negative bacteria are more sensitive.

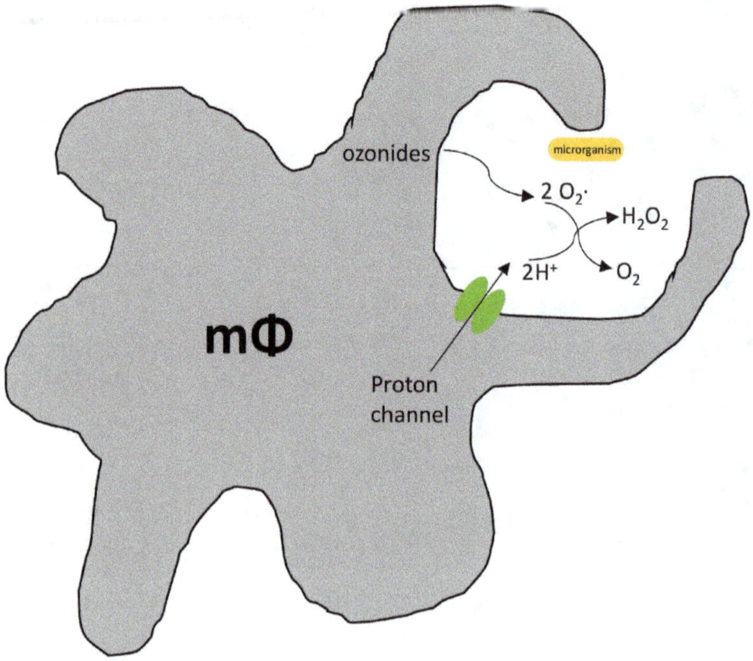

Figure 3. Molecular mechanism of antimicrobial activity of ozonides: the oxygen internalized from ozonides reacts with the proton/protons in order to form H_2O_2 that has a bacteriostatic and bactericidal activity.

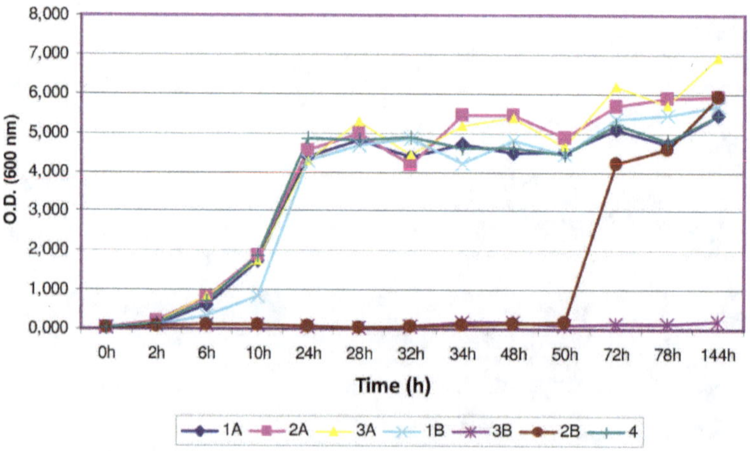

Figure 4. Growth curves of mycete *Epidermophyton floccosum* in liquid culture medium: 1A, 2A, and 3A are the positive controls with 12.5, 25, and 50 mg/ml of nonozonized olive oil, respectively; 1B, 2B, and 3B are ozonized olive oil samples with 12.5, 25, and 50 mg/ml of ozonized olive oil, respectively; 4 is the negative control.

For virus inactivation, a higher gas dosage than that required for bacteria is necessary. The ozone oxidates and subsequently inactivates the specific viral receptors used to bind the cell wall for virus invasion [54]. We tested the antibacterial activity of Bioxoil™ on mycete *Epidermophyton floccosum*, demonstrating its efficacy in the inhibition of mycete's growth in liquid and agar medium; the bacteriostatic effect is obtained in the presence of 5 μl/ml of ozonated olive oil, and the bactericidal effect is obtained in the presence of 15 μl/ml (**Figure 4**).

The antibacterial activity of Bioxoil™ was also tested on *Staphylococcus aureus* and *Staphylococcus epidermidis*, and its efficacy in inhibiting microbes growing both in liquid medium culture and in agar medium was demonstrated. We defined the minimal inhibitory concentration (MIC) of 50 mg·ml^{-1} for *S. aureus* and of 25 mg·ml^{-1} for *S. epidermidis*. This study confirms that ozonated olive oil has antimicrobial properties, which can be exploited for cutaneous infections, by slow release of O_3, which displays effective disinfectant and stimulatory activities that lead to rapid healing.

3.1.2. Biological activity

The ozonides easily penetrate the cell membrane and, thanks to their biological properties, stimulate skin cells and improve the tropism of the skin by promoting wound healing and repair of ulcers of various kinds; from the experiments, it was found that topical application of products based on ozonides has determined a considerable increase of fibroblasts resulting in increased production of collagen, glycosoaminoglycans, and formation of elastic and reticular fibers. The healing of skin lesions includes complex movements like tissue hemorrhage, inflammation, re-epithelialization, granulation tissue, and finally remodeling. These events involve the coordination of many cell types and matrix proteins, which are important for the control of the various stages of tissue repair. Previous studies have shown that endogenous growth factors, such as fibroblast growth factor (FGF), growth factor derived from platelets (PDGF), the TGF-β factor, and vascular endothelial growth factor (VEGF) are important regulators in the healing of wounds [55]. They are released by macrophages, fibroblasts, and keratinocytes at the site of injury and participate in the regulation of re-epithelialization, formation of granulation tissue, collagen synthesis, and neovascularization [56–58]. The beneficial effects of ozone in the treatment of sores are due to the decrease of bacterial infection and the increasing oxygen tension in the wound. In the literature, it is reported that after exposure to ozone transcription factors are activated, such as NF-kB, and these are important regulators of the inflammatory response and tissue repair process [58]. In conclusion, the ozonated olive oil can accelerate acute cutaneous wound repair, by stimulation of dermal fibroblast, and the ozonized oil has shown to be effective against Gram-negative and -positive bacteria, mycetes, and viruses, so it can be used for the cure of infections.

4. Conclusions

The goal of pharmacological research has always been that of finding drugs that can cure diseases or soothe the pain that derives from them, and this research has evolved over the years in an extraordinary way both in the field of medical knowledge and scientific studies that are more and more powerful and sophisticated. Medicinal herbs, long popular in many parts of the world, are increasingly spreading in the western world and represent a large commercial market with an estimated annual growth of 25%, often replacing synthetic drugs. Among the medicinal herbs, particular interest is reserved to olive oil, called "yellow gold" by the Egyptians for its innumerable beneficial properties. Herbal trade today sees many products based on olive oil for both hygiene and personal care. In the field of oil-based products, particular interest is directed to products containing ozonated oil; these products are the result of the union of the beneficial properties of olive oil with those of ozone. Ozonated oil is the most practical, innovative, harmless, and noninvasive of the techniques of application developed in the field of ozone therapy over the last 130 years. It has demonstrated interesting therapeutic results. The biological effects of ozone include antimicrobial activity (antibacterial, antiviral, and antifungal), antalgic action, and improved O_2 metabolism [59]. In this chapter, the possible applications of the Bioxoil™ products, already distributed in pharmacies and herbalist's shops, have been described; its production line includes five different products characterized by different concentrations of ozonides such as to allow the use for the most varied skin affections. Bioxoil with the highest content of ozonides is indicated for the treatment of bedsores at first and second stages, thanks to its anti-inflammatory and cicatrizing properties, Bioxoil with medium concentrations, but different from each other, is indicated for the treatment of herpes labialis, mycosis, and onychomycosis and for acne due to its antimicrobial action. Finally, Bioxoil with the lowest ozonide content is indicated to soothe contact or allergic irritations. The exceptional usability of the product and its completely natural origin offers a vast market.

Abbreviations

ROS	reactive oxygen species
IsoPs	F2-isoprostanes
COX	cyclooxygenase
LDL	low density lipoprotein
3,4-DHPEA	hydroxytyrosol
3,4-DHPEA-EDA	3,4-dihydroxyphenylethanol-elenolic acid dialdehyde
p-HPEA-EDA	2-(4-hydroxyphenyl)ethyl (4E)-4-formyl-3-(2-oxoethyl)hex-4-enoate
COX-1	cyclooxygenase 1
COX-2	cyclooxygenase 2
PI	peroxide index
AI	acidity index
SG	stratum germinativum
SS	stratum spinosum
SGR	stratum granulosum
SC	stratum corneum
GSH	glutathione
LOP	lipid oxidation
MIC	minimal inhibitory concentration

Author details

Elisabetta Carata[1], Bernardetta Anna Tenuzzo[1] and Luciana Dini[1,2*]

*Address all correspondence to: luciana.dini@unisalento.it

1 Department of Biological and Environmental Science and Technology, Lecce, Italy

2 CNR-Nanotech Centro Ecotekne, Lecce, Italy

References

[1] Shenefelt PD. Herbal Treatment for Dermatological Disorders. In: Wachtel-Galor S, editor. Herbal Medicine: Biomolecular and Clinical Aspects. 2nd ed. Boca Raton (FL): CRC Press/Taylor & Francis; 2011. Chapter 18. https://www.ncbi.nlm.nih.gov/pubmed?term=Benzie%20IFF%5BEditor%5D Benzie IFF, https://www.ncbi.nlm.nih.gov/pubmed?term=Wachtel-Galor%20S%5BEditor%5D

[2] Grigg D. Olive oil, the Meditarranean and the world. GeoJournal. 2001;**53**:163-172

[3] Loumou A, Giourga C. Olive groves: The life and identity of the Mediterranean. Agriculture and Human Values. 2002;**20**:87-95

[4] Trichopoulou A, Katsaiyanni K, Giardelles C. The traditional Greek diet. European Journal of Clinical Nutrition. 1993;**47**:576-581

[5] Viola G, Salvador A, Vedaldi D, Fortunato E, Disaro S, Basso G, Queiroz RP. Induction of apoptosis by photoexcited tetracyclic compounds derivatives of benzo[b]thiophenes and pyridines. Journal of Photochemistry and Photobiology B: Biology. 2006;**82**:105-116

[6] Morrow JD, Awad JA, Roberts LJ II, Burk RF. Isoprostanes—Prostaglandin-like compounds formed in vivo independently of cyclooxygenase. Gastroenterology Clinics. 1996;**25**:409-427

[7] Nakae D, Kobayashi Y, Akai H, Andoh N, Satoh H, Ohashi K, Tsutsumi M, Konishi Y. Involvement of 8-hydroxyguanine formation in the initiation of rat liver carcinogenesis by low dose levels of *N*-nitrosodiethylamine. Cancer Research. 1997;**57**:1281-1287

[8] Berliner JA. Atherosclerosis: Basic mechanisms. Circulation. 1995;**91**:2488-2496

[9] Orlando RC. Mechanisms of epithelial injury and inflammation in gastrointestinal diseases. The American Journal of Gastroenterology. 1995;**107**:8-15

[10] Jenner P, Orlando CW. Oxidative stress and the pathogenesis of Parkinson's disease. Neurology. 1996;**47**:161-170

[11] Vissers MN, Zock PL, Katan MB. Bioavailability and antioxidant effects of olive oil phenols in humans: A review. European Journal of Clinical Nutrition. 2004;**58**(6):955-965

[12] Visioli F, Poli A, Galli C. Antioxidant and other biological activities of phenols from olives and olive oil. Medical Research. 2002;**22**:65-75

[13] Martin-Moreno JM, Willet WC, Gorgojo L, Banegas JR, Fernandez Rodriguez JC, Maisonneuve P, Boyle P. Dietary fat, olive oil intake and breast cancer risk. International Journal of Cancer. 1994;**58**:774-780

[14] Fortes C, Forastiere F, Farchi S, Mallone S, Trequattrinni T, Anatra F. The protective effect of the Mediterranean diet on lung cancer. Nutrition and Cancer. 2003;**46**:30-37

[15] Stoneham M, Goldacre M, Seagroatt V, Gill L. Olive oil, diet and colorectal cancer: An ecological study and a hypothesis. Journal of Epidemiology and Community Health. 2000;**54**:756-760

[16] Bosetti C, Negri E, Franceschi S, Talamini R, Montella M, Conti E, Pagona L, Parazzini F, La Vecchia C. Olive oil, seed oils and other added fats in relation to ovarian cancer (Italy). Cancer Causes and Control. 2002;**13**:465-470

[17] Soler M, Chatenoud L, La Vecchia C, Franceschi S, Negri E. Diet, alcohol, coffee and pancreatic cancer: Final results from an Italian study. European Journal of Cancer Prevention. 1998;**7**:455-460

[18] Hodge AM, English DR, McCredie MRE, Severi G, Boyle P, Hopper JL, Giles G. Foods, nutrients and prostate cancer. Cancer Causes and Control. 2004;**15**:11-20

[19] Petroni A, Blasevich M, Papini N, Salami M, Sala A, Galli C. Inhibition of leukocyte leukotriene production by an olive oil-derived phenol identified by mass-spectrometry. Thrombosis Research. 1997;**87**:15-322

[20] Grignaffini P, Roma P, Galli C, Catapano AL. Protection of low-density lipoprotein from oxidation by 3,4-dihydroxyphenyletanol. Lancet. 1994;**343**:1296-1297

[21] Wiseman SA, Mathot JN, De Fouw NJ, Tijburg LB. Dietary nontocopherol antioxidants present in extra virgin olive oil increase the resistance of low-density lipoproteins to oxidation in rabbits. Atherosclerosis. 1996;**120**:15-23

[22] Petroni A, Blasevich M, Salami M, Papini N, Montedoro GF, Galli C. Inhibition of platelet aggregation and eicosanoid production by phenolic components of olive oil. Thrombosis Research. 1995;**78**:151-160

[23] Della Ragione F, Cucciolla V, Borriello A, Della Pietra V, Pontoni G, Racioppi L, Manna C, Galletti P, Zappia V. Hydroxytyrosol, a natural molecule occurring in olive oil, induces cytochrome *c*-dependent apoptosis. Biochemical and Biophysical Research Communications. 2000;**278**:733-739

[24] Fabiani R, De Bartolomeo A, Rosignoli P, Servili M, Selvaggini R, Montedoro GF, Di Saverio C, Morozzi G. Virgin olive oil phenols inhibit proliferation of human promyelocytic leukemia cells (HL60) by inducing apoptosis and differentiation. Journal of Nutrition. 2006;**136**:614-619

[25] Fabiani R, Rosignoli P, De Bartolomeo A, Fuccelli R, Servili M, Montedoro GF, Morozzi G. Oxidative DNA damage is prevented by extracts of olive oil, hydroxytyrosol, and other olive phenolic compounds in human blood mononuclear cells and HL60 cells. Journal of Nutrition. 2008;**138**:1411-1416

[26] Fabiani R, Sepporta MV, Mazza T, Rosignoli P, Fuccelli R, De Bartolomeo A, Crescimanno M, Taticchi A, Esposto S, Servili M, Marozzi G. Influence of cultivar and concentration of selected phenolic constituents on the in vitro chemopreventive potential of olive oil extracts. Journal of Agriculture and Food Chemistry. 2011;**59**:8167-8174

[27] Beuchamp GK, RSJ K, Morel D, Lin J, Pika J, Han Q, Lee CH, Smit AB, Breslin PA. Phytochemistry: Ibuprofen-like activity in extra-virgin olive oil. Nature. 2005;**437**:45-46

[28] Bakthuridze G, Andguladze D, Kobeshavidze G. Using of olive oil for preventing the cardiovascular diseases in Georgia. Chemistry and Physics of Lipids. 2005;**136**:158

[29] Turner R, Etienne N, Garcia AM, De Pascual-Teresa S, Minihane AM, Weinberg PD, Rimbach G, Antioxidant. Anti-atherogenic activities of olive oil phenolics. International Journal for Vitamin and Nutrition Research. 2005;**75**:61-70

[30] Scislowski V, Bauchart D, Gruffat D, Laplaud PM, Durand D. Effects of dietary n-6 or n-3 polyunsaturated fatty acids protected or not against ruminal hydrogenation on plasma lipids and their susceptibility to peroxidation in fattening steers. Journal of Animal Science. 2005;**83**:2162-2174

[31] De Leonardis A, Macciola V. A study on the lipid fraction of Adriatic sardine filets (Sardinapilchardus). Molecular Nutrition. 2004;**43**:209-212

[32] Burlando B, Verotta L, Cornara L, Bottini-Massa E. In: Libro, editor. Herbal Principles in Cosmetics: Properties and Mechanisms of Action. Boca Raton, Fla.: CRC Taylor & Francis Group; 2010. ISBN 9781439812136

[33] Ichihashi M, Ueda M, Budiyanto A, Bito T, Oka M, Fukunaga M, Tsuru K, Horikawa T. UV-induced skin damage. Toxicology. 2003;**189**:21-39

[34] Nullo F, Proserpio C. La FormaciónTaquetrén en Cañadón del Zaino (Chubut) y sus-relacionesestratigráficas en el ambito de la Patagonia, de acuerdo a la flora, República Argentina. Revista de la Asociación Geológica Argentina. 1975;**30**:133-150

[35] Al-Waili NS, Saloom KS. Effects of topical honey on post-operative wound infections due to gram positive and gram negative bacteria following caesarean section and hysterectomies. European Journal of Medical Research. 1999;**4**(3):126-130

[36] Tabassum N, Hamdani M. Plants used to treat skin diseases. Pharmacognosy Reviews. 2014;**8**(15):52-60

[37] Aburjai T, Natsheh FM. Plants Used in Cosmetics. Wiley Online Library; 2003

[38] Al-Waili NS, Saloom KS, Al-Waili TN, Al-Waili AN. The safety and efficacy of a mixture of honey, olive oil, and beeswax for the management of hemorrhoids and anal fissure: A pilot study. The Scientific World Journal. 2006;**6**:1998-2005

[39] Battinelli L, Daniele C, Cristiani M, Bisignano G, Saija A, Mazzanti G. In vitro antifungal and anti-elastaseactivity of some aliphatic aldehydes from Olea europaea L. fruit. Phytomedicine. 2006;**13**:558-563

[40] Baumann LS. Less-known botanical cosmeceuticals. Dermatologic Therapy. 2007;**20**: 330-342

[41] Darmstadt GL, Saha SK, Nawshad Uddin Ahmed ASM, Chowdhury MA, Law P, Ahmed S, Alam MA, Black R, Santosham M. Effect of topical treatment with skin barrier-enhancing emollients on nosocomial infections in preterm infants in Bangladesh: A randomised controlled trial. Lancet. 2005;**365**:1039-1045

[42] Darmstadt GL, Hossain M, Yoonjoung C, Mahfuza S, Luke MC, Maksuda BA, Samir K. Safety and effect of chlorhexidine skin cleansing on skin flora of neonates in Bangladesh. Pediatric Infectious Disease Journal. 2007;**26**:492-495

[43] Budiyanto A, Ahmed NU, Wu A, Bito T, Nikaido O, Osawa T, Ueda M, Ichihashi M. Protective effect of topically applied olive oil against photocarcinogenesis following UVB exposure of mice. Carcinogenesis. 2000;**21**(11):2085-2090

[44] Ichihashi M, Ahmed NU, Budiyanto A, Wu A, Bito T, Ueda M, Osawa T. Preventive effect of antioxidant on ultraviolet-induced skin cancer in mice. Journal of Dermatological Science. 2000;**23**:45-50

[45] Alvarez M, O'Brien RT. Mechanisms of inactivation of poliovirus by chlorine dioxide and iodine. Applied and Environmental Microbiology. 1982;**44**:1064-1071

[46] Legnani PP, Leoni E, Baraldi M, Pinelli G, Bisbini P. Evaluation of disinfection treatment systems for municipal wastewater reclamation and reuse. Zentralblatt fur Bakteríologie Mikrobiologie und Hygiene Series A. Medical Microbiology Infections. 1996;**98**:552-566

[47] Arana I, Santorum P, Muela A, Barcina I. Chlorination and ozonation of waste-water: comparative analysis of efficacy through the effect on *Escherichia coli* membranes. Journal of Applied Microbiology. 1999;**86**:883-888

[48] Alvarez R, Menendez S, Peguera M, Turrent J. Treatment of primary pioderma with ozonized sunflower oil. In: Second International Symposium on Ozone Applications, Havana. Havana, Cuba: National Center for Scientific Research; 1997. p. 76

[49] Morris G, Menendez S. Oleozon in gynecology. In: Second International Symposium on Ozone Applications, Havana, Cuba, March 24-26. Havana, Cuba: National Center for Scientific Research; 1997; p. 73

[50] Uysal B. Ozonated olive oils and the troubles. Journal of Intercultural Ethnopharmacology. 2014;**3**:49-45

[51] Valacchi G, Fortino V, Bocci V. The dual action of ozone on the skin. British Journal of Dermatology. 2005;**153**:1096-1100

[52] Maoz M, Neeman I. Effect of inula viscose extract on chitin synthesis in dermatophytes and Candida albicans. Journal of Ethnopharmacology. 2000;**71**:479-482

[53] Nagayoshi M, Fukuizumi T, Kitamura C, Yano J, Terashita M, Nishihara T. Efficacy of ozone on survival and permeability of oral microorganisms. Oral Microbiology and Immunology. 2004;**19**:240-246

[54] Geweely NSI. Antifungal activity of ozonized olive oil (oleazone). International Journal of Agriculture and Biology. 2006;**8**(5):670-675

[55] Sechi LA, Lezcano I, Nunez N, Espim M, Dupre IÁ, Pinna A, Molicotti P, Fadda G, Zanetti S. Antibacterial activity of ozonized sunflower oil (Oleozon). Journal of Applied Microbiology. 2001;**90**:279-284

[56] Barrientos S, Brem H, Stojadinovic O, Tomic-Canic M. Clinical application of growth factors and cytokines in wound. Wound Repair and Regeneration. 2014;**22**(5):569-578. DOI: 10.1111/wrr.12205

[57] Ballas CB, Davidson JM. Delayed wound healing in aged rats is associated with increased collagen gel remodelling and contraction by skin fibroblasts, not with differences in apoptotic or myofibroblast cell populations. Wound Repair and Regeneration. 2001;**9**(3):223-237

[58] Werner S, Grose R. Regulation of wound healing by growth factors and cytokines. Physiological Reviews. 2003;**83**(3):835-870

[59] Travagli V, Zanardi I, Valacchi G, Bocci V. Ozone and ozonated oils in skin diseases: A review. Mediators of Inflammation. 2010:1-9. DOI: 10.1155/2010/610418

2

Herbal Medicines in African Traditional Medicine

Ezekwesili-Ofili Josephine Ozioma and
Okaka Antoinette Nwamaka Chinwe

Abstract

African traditional medicine is a form of holistic health care system organized into three levels of specialty, namely divination, spiritualism, and herbalism. The traditional healer provides health care services based on culture, religious background, knowledge, attitudes, and beliefs that are prevalent in his community. Illness is regarded as having both natural and supernatural causes and thus must be treated by both physical and spiritual means, using divination, incantations, animal sacrifice, exorcism, and herbs. Herbal medicine is the cornerstone of traditional medicine but may include minerals and animal parts. The adjustment is ok, but may be replaced with –' Herbal medicine was once termed primitive by western medicine but through scientific investigations there is a better understanding of its therapeutic activities such that many pharmaceuticals have been modeled on phytochemicals derived from it. Major obstacles to the use of African medicinal plants are their poor quality control and safety. Traditional medical practices are still shrouded with much secrecy, with few reports or documentations of adverse reactions. However, the future of African traditional medicine is bright if viewed in the context of service provision, increase of health care coverage, economic potential, and poverty reduction. Formal recognition and integration of traditional medicine into conventional medicine will hold much promise for the future.

Keywords: African, traditional, medicine, spirituality, divination, herbalism

1. Introduction

The development and use of traditional herbal medicine (THM) have a very long historical background that corresponds to the Stone Age. In the continent of Africa, the practice of traditional healing and magic is much older than some of the other traditional medical sciences [1] and seems to be much more prevalent compared to conventional medicine. African traditional medicine is a form of holistic health care system that is organized into three levels of specialty, which include divination, spiritualism, and herbalism, though these may overlap in some situations [2, 3].

A traditional healer is one who provides medical care in the community that he lives, using herbs, minerals, animal parts, incantations, and other methods, based on the cultures and beliefs of his people. He must be seen to be competent, versatile, experienced, and trusted [4]. In other definitions, priestesses, high priests, witch doctors, diviners, midwives, seers or spiritualists, and herbalists are included. Traditional medical practitioner (TMP), however, seems to be a modern acceptable concept agreed on by the Scientific Technical and Research Commission (STRC) of the Organization of African Unity (OAU), which is now African Union (AU). In specific cultures, these people go by their local names, depending on their tribe, such as *Sangoma* or *inyanga* in South Africa, *akomfo, bokomowo* in Ghana, *niam-niam, shaman,* or *mugwenu* in Tanzania, *nga:nga* in Zambia, *shaman or laibon* in Kenya, and *babalawo, dibia,* or *boka*, etc. in Nigeria [5]. It is commonplace to see traditional healers dressed in certain peculiar attires, with head bands, feathers, and eyes painted with native chalk.

Figure 1 below is a typically adorned traditional healer from South Africa.

Traditional medicine is viewed as a combination of knowledge and practice used in diagnosing, preventing, and eliminating disease. This may rely on past experience and observations handed down from generation to generation either verbally, frequently in the form of stories, or spiritually by ancestors or, in modern times, in writing [6]. It has also been said that before attaining knowledge in traditional African medicine, one is often required to be initiated into a secret society, as many characteristics of this form of medicine can only be passed down to initiates. The importance of traditional medicine, however, dwindled during the colonial period, whereby it was viewed as inferior to Western medicine. It was thus banned completely in some countries due to its association with witchcraft /voodoo, supernatural, and magical implications, in which case, it was also termed *"juju"* (Nigeria) or "native medicine," since it made use of charms and symbols which were used to cast or remove spells. Some forms of treatment may also involve ritual practices such as animal sacrifices to appease the gods, if the ailment was envisaged to be caused by afflictions from the gods, especially in the treatment of the mentally ill patients.

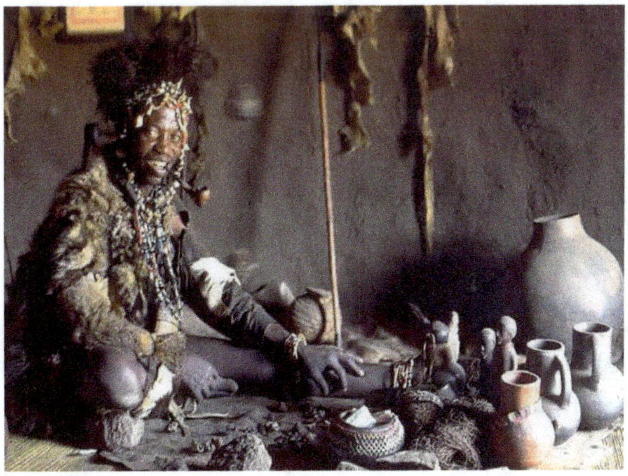

Figure 1. Spiritual healer or *Sangoma* from South Africa (Source—Ancient Origins).

2. Concept of illness and disease

In African traditional setting, there was always an explanation as to why someone was suffering from a certain disease at a particular time. According to Ayodele [7], diseases mostly revolve around witchcraft/sorcery, gods or ancestors, natural, as well as inherited. Illness in the African society is different from the allopathic Western medicine point of view. Illness is believed to be of natural, cultural, or social origin [8]. Cultural or social illness is thought to be related to supernatural causes such as angered spirits, witchcraft, or alien/evil spirits, even for conditions now known to be well understood in modern medicine such as hypertension, sickle-cell anemia, cardiomyopathies, and diabetes. African traditional beliefs consider the human being as being made up of physical, spiritual, moral, and social aspects. The functioning of these three aspects in harmony signified good health, while if any aspect should be out of balance, it signified sickness. Thus, the treatment of an ill person involves not only aiding his/her physical being but may also involve the spiritual, moral, and social components of being as well. Many traditional medical practitioners are good psychotherapists, proficient in faith healing (spiritual healing), therapeutic occultism, circumcision of the male and female, tribal marks, treatment of snake bites, treatment of whitlow, removal of tuberculosis lymphadenitis in the neck, cutting the umbilical cord, piercing ear lobes, removal of the uvula, extracting a carious tooth, abdominal surgery, infections, midwifery, and so on. According to Kofi-Tsekpo [9], the term "African traditional medicine" is not synonymous with "alternative and complementary medicine." African traditional medicine is the African indigenous system of health care and therefore cannot be seen as an alternative.

3. Herbal medicine

Herbal medicine is a part and parcel of and sometimes synonymous with African traditional medicine. It is the oldest and still the most widely used system of medicine in the world today. It is used in all societies and is common to all cultures. Herbal medicines, also called botanical medicines, vegetable medicines, or phytomedicines, as defined by World Health Organization (WHO) refers to herbs, herbal materials, herbal preparations, and finished herbal products that contain whole plants, parts of plants, or other plant materials, including leaves, bark, berries, flowers, and roots, and/or their extracts as active ingredients intended for human therapeutic use or for other benefits in humans and sometimes animals [10, 11].

Herbal medicine is a special and prominent form of traditional medicine, in which the traditional healer, in this case known as the herbalist, specializes in the use of herbs to treat various ailments. Their role is so remarkable since it arises from a thorough knowledge of the medicinal properties of indigenous plants and the pharmaceutical steps necessary in turning such plants into drugs such as the selection, compounding, dosage, efficacy, and toxicity. The use of herbal medicines appears to be universal in different cultures. However, the plants used for the same ailments and the modes of treatment may vary from place to place. The plants used for medicinal purposes are generally referred to as medicinal plants, i.e., any plant in which one or more of its organs/parts contain substances that can be used for therapeutic purposes, or in a more modern concept, the constituents can be used as precursors for the synthesis of drugs. For example, a number of plants have been used in traditional medicine for many years without scientific data to back up their efficacy. In this case, these plants, whole or parts, which have medicinal properties, are referred to as crude drugs of natural or biological origin. They may further be classified as "organized drugs," if such drugs are from plant parts with cellular structures such as leaf, bark, roots, etc., and "unorganized drugs," if they are obtained from acellular portions of plants such as gums, balsams, gels, oils, and exudates. Compared with modern allopathic medicine, herbal medicine is freely available and can easily be accessed by all [12, 13]. As a result, there is limited consultation with traditional healers because there is a fairly good knowledge of common curative herbs especially in the rural areas except in the case of treatment of chronic diseases [12]. Even where consultation is done, there is lack of coherence among traditional healers on the preparation procedures and correct dosage of herbal medicines [14]. However, according to WHO [15], at least 80% of people in Africa still rely on medicinal plants for their health care. In Nigeria, and indeed the entire West Africa, herbal medicine has continued to gain momentum, some of the advantages being low cost, affordability, availability, acceptability, and apparently low toxicity [16, 17].

A detail of plant parts used in herbal medicines is as follows:

1. Roots—i.e., the fleshy or woody roots of many African plant species are medicinal. Most of the active ingredients are usually sequestered in the root bark rather than the woody inner part.
2. Bulbs—A bulb is an underground structure made up of numerous leaves of fleshy scales, e.g., *Allium sativa* (garlic) and *Allium cepa* (onions).
3. Rhizomes—Woody or fleshy underground stem that grows horizontally and brings out their leaves above the ground, e.g., *Zingiber officinale* (ginger), which is used for respiratory problems; *Imperata cylindrica* (spear grass) for potency in men and *Curcuma longa* (turmeric), an antioxidant, anti-inflammatory, and anticancer drug.
4. Tubers—Swollen fleshy underground structures which form from stems/roots, e.g., potatoes and yams such as *Dioscorea dumetorum (ona-(igbo))* for diabetes and *Gloriosa superba* for cancer.
5. Bark—The outer protective layer of the tree stem or trunk. It contains highly concentrated phytochemicals with profound medicinal properties. A host of plants have barks of high medicinal value.
6. Leaves, stems, and flowers of many plants are also medicinal.
7. Fruits and seeds also contain highly active phytochemicals and essential oils.
8. Gums, exudates, and nectars, which are secreted by plants to deter insects and grazing animals and to seal off wounds, are very useful in the pharmaceutical industries.

Sale of herbs in form of dried or fresh plant parts is as lucrative as the prepared medicines. They are usually displayed in markets and sold with instructions on how to prepare them for maximum efficacy.

Figure 2 is a photograph of an herbalist displaying his herbs for sale.

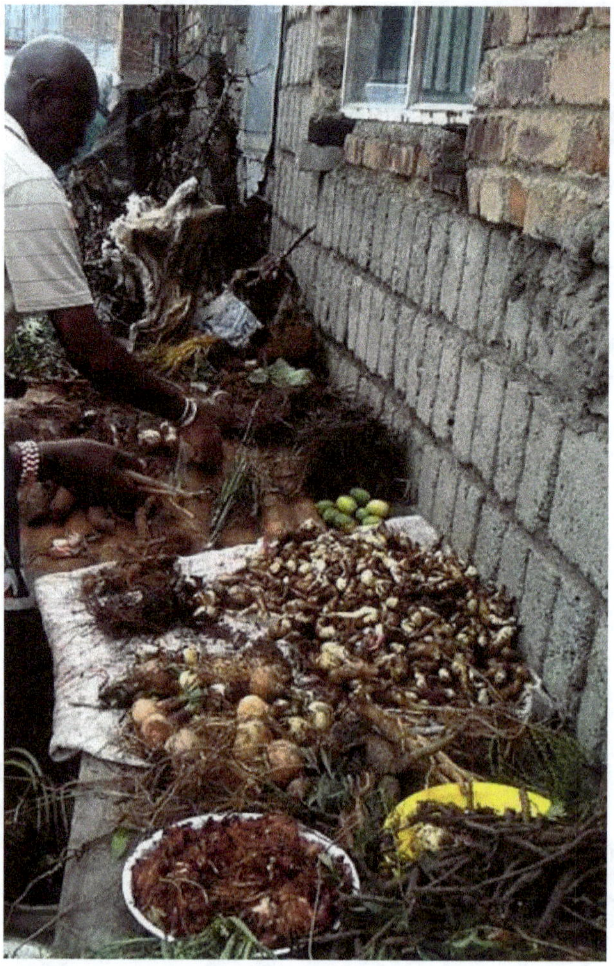

Figure 2. Herbs on display (Source—Ancient Origins).

In many areas of Africa, the knowledge of plant species used and the methods of preparing and administering the medication, especially for serious ailments, still reside with traditional healers. Secrecy and competition still surround the use of these medications, with the healers often being reluctant to hand down their knowledge to anyone but trusted relatives and initiates [18].

3.1. Methods of preparation and dosage forms

Methods of preparation of herbal medicines may vary according to place and culture. The plant materials may be used fresh or dry. With experience, a particular method is chosen to increase efficiency and decrease toxicity. Generally, different methods of preparation include:

1. Extraction—This is prepared with solvent on a weight by volume basis. Sometimes, the solvent is evaporated to a soft mass.
2. Infusions are prepared by macerating the crude drug for a short period of time in cold or hot water. A preservative such as honey may be added to prevent spoilage.
3. Decoctions are made by boiling woody pieces for a specified period of time and filtered. Potash may be added to aid extraction and as preservative.

4. Tinctures are alcoholic infusions which if concentrated may be diluted before administration.

5. Ashing—The dried parts are incinerated to ash, then sieved and added as such to water or food.

6. Miscellaneous—Other types include liniments for external applications in liquid, semi-liquid, or oily forms containing the active substances; lotions which are liquid preparations intended for skin application. Poultices are prepared from macerated fresh part of plant containing the juice from the plant and applied to skin. Snuffs are powdered dried plant inhaled through the nostrils. Dried plants may be burnt, and their charcoal is used as such. Gruels are cereals/porridges made from grains, to which dried powdered plant or its ash is added to be taken orally. Mixtures are sometimes prepared with more than one plant to give synergistic or potentiating effects of the composite plants.

There are also different methods of administration. Apart from the common routes such as oral, rectal, topical, and nasal, other methods include smoking a crudely prepared cigar containing dried plant materials or by passive inhalation. Others are steaming and inhaling the volatile oils exuding from the boiling plant material. These can be used to relieve congestion, headaches, or pulmonary problems. Sitz baths are used for piles [19, 20].

3.2. Ethnobotanical surveys

Information on plants is obtained through ethnobotanical surveys, which involves the study of plants in relation to the culture of the people. Many plants are used in African traditional medicine, but little information is available on their active ingredients/constituents. Ethnobotanical surveys involve the interaction with the people and their environment and are therefore participatory approaches, in which local people are able to contribute their knowledge on the uses of plants within their environment. This may involve the identification, documentation, conservation, and utilization of medicinal plants. Much of the ethnomedicinal information is largely not validated. In Nigeria, a number of authors have published a lot of data on plants with their curative values [16, 20, 21]. These provide a vast array of information for scientific research and validation. Preliminary scientific knowledge is drawn from studies on *in vitro* and *in vivo* bioassays on crude extracts of various plants.

Using plants as medicine provides significant advantages for treating many chronic conditions. For example, information from folklore medicine in Nigeria has it that *Rauvolfia vomitoria* is used for treating hypertension and other nervous conditions while *Ocimum gratissimum* is used for treating diarrheal diseases. Others include *Citrus paradise* seeds for resistant urinary tract infections, pure honey for chronic wound treatment, *Carica papaya* seeds for intestinal parasites, *Garcinia kola* seeds for pain and inflammation, and *Aloe vera* for skin diseases. The same is also true for plants from other African countries [22]. Knowledge of most of these curative properties was accumulated over time from evidence-based observations. A few examples of some Nigerian plants and their uses are shown in **Table 1**.

Table 1 shows some selected Nigerian medicinal plants and their uses.

The curative properties of herbal medicine are validated through scientific investigations, which seek to understand the active chemistry of the plants [23]. The therapeutic activity of a plant is due to its complex chemical nature with different parts of the plant providing

Family	Specie	Local name	Part used	Medicinal uses
Acanthaceae	*Acanthus montanus*		Stem, twig	Syphilis, cough, emetic, vaginal discharge
Amaranthaceae	*Amaranthus spinosus*		Whole plant	Abdominal pain, ulcers, gonorrhea
Apocynaceae	*Alstonia boonei*		Root, bark, leaves	Breast development, filarial worms
Bombacaceae	*Adansonia digitata*		leaves, fruit, pulp, bark	Fever, antimicrobial, kidney, and bladder disease
Combretaceae	*Combretum grandiflorum*	Ikedike	leaves	Jaundice
Euphorbiaceae	*Bridelia ferruginea*	iri, kirni	leaves, stem, bark, root	insomnia, mouth wash, gonorrhea
Hypericaceae	*Harungana madagascariensis*	Otoro, alilibarrafi	Stem, bark, root bark	piles, trypanosomiasis
Fabaceae	*Afzelia africana*	Apa-igbo, akpalata	leaves, roots, bark, seeds	gonorrhea, hernia
Liliaceae	*Gloriosa superba*	mora, ewe aje, baurere	tubers, leaves	gonorrhea, headlice, antipyretic

Table 1. Some selected Nigerian medicinal plants and their uses. Source: Abd El-Ghani [51].

certain therapeutic effects. Chemical components or phytochemicals found in plants that are responsible for the various therapeutic effects include alkaloids, glycosides, tannins, acids, coumarins, sterols, phenols, etc. Many modern pharmaceuticals have been modeled on or were originally derived from these chemicals, for example, aspirin is synthesized from salicylic acid derived from the bark of *Salix alba* and the meadowsweet plant, *Filipendula ulmaria*. Quinine from *Cinchona pubescens* bark and artemisinin from *Artemisia annua* plant are antimalarial drugs. Vincristine and vinblastine are anticancer drugs derived from Madagascar periwinkle (*Catharanthus roseus*), used for treating leukemia. Morphine and codeine, derived from the opium poppy (*Papaver somniferum)*, are used in the treatment of diarrhea and pain relief, while digitoxin is a cardiac glycoside derived from foxglove plant (*Digitalis purpurea*) [22, 24]. Medicinal plants are also important materials for the cosmetic industries.

The use of herbal drugs dwindled toward the end of the 19th century due to the advent of synthetic chemistry. However, there was a resurgence of interest in plant medicines in more recent years, as synthetic drugs became less effective due to high levels of resistance and also due to higher toxicity and cost. It is estimated that more than half of all synthetic drugs in use are derived from plants [25].

4. Clinical practice of African traditional/herbal medicine

In African traditional medicine, the curative, training, promotive, and rehabilitative services are referred to as clinical practices Clinical practice can also be viewed as the process of evaluating conditions of ill-health of an individual and its management. These traditional health care services are provided through tradition and culture prescribed under a particular philosophy, in which the norms and taboos therein are strictly adhered to and form the basis for the acceptability of traditional health practitioners in the community they serve [26].

According to the World Health Organization (WHO), health is defined as "a state of complete physical, mental and social well-being and not merely the absence of disease or infirmity" [15, 27] and views health as one of the fundamental rights of every human being. The combination of physical, mental/emotional, and social well-being is commonly referred to as the health triangle.

The recognition of disease and illnesses in traditional Africa meant that every society needed to devise means of containing its problem. Worldwide, different societies have different herbal traditions that have evolved over a long period of time. Similar to modern day Western treatment patterns, African traditional societies also involved herbalism, surgery, dietary therapy, and psychotherapy, in addition to traditional exorcism, rituals, and sacrifice [28]. These medical technologies had evolved even before the coming of the "white man" (Arabs and Europeans). Successful treatments became formalized, sometimes with prescriptions of correct methods of preparation and dosage. In addition, the ingredients and the manner of preparation varied with the ailment but were also dependent on various factors such as geographical, sociological, and economic, but the significant point was that in many cases, patients were cured of their physical or psychological ailments [29]. In African traditional medicine, traditional health practitioners (THP) assess patients in order to diagnose, treat, and prevent disease using their expertise by the following methods:

4.1. Divination

Divination means consulting the spirit world. It is a method by which information concerning an individual or circumstance of illness is obtained through the use of randomly arranged symbols in order to gain healing knowledge. It is also viewed as a way to access information that is normally beyond the reach of the rational mind. It is a transpersonal technique in which diviners base their knowledge on communication with the spiritual forces, such as the ancestors, spirits, and deities [30]. It is, therefore, an integral part of an African traditional way of diagnosing diseases. The "spirit world" is consulted to identify the cause of the disease or to discover whether there was a violation of an established order from the side of the sick person. This is established through the use of cowry shells, throwing of bones, shells, money, seeds, dice, domino-like objects, or even dominos themselves, and other objects that have been appointed by the diviner and the spirit to represent certain polarities on strips of leather or flat pieces of wood. The divining bones that form the large majority of the objects include bones from various animals such as lions, hyenas, ant-eaters, baboons, crocodiles, wild pigs, goats, antelopes, etc. The bones represent all the forces that affect any human being anywhere, whatever their culture [31]. Because of the revealing powers of divination, it is usually the first step in African traditional treatment and medicine [32].

4.2. Interviews and medical reports

Oral interviews are sometimes used by some traditional healers to find out the history behind the sickness, where they have been for treatment and how long the person has been in that condition. This approach enables them to know how to handle the matter at hand. In some cases, the healer might require other family members to speak on behalf of the sick person in cases where the patient is not able to express him/herself. In modern times, after the healing process, they also advise their clients or patients to go for medical diagnoses to confirm that they are healed, and the medical reports sometimes serve for record keeping for future reference and are a way of assuring other clients of their ability and credibility. Due to the holistic approach of the healing process, the healers do not separate the natural from the spiritual or the physical from the supernatural [33]. Thus, health issues are addressed from two major perspectives—spiritual and physical.

4.3. Spiritual perspective

Spiritual-based cases are handled in the following manner:

i. **Spiritual protection**: If the cause of the disease is perceived to be an attack from evil spirits, the person would be protected by the use of a talisman, charm, amulets, specially designed body marks, and a spiritual bath to drive the evil spirits away. These are rites aimed at driving off evil and dangerous powers, spirits, or elements to eliminate the evils or dangers that may have befallen a family or community [34].

ii. **Sacrifices**: Sacrifices are sometimes offered at the request of the spirits, gods, and ancestors. Sometimes, animals such as dogs and cats are slaughtered or buried alive at midnight to save the soul of the one at the point of death, with the belief that their spirits are strong enough to replace life [30]. There is also the view that because they are domestic animals and are very close to people, sometimes when they see that someone very close to them is about to die, they offer their lives for that person to live. This is true especially where the animal dies mysteriously; thus, it is believed that it had offered its life in place of the life of its owner. Rituals are sometimes performed in order to consecrate some herbs without which the medicine is meaningless. Divine and ancestral sanctions are considered necessary before and during the preparation and application of medicine [35].

iii. **Spiritual cleansing**: Spiritual cleansing may be required of the sick person to bathe at specific times for a prescribed number of days either with water or animal blood poured from head to toe. This practice is common among some communities in Ghana [34].

iv. **Appeasing the gods**: If a disease is perceived to be caused by an invocation of a curse or violation of taboos, the diviner appeases the ancestors, spirits, or the gods according to the severity of the case. The individual is often required to provide certain items for sacrifice and/or libation, such as spotless animals (dove, cat, dog, goat, and fowl), local gin, cola nut, eggs, and plain white, red, or black cloth. These items are usually specified by the gods. The used items may be thrown into the river, left to rot, or placed at strategic places, usually at cross roads at the outskirts of the community, depending on the nature and severity of the case [36].

v. **Exorcism**: This is a practice of expelling demons or evil spirits from people or places that are possessed or are in danger of being possessed by them. Many of the traditional communities believe that illness, especially mental illness, is mostly caused by evil spirits. Exorcism can only be performed by a religious leader or a priest who has the authorities and powers to do so. Sometimes, an effigy made of clay or wax would be used to represent the demon and would ultimately be destroyed. Exorcism may be accompanied by dancing to the beating of drums, singing, and sometimes flogging the individual or touching him/her with strange objects such as animal tails and other objects to chase out the spirit. The possessed individual would be somewhat agitated but would only calm down as soon as the spirit is removed from the body. Exorcism is practiced, not only in Africa but also in ancient Babylonian, Greek, and other ancient cultures of the Middle East. This practice is also performed for those who are mentally challenged. In their view, until the possessed person is delivered from the power of that evil spirit, the person will not have his or her freedom. Hence, the practice of exorcism is considered necessary [37].

vi. **Libation**: Libation involves pouring of some liquid, mostly local gin on the ground or sometimes on objects followed by the chanting or reciting of words. It is usually regarded as a form of prayer. The liquid could also be water or in modern times, wine, whisky, schnapps, or gin. Some cultures also use palm wine, palm oil, and coconut water, while some others use corn flour mixed with water [38]. Libation pouring as is practiced in some communities has three main parts, namely invocation, supplication, and conclusion.

- **Invocation:** They first invoke the presence of the almighty God, mother earth, and the ancestors. According to the practitioners of libation pouring, offering the ancestors and spirits drink is a way of welcoming them
- **Supplication:** After invocation, requests are made to the invoked spirits, gods, or ancestors to intercede on their behalf for mercy and forgiveness of offenses such as taboo violations and to seek for spiritual consecration (cleansing) of either the community or individual(s). The content of the prayer is usually case specific [38].
- **Conclusion:** At the end of the libation pouring, they thank the invoked ancestors and spirits. They finally invoke curses on those who wish them evil or failure, meaning that in the process of prayer, it would be unwise to seek the welfare of one's enemy. Therefore, those who wish evil (i.e., enemies, witches, and people with evil powers) on them should fall and die [8]. In this process, the person pouring the libation would be pouring the drink or liquid on the ground as he is reciting the prayers, followed by responses to each prayer point by observers.

4.4. Physical perspectives

If the illness is of a physical nature, the following approaches are exploited:

a. **Prescription of herbs**: Herbs are prescribed to the sick person according to the nature of the illness. Each prescription has its own specific instructions on how to prepare the herb, the dose, dosing regimen, and timeframe

b. **Clay and herbs application:** Application of a mixture of white clay with herbs may be relevant in some of the healing processes. The mixture is applied to the entire body for a number of days, especially in the case of skin diseases. The view is that the human body is made out of the dust or ground; therefore, if the body has any problem, you would have to go to where it came from to fix it. The use of clay with some special herbs is also sometimes used for preventive rituals to ward off the evil spirits responsible for illness.

c. **Counseling:** The sick person is sometimes counseled on the dos and don'ts of treatment, the foods to eat or avoid, to be generally of good behavior as established by society and culture, failure of which the good spirits would withdraw their blessings and protection and therefore, open doors for illness, death, drought, and other misfortunes. This is mostly done when it is an issue of a violation of a taboo [39].

The THPs use experience, added to the accumulated knowledge handed down by their ancestors in order to provide effective and affordable remedies for treating the main ailments (such as malaria, stomach infections, respiratory problems, rheumatism, mental problems, bone fracture, infertility, complications of childbirth, etc.) that afflict populations of the African region and in addition offer counseling/advice and solutions to prevent future reoccurrence.

5. Peculiarities in traditional herbal medicine practice from selected African countries

As there is an African way of understanding God, in the same way, there is an African way of understanding the visible world around us—the cattle, trees, people, and cities, as well as the unseen world, the supernatural world of spirits, powers, and diseases [40, 41]. People developed unique indigenous healing traditions adapted and defined by their culture, beliefs, and environment, which satisfied the health needs of their communities over centuries [15]. Different ethnic groups and cultures recognize different illnesses, symptoms, and causes and have developed different health-care systems and treatment strategies. In spite of these, profound similarities exist in the practice of traditional medicine in different African countries. The increasing widespread use of traditional medicine has prompted the WHO to promote the integration of traditional medicine and complementary and alternative medicine into the national health care systems of some countries and to encourage the development of national policy and regulations as essential indicators of the level of integration of such medicine within a national health care system. The peculiar practices of some countries are described below:

5.1. Ghana

In Ghana, herbal medicine is usually the first approach to treat any illness, especially in the rural areas. Lack of access to medical facilities, poor roads/infrastructure, and affordability of treatment are some of the main reasons for the prevalent use of traditional healers. Besides, ratio of medical doctors to the patients is about 1:20000, while for traditional healers, the ratio is 1:200. This plays a major role in health care decision making. Other influencing factors, such as financial situation, education, and advice from friends and family, contribute to choice of type of health care [42]. Traditional medicine has a long history in Ghana. This knowledge is typically in the hands of spiritual healers, but the vast majority of families have some knowledge of traditional medicine, which is often inherited and passed down through the generations via folklore.

Most people in Ghana fully accept modern science-based medicine, but traditional medicine is still held in high regard. They believe in the physical and spiritual aspects of healing. Herbal spiritualists collectively called "*bokomowo*" indulge in occult practices, divinations, and prayers and are common all over the country. Tribal vernacular names of traditional healers include "*gbedela*" (Ewe), "*kpeima*" (Dagomba), "*odunsini*" (Akan), and "*isofatse*" (Ga).

In some Ghanaian communities, especially in the Akan communities, traditional healers and practitioners are of the opinion that disobeying taboos is one of the ways that could lead to severe illness to the person(s) or community involved [43]. Taboos form an important part of African traditional religion. They are things, or a way of life, that are forbidden by a community or a group of people. One could also become sick through invocation of curses in the name of the river deity, *Antoa*, upon the unknown offender.

In today's Ghana, a traditional Medical Directorate has been established in the ministry of health to provide a comprehensive, recognizable, and standardized complementary system of health based on excellence in traditional and alternative medicine. Establishing centers for integrating scientific research into plant medicines and incorporating traditional medicine into university curricular are now the current status in Ghana [44]. Also, degree-awarding traditional medical schools now train and graduate traditional medical doctors.

5.2. Zambia

The first principle is diagnosis followed by complex treatment procedures using plants from the bush, followed by many rituals, the ultimate aim being to cure disease. Serious or chronic illnesses require "chizimba," which means sealing a disease or illness away forever. This involves killing a lizard and burning the heart with roots of certain trees and grinding with charcoal. Tiny cuts are made on the ailing area and left breast and the mixture rubbed into the cuts.

Plants may be used singly or in combination with other plants. The plant parts are harvested fresh, pulverized, and left to dry first, then soaked in water or other solvents like local gin. Some plant materials are burnt as charcoal and used as powder. Six major types of treatment common to the 72 or more ethnic groups in Zambia include drinking, eating, drinking as porridge, making small cut on skin and applying, bathing with herbs, dancing to exorcize spirits, and steaming with boiling herbs. The Zambian traditional healer is called *Nga:nga* [45].

5.3. Tanzania

In Tanzania, traditional medicine has been practiced separately from allopathic medicine since colonial period but is threatened by lack of documentation, coupled with the decline of biodiversity in certain localities due to the discovery of natural resources and excessive mining, climate change, urbanization, and modernization of agriculture. Traditional medicine in Tanzania is used by people of all ages in both urban and rural areas for both simple and chronic diseases. The traditional healers are of four different types: diviners, herbalists, traditional birth attendants, and bone setters. Erosion of indigenous medical knowledge occurred as most of the traditional health practitioners were aging and dying, and the expected youths who would inherit the practice were shying away from it and those in the rural areas dying of

AIDS. Another constraint to the development of traditional medicine in Tanzania was lack of data on seriously threatened or endangered medicinal plant species [46]. As it stands today, the traditional medical practice is under the Ministry of health. Efforts are being made to scale up traditional medical practice by creating awareness of the importance of traditional medicine and medicinal plants in health care and training of traditional health practitioners on good practice, conservation, and sustainable harvesting [47].

5.4. South Africa

Traditional medicine features in the lives of thousands of people in South Africa every day. In fact, it is estimated that 80% of the population uses traditional medicines that are collectively called muti. Muti is a word derived from medicinal plant and refers to traditionally sourced plant, mineral, and animal-based medicines.

In addition to herbs, traditional medicine may use animal parts and minerals. However, only plant muti is considered a sustainable source of medicines. South African traditional plant medicines are fascinating with so many colors, forms, and effects. It is an art to know these and to use them correctly to bring about health and harmony, which is the aim of all true traditional healers. The plant muti is commonly sold in specific sections of the open markets in South Africa, as shown in **Figure 3**.

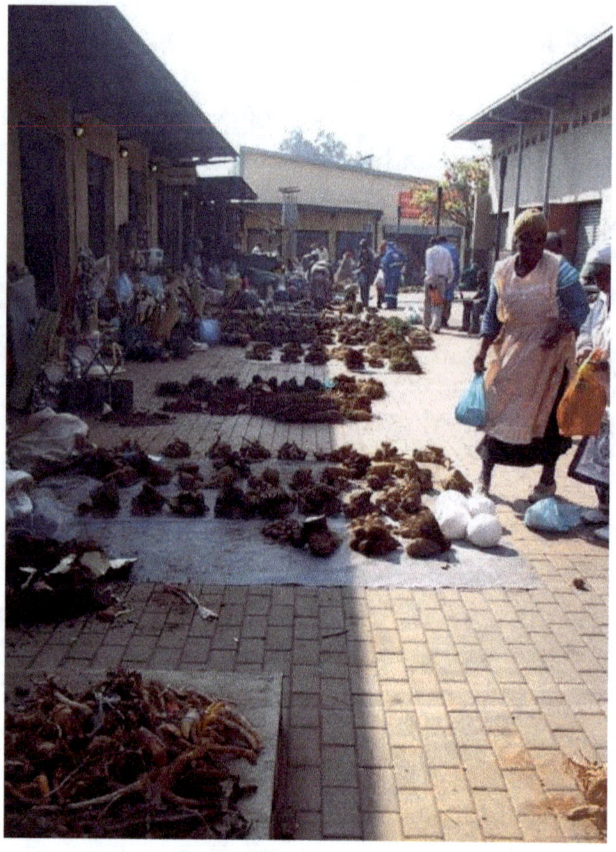

Figure 3. *Muti* market in Johannesburg (Source—Ancient Origins).

Figure 3 shows a muti market in Johannesburg.

The traditional healers known as the *Sangoma or Inyanga* are holders of healing power in the southern Bantu society. In a typical practice with a female traditional practitioner, the methods used depended on the nature of the complaint. For example, headaches are cured by snuffing or inhaling burning medicines, bitter tonics are used to increase appetite, sedative medicines for depression, vomiting medicines to clean the digestive system, and antibiotic or immune boosting medicines for weakness or infection. She often counseled patients before administering appropriate healing herbal medicines [48].

5.5. Kenya

As in many countries in Sub-Saharan Africa, Kenya is experiencing a health worker shortage, particularly in rural areas. Anecdotal evidence suggests that globally, traditional medical practitioners (THMPs) are the only point of contact for at least 80% of the rural poor [10]. In Kenya, very little quantitative evidence or literature exists on indigenous medicine and the health practices of alternative healers or the demand for traditional medical practitioners or on the role that they play in providing particular health services for the rural poor. As a result, TMPs currently do not have sufficient formal government recognition and are often sidelined in Human Resources in Health (HRH) planning activities; further, their activities remain unregulated. Community-derived data show that hospitals are preferred if affordable and within reach. There is also significant self-care and use of pharmacies, although THMPs are preferred for worms, respiratory problems, and other conditions that are not as life threatening as infant diarrhea and tuberculosis [49].

Traditional Medicine Practitioners in Kenya generally known as *"laibon"* far outnumber conventional or allopathic providers. Their practices are no different from other African countries. In many cases, they combine both modern and herbal medicines, especially if they are afflicted by chronic ailments such as HIV/AIDS, hypertension, cancer, and diabetes [50].

5.6. Nigeria

The various ethnic groups in Nigeria have different health care practitioners aside their western counterparts, whose mode of practice is not unlike in other tribes. The Yorubas call them "babalawos," the Igbos call them "dibia," while the Northerners or Hausas call them "boka" [5]. Traditional/herbal medicines have impacted the lives of people, especially in the rural areas where access to orthodox medicare is limited [51]. Apart from the lack of adequate access and the fear of expired or fake drugs, the prohibitive cost of western medicine makes traditional medicine attractive. Various training schools exist for both herbal medicine and homeopathy, and as such, most modern traditional health practitioners have great knowledge of pharmaceutical properties of herbs and the shared cultural views of diseases in the society and they combine their knowledge with modern skills and techniques in processing and preserving herbal medicines, as well as in the management of diseases. In oral interviews with two modern traditional medicine practitioners, Dr. Anselm Okonkwo of Saint Rita's Ethnomedical Research Center, Enugu, Nigeria, a Veterinary doctor, and Mr. Uche Omengoli of CGP Herba-Medical

Consultancy and Research, Enugu, Nigeria, a medical laboratory technologist, both revealed that their knowledge and 'gift' of medical practice were handed down by aged relatives who were also in the practice by both tutelage and supernatural means. Knowledge was however improved by further training, interaction, and discussion with colleagues, consultation of books on herbal medicine, and the Internet. They claimed that the practice was very lucrative, especially since some ailments that defied orthodox medicine such as epilepsy and madness could be completely treated by traditional medicine. The two men divulged that the old concept of secrecy and divination is gradually fading away and being taken over by improved skills, understanding, and use of modern equipment where necessary. Both however agreed to the "mystic" or esoteric power of plants, which they sometimes employ in their diagnosis and treatment. An Enugu, Nigeria-based nonprofit organization, the Association for Scientific, Identification, Conservation and Utilization of Medicinal Plants of Nigeria (ASICUMPON), of which the writer is a member, is committed to "highlighting the usefulness of medicinal plant resources and scientific assessment, preparation and application of these for the betterment of humanity and as Africa's contribution to modern medical knowledge," under the chairmanship of Reverend Father Raymond Arazu. Another prominent member of the association, Professor J.C. Okafor, who is a renowned silviculturist and plant taxonomist, is helping members to identify and classify plants. The group also shares and documents evidence-based therapeutic knowledge. Such groups and training schools exist all over Nigeria. ASICUMPON has published a checklist of medicinal plants of Nigeria and their curative values [19]. Other books have likewise produced useful information [16, 21]. The greatest problem still facing herbal medicine in Nigeria is lack of adequate standardization and safety regulations [52]. However, the interest and involvement of educated and scientific-minded people in herbal medicine practice have to a great extent demystified and increased the acceptability of these medicines by a greater percentage of would-be skeptical populace. A photograph of Dr. Anselm Okonkwo is shown here in **Figure 4**, who is a veterinary doctor and a typical educated and knowledgeable herbal practitioner with the writer after interviewing him.

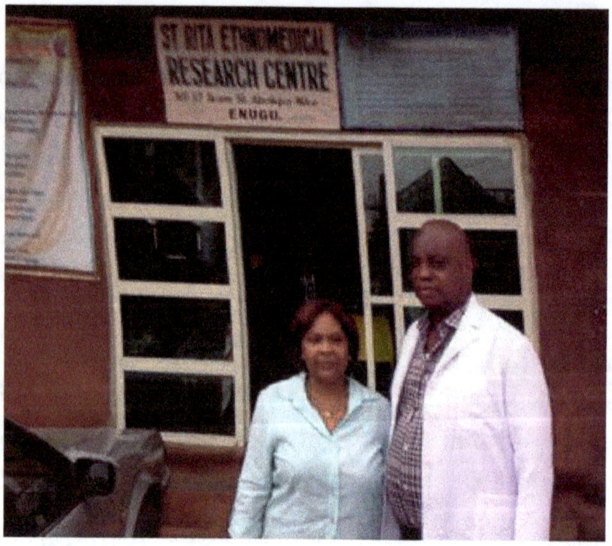

Figure 4. The writer with Dr. Okonkwo of St Rita's Ethnomedical Research Center, Enugu, after the interview.

6. Adverse effects of herbal medicines

An adverse drug reaction is defined as "a harmful or troublesome reaction, due to intervention related to the use of a healing substance, which envisages risk from future administration and requires prevention or explicit treatment, or alteration of dose and method of administration, or withdrawal of the medical substance." Any substance with a healing effect can generate unwanted or adverse side reactions. As with synthetic drugs, the quality, efficacy, and safety of medicinal plants must also be assured. Despite the widespread use of herbal medicines globally and their reported benefits, they are not completely harmless. In as much as medicinal herbs have established therapeutic effects, they may also have the potential to induce adverse effects if used incorrectly or in overdose. The likelihood of adverse effects becomes more apparent due to indiscriminate, irresponsible, or nonregulated use and lack of proper standardization. These concerns have been the focus of many international forums on medicinal plants research and publications [53]. The rich flora of Africa contains numerous toxic plants, though with interesting medicinal uses. The toxic constituents (e.g., neurotoxins, cytotoxins, and metabolic toxins) from these plants can harm the major systems of the human body (cardiovascular system, digestive system, endocrine system, urinary system, immune system, muscular system, nervous system, reproductive system, respiratory system, etc.) [25].

In a survey in Lagos metropolis, Nigeria, among herbal medicine users, it was found that herbal medicine was popular among the respondents but they appeared to be ignorant of its potential toxicities [22]. Several herbal medicines have been reported to have toxic effects. Current mechanisms to track adverse effects of herbal medicines are inadequate [15, 54, 55]. Consumers generally consider herbal medicines as being natural and therefore safe and view them as alternatives to conventional medications. Only very few people who use herbal medicines informed their primary care physicians. It is therefore likely that many adverse drugs reactions go unrecorded with either patients failing to divulge information to health services, and no pharmacovigilance analyses are being carried out, or the observations are not being reported to appropriate quarters such as health regulatory bodies. Establishing a diagnosis of herbal toxicity can be difficult. Even when herbal-related toxicity is suspected, a definitive diagnosis is difficult to establish without proper analysis of the product or plant material. Very few adverse reactions have been reported for herbal medicines, especially when used concurrently with conventional or orthodox medicines [15]. The results of many literature reviews suggest that the reported adverse drug reactions of herbal remedies are often due to a lack of understanding of their preparation and appropriate use.

In a research of liver and kidney functions in medicinal plant users in South-East Nigeria, it was found that liver problems were the most prominent indices of toxicity as a result of chronic use [56]. **Figures 5** and **6** refer to the effect of consumption of herbal medicines and length of usage respectively, on serum enzymes, as an index of liver function. Toxic components in these herbs such as alkaloids, tannins, oxalates, etc., may likely be responsible for such observed toxicities.

Another important source of toxicity of herbal medicines worth mentioning is microbial contamination due to poor sanitary conditions during preparation [57]. Toxicity may also arise as a result of herb-drug interaction in situations where there is co-administration of herbal

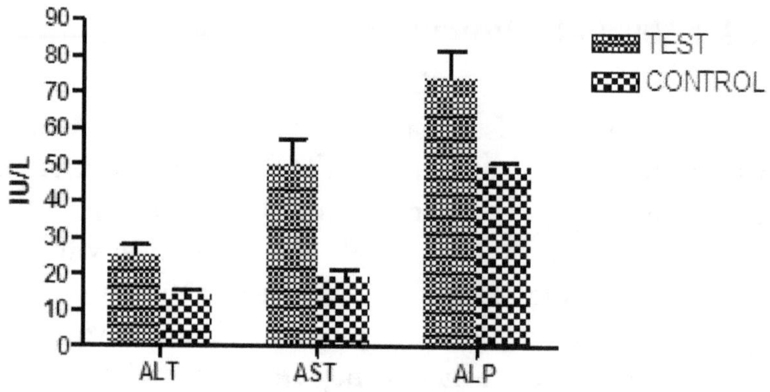

Figure 5. Serum enzyme levels in herbal medicine users (test group) and nonusers (control).

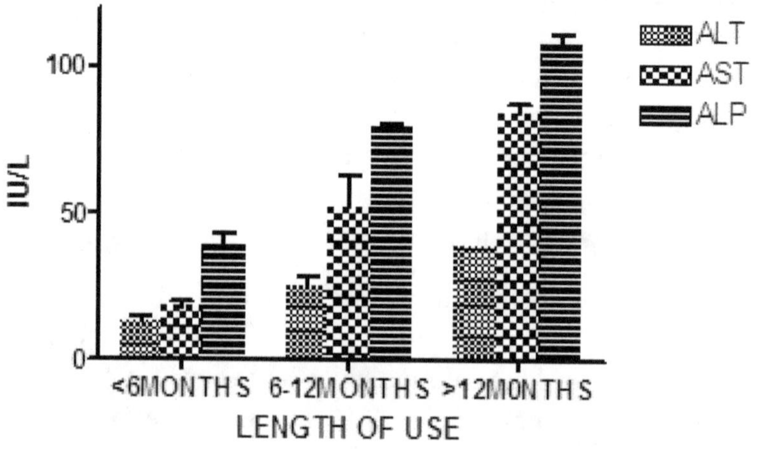

Figure 6. Effect of length of use of herbal medicine on serum enzyme levels.

medicines with some conventional drugs or supplements [11]. Incorrect identification and misuse of plants may also lead to toxicity.

It is therefore pertinent at this time to present correct, timely, and integrated communication of emerging data on risk as an essential part of pharmacovigilance, which could actually improve the health and safety of patients. This calls for improved collaboration between traditional practitioners and modern health care professionals, researchers, and drug regulatory authorities. The latency period between the use of a drug and the occurrence of an adverse reaction, if determined, can also help in its causality assessment in pharmacovigilance management [25]. Such information can be invaluable in the interpretation of drug safety signals, and facilitate decisions on further protective actions to be taken concerning future use.

7. Traditional African medicine and its relationship with modern medicine

Plants have been the primary source of most medicines in the world, and they still continue to provide mankind with new remedies. Natural products and their derivatives represent more than 50% of all drugs in clinical use, of which higher plants contribute more than 25%. These are no doubt more important in developing countries but quite relevant in industrialized world in the sense that pharmaceutical industries have come to consider them as a source or lead in the chemical synthesis of modern pharmaceuticals [24, 58]. A number of African plants have found their way in modern medicine. These plants which had been used traditionally for ages have through improved scientific expertise been the sources of important drugs. Examples of such drugs and their sources include:

Ajmalicine for the treatment of circulatory disorders and reserpine for high blood pressure and mental illness both from *Rauvolfia serpentina,* L-Dopa for parkinsonism is obtained from *Mucuna* species, vinblastine and vincristine used for the treatment of leukemia from *Catharanthus roseus,* physostigmine from *Physostigma venenosum,* or "Calabar bean," used as a cholinesterase inhibitor, strychnine from the arrow poison obtained from the plant *Strychnos nux-vomica,* atropine and hyoscine from *Atropa belladonna* leaves. A host of other African plants with promising pharmaceutical potentials include *Garcinia kola, Aframomum melegueta, Xylopia aethiopica, Nauclea latifolia, Sutherlandia frutescens, Hypoxis hemerocallidea* (African wild potato), and *Chasmanthera dependens* as potential sources of antiinfective agents, including HIV, with proven activities [59], while *Cajanus cajan, Balanites aegyptiaca, Acanthospermum hispidum, Calotropis procera, Jatropha curcas,* among others, as potential sources of anticancer agents [60]. Biflavonoids such as kolaviron from *Garcinia kola* seeds, as well as other plants, have antihepatotoxic activity [61].

8. Advantages and disadvantages of traditional herbal medicine

Both Western or traditional medicine come with their own challenges. Currently, there are many western drugs on the market which have several side effects, in spite of their scientific claims. In like manner, African traditional herbal medicine or healing processes also have their own challenges. The following are reported as some of the advantages and disadvantages:

8.1. Advantages

African herbal medicine is "holistic" in the sense that it addresses issues of the soul, spirit, and body. It is cheap and easily accessible to most people, especially the rural population. It is also considered to be a lot safer than orthodox medicine, being natural in origin.

8.2. Disadvantages

Some of the disadvantages include improper diagnosis which could be misleading. The dosage is most often vague and the medicines are prepared under unhygienic conditions, as evidenced by microbial contamination of many herbal preparations sold in the markets [57]. The knowledge is still shrouded in secrecy and not easily disseminated. Some of the practices which involve rituals and divinations are beyond the scope of nontraditionalists such as Christians who find it incomprehensible, unacceptable, and difficult to access such services [8, 62].

9. Conclusion

Long before the advent of Western medicine, Africans had developed their own effective way of dealing with diseases, whether they had spiritual or physical causes, with little or no side effect [63]. African traditional medicine, of which herbal medicine is the most prevalent form, continues to be a relevant form of primary health care despite the existence of conventional Western medicine. Improved plant identification, methods of preparation, and scientific investigations have increased the credibility and acceptability of herbal drugs. On the other hand, increased awareness and understanding have equally decreased the mysticism and "gimmicks" associated with the curative properties of herbs. As such, a host of herbal medicines have become generally regarded as safe and effective. This, however, has also created room for quackery, massive production, and sales of all sorts of substandard herbal medicines, as the business has been found to be lucrative.

African traditional herbal medicine may have a bright future which can be achieved through collaboration, partnership, and transparency in practice, especially with conventional health practitioners. Such collaboration can increase service and health care provision and increase economic potential and poverty alleviation. Research into traditional medicine will scale up local production of scientifically evaluated traditional medicines and improve access to medications for the rural population. This in turn would reduce the cost of imported medicines and increase the countries' revenue and employment opportunities in both industry and medical practice. With time, large scale cultivation and harvesting of medicinal plants will provide sufficient raw materials for research, local production, and industrial processing and packaging for export.

The scope of herbal medicines in Africa in the near future is very wide, but the issue of standardization is still paramount [64].

This therefore calls for ensuring that the raw materials should be of high quality, free from contaminations and properly authenticated, and samples deposited in University, National, and Regional herbaria. There is need for pharmacopeia to provide information on botanical description of plants, microscopic details, i.e., pharmacognosy, origin, distribution, ethnobotanical information, chemical constituents and structures, methods of quality control, pharmacological profile and clinical studies, including safety data, adverse effects, and special precautions [21, 62]. Such wealth of information will no doubt bring about uniformity in production quality. Rather than viewing African herbal medicine to be inferior, it may yet turn out to be the answer to the treatment of a host of both existing and emerging diseases such as malaria, HIV/AIDS, ebola, zika, etc., that may defy orthodox medicine.

9.1. Future perspectives

Future perspectives in this area include:

a. All countries in the African region must seek to recognize traditional medical practice by putting out regulations and policies that will be fully implemented to ensure that the

THPs are qualified and accredited but at the same time respecting their traditions and customs. They must also be issued with authentic licenses to be renewed frequently.

b. Incorporation of systems that will provide an enabling environment to promote capacity building, research, and development, as well as production of traditional herbal medicines of high standards.

c. Harnessing the importance of traditional herbal medicine and integrating the conventional medicine to combat priority diseases such as malaria, HIV/AIDS, diabetes, sickle cell anemia, hypertension and tuberculosis.

d. Raising the standards of African traditional herbal medicine to international standards through intercountry collaboration.

These if achieved would put African herbal medicine in an admirable position in the World health care system.

Author details

Ezekwesili-Ofili Josephine Ozioma* and Okaka Antoinette Nwamaka Chinwe

*Address all correspondence to: ezekjojo@yahoo.com

Department of Applied Biochemistry, Nnamdi Azikiwe University, Awka, Nigeria

References

[1] Natako L: "Honouring the African Traditional Herbalist" African Traditional Herbal Research Clinic Newsletter. Special Edition—HIV/AIDS.25 years. 2006;**1**(10).

[2] Chavunduka EL: Christianity, African Religion and African Medicine in World Council of Churches. 1990. Available from: http://wcc.coe.org/wcc/what/interreligions/cd33-02.htm [Accessed: November 18, 2017]

[3] Mahomoodally MF. Traditional Medicine in Africa: An Appraisal of Ten Potent African Medicinal Plants Evidence Based Complementary and Alternative Medicine. Epub December 3, 2013. DOI: 10.1155/2013/617459 [Accessed: October 30, 2017]

[4] Sofowora EA. Medicinal Plants and Traditional Medicine in Africa. 1st ed. Somerset, New Jersey: John Wiley and Sons Ltd; 1982. pp. 55-62

[5] Abdullahi AA. Trends and challenges of traditional medicine in Africa. African Journal of Traditional, Complementary, and Alternative Medicines. 2011;**8**(5 Suppl):115-123. DOI: 10.4313/ajtcam.v8i5S.5 [Accessed: November 12, 2017]

[6] Mokgobi MG. Understanding traditional African healing. Afr J Phys Health Educ Recreat Dance. 2014;**20**(Suppl 2):24-34

[7] Ayodele SJ. The Yoruba cultural construction of health and illness. Nordic Journal of African Studies. Nigeria: University of Ibadan Press; 2002;**11**(3):322-335

[8] White P. The concept of disease and healthcare in African traditional religion in Ghana. HTS Theological Studies. 2015;**71**(3):5

[9] Kofi-Tsekpo M. Institutionalization of African traditional medicine in healthcare systems in Africa. African Journal of Health Sciences. 2004;**11**(1-2):i-ii

[10] World Health Organization. Legal Status of Traditional Medicine and Complementary/Alternative Medicine: Worldwide Review. Geneva: WHO; 2001

[11] Phua DH, Zosel A, Heard K. Dietary supplements and herbal medicine toxicities—When to anticipate them and how to manage them. International Journal of Emerging Medicine. 2009;**2**(2):69-76

[12] Tabuti JZRS. Herbal medicine used in the treatment of malaria in Budiope County, Uganda: A case study of Budiope County. Journal of Ethnopharmacology. 2006;**116**:33-42. The Garden Club of America/Makerere University Anne S. Catham Fellowship in Medicinal Botany, Makerere University

[13] Anoka AN. Herbal medicine used in the treatment of Malaria: *Vernonia amygdalina*: An overview of evidence and pharmacology. In: Acree B, editor. Toxicity and Drug Testing. Croatia: InTech; 2012

[14] Wilcox MI, Bodeker G. Traditional herbal medicine for malaria. British Medical Journal. 2004;**13**:1156-1159

[15] World Health Organization. WHO Traditional Medicine Strategy 2002-2005. Geneva: WHO Press; 2002

[16] Sofowora EA. Medicinal Plants and Traditional Medicine in Africa. 2nd ed. Ibadan, Nigeria: John Wiley and Sons Ltd, Spectrum Books; 1993. pp. 55-62

[17] Parmer V. Herbal Medicine: Its Toxic Effect and Drug Interactions. The Indian Anaesthetics' Forum; 2005. pp. 1-9

[18] Okafor JC, Ham R. Identification, utilization and conservation of medicinal plants in Southeastern Nigeria. Issues in African Biodiversity. The Biodiversity Support Program 1999. No. 3

[19] ASICUMPON. Checklist of Medicinal Plants of Nigeria and their Uses. Enugu, Nigeria: Trinity-Biz Publishers; 2005

[20] Okafor JC. Tropical Plants in Healthcare Delivery in Nigeria: A Guide in the Treatment of Common Ailments and Conditions. Ibadan, Nigeria: Book Builders Publishers; 2013

[21] Iwu MM. Handbook of African Medicinal Plants. 2nd ed. London, New York, Washington DC: CRC Press; 2014

[22] Oreagba IA, Oshikoya KA, Amachree M. Herbal medicine use among residents in Lagos, Nigeria. BMC Complimentary and Alternative Medicines. 2011;**11**:117-124. DOI: 10.1186/1472-6822-11-117

[23] Dawang DN, Mashat MV, Nyam DB, Pam PG, Tongwring DP. Ethnobotanical studies of medicinal plants in Barkin Ladi Local Government Area, Plateau State, Nigeria. IOSR Journal of Pharmacy and Biological Sciences. 2016;**11**(1):18-22

[24] Akerele O. Traditional medicine: Nature's medicinal Bounty: Don't throw it away. World Health Forum. 1993;**4**:390-395

[25] Kamsu-Foguem B, Foguem C. Adverse drug reactions in some African herbal medicine: Literature review and stakeholder interviews. Integrative Medicine Research. 2014; **3**(3):126-132

[26] Mhame PC, Busia K, Kasilo MJK. Clinical practice of African traditional medicine. African Health Monitor. 2010. Issue 13. Available at: www.aho.afro.int/en/ahm/issue/3 [Accessed: December 2, 2017]

[27] World Health Organization. National Policy on Traditional Medicine and Regulation of Herbal Medicine: Report of a WHO Global Survey. Geneva: WHO; 2005

[28] Tasha D. Traditional African Healing. 2012 12.07.2015. Available at: www.africanholocaust.netnews-ah/trad/healing.html [Accessed: November 2, 2017]

[29] Andah BW. Nigerian Indigenous Technology. Nigeria: Ibadan University Press; 1992. pp. 11-12

[30] Olupona JK. Owner of the day and regulator of the universe: Ifa divination and healing among the Yorubas of South-Western Nigeria. In: Winkelman M, Peeks PM, editors. Divination and Healing: Potent Vision. Tucson, Arizona: University of Arizona Press; 2004

[31] Cumes D. Divination_bones. 2014. Available at: http://davidcumes.com/divining_bone.html [Accessed: November 20, 2017]

[32] Omonzejele PF. African concepts of health, disease and treatment: An ethnic inquiry. Explorer. 2008;**4**(2):120-123. DOI: 10.1016/j.explore.2007.12.001

[33] Thorpe SA. African Traditional Religion. Pretoria: University of South Africa Press; 1993

[34] Westerlund D. African Indigenous Religious and Disease Causation. Leiden: Brill N.V.; 2006

[35] Idowu B. African Traditional Religion: A Definition. London: Orbis Books; 1973. SCM

[36] Insoll T. Talensi animal sacrifice and its archeological implications. World Archeology. 2010b;**42**:231-244

[37] Avorgbedor D. Bildung Dee Hoo! Sonic articulations in healing and exorcism practices of the Anio-Ewe. The World of music. 2000;**42**(2):9-24

[38] Adjaye JK. The performativity of Akan libations: An ethnopoeitic construction of realty. Ghana Studies. 2001;**4**:107-138

[39] Sundermeier T. The Individual and Community in African Traditional Religions. Munster: LIT Verlag; 1998

[40] Dime CA. African Traditional Medicine: Perculiarities. Ekpoma: Edo State University Press; 1995

[41] Oduro T, Hennie P, Nussbaum S, Brain B. Mission in an African Way: A Practical Introduction to African Instituted Churches and Their Sense of Mission. Wellington: Christian Literature Fund and Bible Media; 2008

[42] Tabi MM, Powell M, Hodnicki D. Use of traditional healers and modern in Ghana. International Nursing Review. 2006;**53**:52-58

[43] Gyekye K. An Essay of African Philosophical Thought: The Akan Conceptual Scheme. Philadelphia: Temple University Press; 1995

[44] Adusi-Poku Y, Okire LKN, Lortsi-Akakpo FK, Fleischer TC, Mensah MLK, Arhin P, et al. Assessing herbal medical practitioners in professional qualifying examination in Ghana, a model. African Journal of Traditional, Complementary, and Alternative Medicines. 2010;**7**(1):85-87

[45] Tembo M. Principles and Methods of African Traditional Medicine. 2016. Available at: www.hunger for culture.com [Accessed: November 6, 2017]

[46] Tambwe M. Tanzania: Traditional medicine has place in health. Tanzania Daily News (Dar-es Salaam). Available at: allafrica.com/stories/201211040038.html [Accessed: November 4, 2017]

[47] Kayombo EJ, Mahunnah RLA, Uiso FC. Prospects and challenges of medicinal plants conservation and traditional medicine in Tanzania. Anthropology. 2013;**1**:108. DOI: 10.4172/2332-0915.1000108

[48] Ancient Origins: Reconstructing the Story of Humanities Past: Traditional Medicine and Its Role in Healing in a Modern World. Available from: https://en.wikipedia.org/wiki/file [Accessed: November 6, 2017]

[49] Lambert J, Leonard K, Mungai G, Ominde-Ogaja E, Gatheru G, Mirangi T, Owara J, Herbst CH, Ramana GNV, Lemiere C. The contribution of traditional herbal medicine practitioners to Kenyan health care delivery: Results from community health-seeking behavior vignettes and a traditional herbal medicine practitioner survey. Health, Nutrition and Population (HNP) Discussion Paper. 2011. The International Bank for Reconstruction and Development/The World Bank NW Washington, DC

[50] Kigen GK, Rono HK, Kikpore K, Rotich J. Current trends of traditional herbal medicine oractice in Kenya: A review. African Journal of Pharmacology and Therapeutics. 2013;**2**(1):32-37

[51] Abd El-Ghani MM. Traditional medicinal plants in Nigeria: An overview. Agriculture and Biology Journal of North America. 2016;**7**(5):220-247

[52] Ekeanyanwu CR. Traditional medicine in Nigeria: Current status and the future. Research Journal of Pharmacology. 2011;**5**(6):90-94

[53] Angell M, Kassier JP. Alternative medicine—The risk of untested and unregistered remedies. New England Journal of Medicine. 1998;**339**:839-841

[54] Bury RW, Fullinfaw RO, Barraclough D, Muirden KD, Moulds RF, Anghie T. Problem with herbal medicines. Medical Journal of Australia. 1987;**146**:324-325

[55] Oshikoya KA, Njokunma OF, Chukwura HF, Ojo OI. Adverse drug reactions in Nigerian children. Paediatric and Perinatal Drug Therapy. 2007;**8**:81-88

[56] World Health Organization: WHO traditional medicine Strategy 2002-2005; 2002. WHO Geneva. WHO, 2002

[57] Ezekwesili-Ofili JO, Onyemelukwe NF, Asogwa P, Orji I. The bioload and aflatoxin content of herbal mediines from seleted states in Nigeria. African Journal of Traditional, Complementary, and Alternative Medicines. 2014;**11**(3):143-147

[58] Hamman O. The Joint ICUN-WWF plants conservation programme and its interest in medicinal plants. In: Akerele et al., editors. Conservation of Medicinal Plants. Cambridge: Cambridge University Press; 1991. pp. 199-212

[59] Street RA, Prinsloo G. Commercially important medicinal plants of South Africa: A review. Journal of Chemistry. 2013:205048. DOI: 10.1155/2013/205048

[60] Mbele M, Hull R, Dlamini Z. African medicinal plants and their derivatives: Current efforts towards potential anti-cancer drugs. Experimental and Molecular Pathology. 2017;**103**:121-134

[61] Iwu MM, Igboko OA, Onwuchekwa AA, Okonji CO. Evaluation of the antihepatotoxic activity of the bioflavonoids of garcinia kola seeds. Journal of Ethnopharmacology. 1967; **21**:127-238

[62] Asamoah-Gyadu JK. Therapeutic strategies in African religion: Health, herbal medicinal and indigenous Christian spirituality. 2014;**20**(11):83

[63] Trinter I. African traditional healers: Cultural and religious beliefs intertwined in a holistic way. South African Pharmaceutical Journal. 2007;**74**(8):56-60

[64] Brendler T, Eloff JN, Gurib-Fakim A, Philips LD. African Herbal Pharmacopoeia. Mauritius: Association for African Medicinal Plants Standards; 2010

3

Toxicity and Safety Implications of Herbal Medicines

Merlin L.K. Mensah, Gustav Komlaga,
Arnold D. Forkuo, Caleb Firempong,
Alexander K. Anning and Rita A. Dickson

Abstract

The use of herbal medicines has seen a great upsurge globally. In developing countries, many patronize them largely due to cultural acceptability, availability and cost. In developed countries, they are used because they are natural and therefore assumed to be safer than allopathic medicines. In recent times, however, there has been a growing concern about their safety. This has created a situation of ambivalence in discussions regarding their use. Some medicinal plants are intrinsically toxic by virtue of their constituents and can cause adverse reactions if inappropriately used. Other factors such as herb-drug interactions, lack of adherence to good manufacturing practice (GMP), poor regulatory measures and adulteration may also lead to adverse events in their use. Many *in vivo* tests on aqueous extracts largely support the safety of herbal medicines, whereas most *in vitro* tests on isolated single cells mostly with extracts other than aqueous ones show contrary results and thus continue the debate on herbal medicine safety. It is expected that toxicity studies concerning herbal medicine should reflect their traditional use to allow for rational discussions regarding their safety for their beneficial use. While various attempts continue to establish the safety of various herbal medicines in man, their cautious and responsible use is required.

Keywords: traditional medicine, herbal medicine, medicinal plants, toxicity, safety

1. Introduction

This chapter is primarily to appraise the pertinent determinants of the safety of medicinal plants or herbal medicines used in African traditional medicine and the implications of their toxicity. In view of the current global upsurge in their usage, it has become necessary to review issues related to herbal medicines toxicity within appropriate contexts to allow for their beneficial use. In this regard, the safety implications of medicinal plants used in traditional medicine and or in diets are discussed and some literature on animal toxicity, acute and chronic toxicities, and cytotoxicity of some African medicinal plants are reviewed.

Plants have been used since time immemorial for diverse purposes in the life of mankind particularly as food, and medicines for nutrition and the treatment of diseases, respectively, in both humans and animals. They are used in all cultures of the world and have been relied upon for several millennia to support, promote and restore human health. They form a vital component of traditional medicine (TM) and their use for the maintenance of health and well-being is a common practice in all African societies. They are used as remedies for the prevention and treatment or management of a plethora of disease conditions including relatively new ones such as HIV/AIDS [1].

Traditional medicine used to be the only health-care system available to the whole of the African population prior to the introduction of allopathic or conventional medicine [2]. The practice received international recognition after the 1978 Alma Ata Conference Declaration, which aimed to achieve primary health care for all by the year 2000 through the use of traditional medicine [3]. TM, especially herbal medicine, still forms the backbone of rural health care in Africa, supporting an estimated 80–90% of the population.

2. Justification for the use of herbal medicines

There exist diverse reasons for the continuing use of herbal medicines for health care in Africa; these include cultural acceptability, easy accessibility and affordability, and in some instances, non-availability and prohibitive cost of allopathic medicines [4]. Some people also employ herbal medicines under other circumstances, for example, in health conditions that had failed to respond to orthodox treatment or which allopathic medicines are deemed not to treat adequately and less safely [5]. Other health conditions believed to have spiritual origins [2] and those thought to need holistic therapies are also managed with herbal medicines.

3. Evolution of herbal medicine in traditional medicine

The practice of herbal medicine is embedded in traditional medicine which origins may be implied in varied anecdotes. It is claimed that its beginnings in humans were instinctive, as seems to be the case in animals. As humans were afflicted by various illnesses over time, they learned to pursue remedies from various formulations from plant and animal parts, and mineral substances. Over time, the therapeutic properties of medicinal plants for the treatment of certain diseases have been validated through scientific experiments; thus, medicinal plants usage gradually abandoned the anecdotal framework and became founded on empirical and explicatory facts [6].

Other diverse claims have been made in relation to the origin of herbal medicines used in traditional medicine in Africa. Some claimed the medicines originated from the deities or superior beings as a gift to man through the medium of dwarfs or spirit beings who 'abducted' some individuals and took them away from human habitation into the spirit world either in the forest or in the water bodies. Such persons returned to human habitation trained and equipped to fight the diseases that threaten the well-being of not only individual sufferers but also the entire family or community. Some other knowledge of medicines is claimed to have come by revelation through dreams, visions and extrasensory perception. The above postulates on the origin of herbal medicines formed the basis of a sophisticated traditional medical system in Africa, a time-tested system where information on medicinal plants use was methodically collected over several years, and which provides remedies for most diseases today in Africa. The African Traditional Medicine practitioners' own experience, added to the accumulated knowledge passed on, usually orally, through generations, allow them to offer effective remedies for treating ailments that afflict the community [5].

Lately, the knowledge and use of traditional medicine have also been acquired through apprenticeship by individuals understudying a recognized practitioner over defined periods of time. More recently, with increased access to information, some practitioners, especially those outside the indigenous cultures, acquire the knowledge about medicinal plants and their uses from Internet sources including online scientific journals and books including e-books. Another avenue of knowledge acquisition has been through formal education and training in exclusively scientific settings as at colleges or universities where degrees or diplomas are awarded on graduation.

4. Attitudes toward traditional medicine

Ever since the dawn of the scientific era, prejudice against traditional medicine has been noted [7]. This has resulted in a situation described as 'passionate ambivalence' toward TM, fuelled by the influence of Western religion and education, urbanization and globalization phenomena in Africa [2]. The result has been continued as negative pronouncements from some segments of western-educated African elites concerning the use of TM especially concerning the quality, efficacy and safety of African medicinal products, creating doubts about the benefits of the medicines. This is in spite of the fact that TM still plays an important role in health-care delivery in Africa and had rarely witnessed major reported cases of adverse effects even after hundreds of years of practice [2].

Besides, some persons with little or no knowledge of herbal medicines tend to focus on reported toxicities and criticize the practice often out of context. Moreover, mass media reports of adverse events tend to be sensationalized and give a negative impression about the outcomes from the use of herbal medicines, instead of identifying the causes of these events, which may relate to a variety of issues [8]. Several scientific studies conducted on the biochemical properties of medicinal plants used in traditional medicines to treat various illnesses have confirmed their efficacy and safety especially in animals. As seen in several publications, the efficacy [9] and sometimes the safety of some medicinal plants and herbal medicines have been validated through research [10–12].

5. Toxicity of chemicals

Toxicity refers to the relative ability of a substance to cause adverse effects in living organisms [13]. It may also be defined as the extent to which an exposed tissue is damaged by a chemical substance and covers the effect on a whole organism and sub-structural component of an organism such as the cell (cytotoxicity) or organ (organotoxicity). Toxicity may further be defined to cover the study of the adverse effects of chemicals on living organisms as well as their symptoms, mechanisms and treatments. Toxicity studies may be classified as acute, subacute/subchronic and chronic effects depending upon the quantity and duration of administration of the agents [14].

5.1. Acute toxicity

Acute toxicological studies investigate the toxic effects produced by a single large-dose exposure to a toxicant lasting no longer than 24 h. This may result in severe biological effects (harm or death) to the organism. The results of acute toxicity are not only important in the consideration of accidental poisoning with a chemical but also are used for the planning of chronic toxicological studies [15]. The development of tolerance is usually revealed by an acute exposure. The starting point for toxicological classification of chemicals uses the LD_{50} value, which is the dose administered in acute toxicity testing that causes death in 50% of experimental animals [16].

5.2. *Chronic* toxicity

Chronic exposure refers to the administration of a toxin over an extended period of time, usually measured in months or years; this can cause irreversible toxicity. Periods between acute and chronic exposure could be referred to as subacute or subchronic. The results of chronic and acute toxicological studies help in the evaluation of any possible hazardous effect of a new drug or a drug which is in use with little or no documentation of its systemic toxicity.

6. Toxicity of medicinal plants

Generally, medicinal plants contain bioactive compounds which demonstrate both intra- and inter-species variation in type and content. Plants by virtue of their chemical constituents are potentially toxic; thus, some plants used in traditional medicine are intrinsically toxic. Some plants well known in traditional medicine to be toxic or poisonous include *Atropa belladonna*, *Datura* spp., *Digitalis* spp. [17].

Many plants used in traditional medicine or used as food have demonstrated some toxicity (mutagenic and carcinogenic) effects [18]. The issue of the possible toxic, genotoxic and/or mutagenic effects of plants used in traditional medicine has been highlighted in the review by Fennell et al. [19]. However, some of the toxic plants are useful to man as medicines and also as poisons for hunting and for use as pesticides, for example, Datura (tropane alkaloids), Digitalis (cardiac glycosides) and Pyrethrum (pyrethrin insecticides). Well-known medicinal plants have demonstrated toxicity in laboratory studies and field observations. For example, *Lantana camara* used in the management of malaria and other diseases has been reported to be hepatotoxic in several animal species which could be of concern regarding its chronic use in man [20].

Similarly, *Momordica charantia*, a known anti-diabetic and antimalarial plant but also used in Ghana as an abortifacient [21, 22], has reportedly caused deadly hypoglycemia in children [23].

7. Medicinal plant use in therapy

The basis for the medicinal use of the plants is the presence of mixtures of different biologically active plant constituents or phytochemicals (secondary metabolites) such as alkaloids, glycosides, terpenoids, and so on that may act individually, additively or in synergy to demonstrate an effect which may be useful or harmful to health. Some of these plants have been designated as poisonous plants because of their effects in impacting biological functions in other organisms which are harmful [24]. They are therefore damaging to either the survival or the normal function of the individual. The dose received may be due to either acute (short) or chronic (long-term) exposure. However, in TM, plants with toxic constituents are known and are avoided or used cautiously in herbal product formulations. Even if these are employed in medicinal products, they are employed below toxic levels and hence, if at all, hardly result in any fatality when administered by professional practitioners or experienced persons.

8. Safety of medicinal plants and herbal medicines used in traditional medicine

Generally, plants used in traditional medicines have been considered safe as a result of the long history of use in the treatment of diseases based on knowledge accumulated over several centuries. In many cultural settings, toxic fatalities have been rare due to systematic selection of medicinal plants for use. While thousands of people die each year from even supposedly 'safe' over-the-counter remedies, deaths or hospitalizations due to herbs are so rare that they are hard to find; not even the United States National Poison Control Centers have a category in their database for adverse reactions to herbs [17].

When used appropriately as dietary supplements, food supplements or medicines, traditional medicines are generally regarded as safe. However, there are instances where adverse events ascribed to herbal medicines used have been reported in both humans and animals. For example, Barbosa et al. [25] reported clinical and pathological neurological disorders in horses following a large intake of fresh *Bambusa vulgaris* leaves. Paradoxically, the aqueous decoction is a popular antimalarial medicine in Ghana [11, 21] and this has been used without any report of adverse reaction. Besides, the aqueous extract of the leaves did not cause cytotoxicity in normal human cells [11, 21]. In these situations, the dose of the constituents administered is of great importance; as stated by Paracelsus that, 'All substances are poisons; there is none, which is not a poison. The right dose differentiates a poison and a remedy' [26]. This is to say that the toxicity of any substance, including medicinal plants and even food, is largely dependent on the amount or dose used. A non-toxic substance can be toxic at a high dose, and a very toxic substance can be considered safe if the dose is low [27]. Over-dosage in the course of treatment is bound to pose safety problems. The dose-toxicity relationship was illustrated by the toxicity of *Bupleuri chinense* in which the toxic dose was about 21 times than the common clinical dose of 9 g/60 kg [28].

Apart from an overdose, adverse events may also arise from the misidentification of medicinal plants, errors in the use of herbal medicines both by health-care providers and by consumers, and misuse and use over long periods even at tolerable dose [8, 29].

Interactions between herbs (herbal medicines) and drugs (allopathic medicines) may increase or decrease the pharmacological or toxicological effects of either component. Thus, synergistic therapeutic effects may complicate the administration of medications for chronic diseases, for example, herbs traditionally used to treat diabetes could theoretically lead to hypoglycemia if taken concomitantly with conventional antihyperglycaemic drugs [30].

In the formal herbal industry, the toxicity problems of medicinal plants could be attributable to insufficient quality assurance and non-compliance with the standards of good manufacturing practice [8, 31], and also inadequate access to the information required for the effective use of herbal medicines and inappropriate approaches to their use. Furthermore, the problem could be complicated by adulteration of herbal remedies by the addition of synthetic drugs and other potentially toxic compounds such as other botanicals, pathogenic microorganisms, toxins, pesticides and fumigants agrochemical residues or heavy metals [8, 29, 32]. The majority of adverse events related to the use of herbal products are attributable to weak quality control systems leading either to poor product quality [8]. According to WHO [8], poor regulatory measures and largely uncontrolled distribution channels could partly account for such events. These give rise to poor quality products arising from such situations as adulteration of herbal products with other undeclared medicines and potent pharmaceutical substances, such as corticosteroids and non-steroidal anti-inflammatory agents [8].

Usually, it is difficult to identify genuine adverse reactions to herbal medicines and herbal products until the cause of such events has been established. When appropriately employed, herbal medicines are relatively safe. Long historical including experience passed on from generation to generation has demonstrated their safety and efficacy [33].

It is worth noting that toxicity results of many medicinal plants are very often misinterpreted and wrong conclusions drawn with regard to traditional practices. Many toxicity studies were conducted on medicinal plants extracted in organic solvents such as methanol, dichloromethane, and so on other than aqueous extracts as used in traditional medicine practice. This was the case as reported in the degree of hepatotoxicity damage caused by the alcohol extracted *B. chinense* which proved more serious than that caused by the water extract [28].

9. Challenges of contemporary herbal medicine practice in Africa

Traditional medicines are increasingly being used outside the confines of traditional cultures and far beyond geographical areas without proper knowledge of their use and the underlying principles [8]. They are therefore practiced in ways that deviate from the traditional norm of practice within the specific traditional setting. Such deviations include the method of extraction—where highly efficient and sophisticated technological tools are frequently used for extracting medicinal plants and then reformulating the extract into a final product. Such an approach is entirely different from the hitherto traditional approaches of macerating the plant materials either dried or fresh often in boiling water to produce decoctions, which are then administered. This traditional approach therefore tends to make the herbal medicine safe since potentially toxic compounds are not extracted due to the inherent inefficiency in the aqueous extraction method (preparation of the decoction). Also, doses employed in contemporary practice often tend to be different from the traditional doses, which were systematically established over several years of practice and proven to be safe. Besides, herbal medicines are used for non-traditional indications in recent years. A typical example is the use of herbal medicines for relieving constipation but abused as an abortifacient by the youth due to its induced contractive effect on smooth muscles such as the endometrial muscles. The concomitant use of traditional medicines with other types of medicines is quite outside the traditional context and has become a matter of particular safety concern [8].

Another challenge posed to the practice is the lack of appropriate foundational knowledge in traditional medicine practice and the herbal medicines used to treat diseases. This is a common occurrence among many contemporary practitioners, especially those in urban and cosmopolitan areas. The work of such practitioners is based on information gathered from indirect sources such as the Internet or from reading books and therefore lacking in specific knowledge. These 'neo-herbalists' most often lack the expertise and basic principles necessary for the use of herbal medicines. Their practice may therefore not be entirely safe and can put patrons at risk of adverse reactions.

Besides, documented knowledge about medicinal plants and their uses within cultural settings rarely contains information on potential toxicity of the plants. This is because many ethnopharmacologists tend to focus more on the therapeutic property of the plants and hence do not inventory their toxicological information. This failure to document and contextualize potential toxicity of plants in the perspective of local healing traditions and healing practitioners' methods and approaches to treatment does not promote the safe use of medicinal plants outside the boundaries of the cultures where the medicinal plants are used.

10. Cytotoxicity of African medicinal plants

Cytotoxicity refers to the ability of a substance to interfere with cell attachment, alter its growth, proliferation and or cause death [34]. Accurate determination of cytotoxicity is necessary to identify compounds or effective parts that might pose health risks to humans. Surprisingly, most cytotoxic assays are geared toward screening only bioactive compounds that can kill rapidly dividing cancer cells. Cytotoxic substances may destroy living cells via either necrosis/lysis (i.e. accidental cell death) or apoptosis (i.e. programmed cell death) [35]. In cancer drug discovery, for example, potential cytotoxic agents induce apoptosis instead of necrosis with very low or no toxicity toward normal cells. Only few case studies have investigated normal cells to determine the cytotoxicity of especially African medicinal plants.

Toxicity studies on most medicinal plants using animal models have provided results that strengthen their use among humans; however, many such plants could be associated with some cytotoxicity (**Table 1**). As a consequence, researchers have supported the use of human cell lines for *in vitro* cytotoxicity assays in predicting human acute toxicity as alternatives

Species	Normal cell type	Popular medicinal use	Plant part	References
Low cytotoxicity (>50 μg/ml)				
Afrostyrax lepidophyllus	MRC-5 cells	Anthelmintic, vomiting, urinary infections	Stem bark	[41]
Drypetes gossweileri	MRC-5 cells	Anthelmintic, purgative, tonic, bronchitis, cough, pains, relieve urethral discharge, diarrhea	Stem bark	[41]
Napoleona vogelii	MRC-5 cells	Dermatosis, sexual asthenia, stomach aches, diarrhea	Stem bark	[41]
Tectona grandis	HUVECs	Bronchitis, hyperacidity, dysentery, verminosis, diabetes, leprosy, inflammation, skin diseases, pruritus, stomatitis, ulcers, hemorrhages, constipation, piles, leucoderma, headache, biliousness, anuria, urethral discharges, body swellings, menstrual disorders	Leaf	[11]
Moderate cytotoxicity (30–50 μg/ml)				
Cryptolepis sanguinolenta	V79 cells	Fever, hepatitis, malaria, hypertension, urinary and upper respiratory tract infections, colic, stomach complaints, amoebic dysentery, diarrhea, wounds, measles, hernia, snakebites, rheumatism, insomnia, antiplasmodial activity, anticancer, antifungal, antibacterial, hypotensive, antipyretic, anti-inflammation, antihyperglycemia	Root	[42]
Isolona hexaloba (Rb)	MRC-5 cells	Pains, sexual weakness, headache, intestinal cramps, malaria, rheumatism	Root back	[41]
Mammea africana (Sb)	MRC-5 cells	Wounds, filariasis, mycosis, skin diseases	Stem back	[41]
Phyllanthus fraternus	HUVECs	Malaria, chronic pyrexia, chills, intermittent fever, painful joints, diarrhea, ulcer, dysmenorrhea and edema	Whole plant	[11]
Psidium guajava	MRC-5 cells	Antispasmodic, astringent, febrifuge, vulnerary, astringent, dysentery, diarrhea, constipation, diabetes, hepatitis, gonorrhea, diarrhea.	Leaf	[41]
High cytotoxicity (10–30 μg/ml)				
Terminalia ivorensis	HUVECs	Wounds, hemorrhoids, infections, gonorrhea, kidney disease, aphrodisiac	Leaf	[11]
Tetrapleura tetraptera	MRC-5 cells	Enema, malaria, fungal infections, arthritis, filariasis, gastritis, epilepsy	Fruit	[41]
Harungana madagascariensis	MRC-5 cells	Anemia, venereal diseases, nephrosis, gastrointestinal disorders, malaria.	Stem bark	[41]
Very high cytotoxicity (<5 μg/ml)				
Enantia chlorantha	MRC-5 cells	Intestinal worms, spasms malaria, sexual asthenia.	stem bark	[41]
Piptadeniastrum africanum	MRC-5 cells	Sexual asthenia, Constipation, intestinal cramps, pain.	stem bark	[41]

Species	Normal cell type	Popular medicinal use	Plant part	References
Quassia africana	MRC-5 cells	Malaria, blenorragia, hypertension, scabies, gastrointestinal affections, hernia, febrifuge, anti-rheumatic, anthelmintic, antalgic, tonic, stomach pains, gastric hemorrhoids, diarrhea, antiwounds	root bark	[41]

Table 1. Cytotoxic activities of aqueous extracts of African medicinal plants.

to acute lethality studies in rodents [36]. The selectivity exhibited by cytotoxic plants also underscores the need to distinguish highly active but toxic extracts from those that are selectively active against certain pathogens, diseased conditions and even cancerous cells. This provides good leads for continuous research on promising extracts, the sources of interesting biologically active and therapeutically useful compounds with excellent activity and low toxicity [37]. Toxicity testing at the cellular level is therefore very useful and recommended for all bioactive medicinal plants. Clearly, information on cytotoxicity of plants commonly used in traditional medicine in Africa is essential for assessing the quality, efficacy and safety of their preparations. Such knowledge is also critical in developing new therapeutic products to ensure the safety of end users of herbal medicine.

In spite of the assumed safety of African medicinal plants, studies have shown that many plants used as food or traditional medicines are also potentially cytotoxic, mutagenic and carcinogenic [38–40]. A comprehensive survey by [37], for instance, recorded 400 plants of African origin with cytotoxic effects. These plant species, according to the study, are used to treat diseases of considerable economic burden to the African continent, of which malaria, leishmaniasis and sleeping sickness received much attention. The study, however, identified approximately 14 or 56% of the listed plant species as having significant cytotoxic activities (IC_{50} < 30 μg/ml) against some normal cells such as human normal lung fibroblast (MRC-5), human kidney epithelial and human monocytes. While the list compiled by McGaw et al. [37] comprised many species with high efficacy against cancerous cells or pathogens, it indicated that at least 14% of these African medicinal plants may be harmful to humans.

Although the above observation calls for great care in plant use and close monitoring of their potential side effects, there are also clear reasons why cytotoxicity results could not always be wholly extrapolated into safety prediction in TM: except when organotypic cultures are used [37].

11. Drawbacks of using cytotoxicity to predict safety of herbal medicines in TM

There are some shortcomings to extrapolating cytotoxicity studies to the safety of herbal medicine used in traditional medicine. Among this is the fact that tissue responses due to *in vivo* toxicity cannot be addressed by toxic responses in cells [37]. According to McGraw et al. [37], a critical factor in toxicology is metabolism *in vivo*, as some substances lacking toxicity initially may produce toxic metabolites after being exposed to liver enzymes, while other substances that are toxic in vitro may become detoxified. Other factors such as the capacity of the substance to penetrate the tissue, and clearance and excretion of the product cannot be accounted for using the cellular model. The time of exposure and the rate of change for these extracts are not the same in both *in vitro* and *in vivo* studies. Notwithstanding these limitations of cytotoxicity assay, it still needs to be an integral part of evaluating the safety of medicinal plants because they provide direct information at the cellular level which may be important in assessing the true toxicity of such plants.

Other limitations in cytotoxicity studies with regard to safety prediction for herbal medicines is the use of organic solvent such as methanol, dichloromethane, petroleum ether, ethyl acetate, and so on extracts as against water decoctions/extracts. In situations like this, it is not reasonable to compare the cytotoxicity results of the organic solvent extract with what pertains in TM. Such studies are common because the focus of most cytotoxicity studies has not been the safety assessment of the plants as used in TM but to determine the fractions which contain the potentially safe and efficacious compounds. In some cases, while efficacy study was conducted for both organic solvent and aqueous extracts, cytotoxicity was determined for only the organic solvents. This makes it difficult to relate the toxicity of the plant to safety in traditional use. In most cases, the organic extracts tend to be more efficacious than the aqueous extracts. This could imply that the organic extracts are more cytotoxic than the aqueous extracts since, generally, they (organic extracts) tend to extract more active compounds, which are both efficacious and cytotoxic.

12. Some herbal medicine products clinically evaluated for safety

There have been few reports of the clinical safety of herbal product used in TM. A coded herbal medicine made of *Saraca indica,* Foeniculum vulgare, Juniperus communis, *Mentha piperita* and Zingiber officinale used to treat dysmenorrhea was found to be safe from such toxic effects as hepatotoxicity, nephrotoxicity and other side effects such as menorrhagia, gastro-intestinal disturbance and palpitation in a random-controlled clinical trial [43]. Also an unnamed herbal product made of Capparis spinosa root, Cichorium intybus seed, whole plant of Solanum nigrum, *Terminalia arjuna* bark, Cassia occidentalis seed, aerial part of *Achillea millefolium* and whole plant of Tamarix gallica and used for the management of liver disorders evaluated clinically was well tolerated and did not produce any adverse event in participants [44]. Tetteh et al. [12] reported that a Ghanaian polyherbal medicine, Adutwumwaa malamix, used in the treatment of malaria did not show any hepatotoxic or hematotoxic effects nor any adverse complaint in the populations studied for its clinical effectiveness and safety. Turkson et al. also reported the safety of another Ghanaian herbal medicine for the treatment of malaria and indicated that kidney and liver function tests and full blood count were within normal range at the end of the study, an indication that the product is clinically safe [45]. The tea bag formulation of the root powder of C. sanguinolenta has effectively treated acute uncomplicated malaria on relatively short treatment regimens and did not show any toxicity in man [46]. This was against the fact that the aqueous extract of the root is genotoxic in the Chinese hamster lung fibroblast (V79) cell line [42, 47] and the ethanolic extract of the stem increased platelet counts in albino rats [48].

13. Toxicity studies on some African medicinal plants

13.1. *Cryptolepis sanguinolenta* (Lindl.) Schltr

C. sanguinolenta (Apocynaceae) is a West African climbing shrub. The aqueous extract of the root has been used for centuries in African traditional medicine for the treatment of diseases including malaria, bacterial infections, hepatitis and rheumatism. It is also used as a spasmolytic and tonic [49]. In Ghana, several cryptolepis-based products are prescribed in herbal medicine clinics, sold in pharmacies, licensed chemical and herbal medicine shops for the treatment of malaria [21].

13.1.1. Animal and cell toxicity

Acute and sub-acute oral toxicity evaluation of the aqueous extract of the root suggested general safety at oral dosages below 500 mg/kg in Sprague Dawley rats. The extract did not exhibit either physiological or behavioral abnormality [50]. However, the ethanolic extract of the stem demonstrated localized systemic acute and sub-chronic toxicity by selectively stimulating the bone marrow leading to an increase in platelet counts in albino rats [48]. On the other hand, the aqueous extract of the root demonstrated genotoxicity against the Chinese hamster lung fibroblast (V79) cell line inducing mutagenicity at high concentrations and causing DNA damage [42, 47]. The ethanolic extract of the stem thus poses hematological challenges to white blood cells and platelets and showed localized systemic toxicity by selectively stimulating the bone marrow.

13.2. *Artemisia afra* (Jacq. Ex. Willd), 'African wormwood'

A. afra has been used for coughs, colic, fever, loss of appetite, earache, headache, malaria and intestinal worms [51]. Several studies have been conducted to substantiate the traditional use of this herb; it is also being investigated in diseases like diabetes, cancer and respiratory diseases among others [51].

In acute toxicity studies of aqueous extract of *A. afra* in mice administered doses (i.p., 1.5–5.5 g/kg) caused a regular dose-dependent increase in the death rate and also of general adverse behavior, but with single doses (2–24 g/kg) administered orally, the previous observed increases in the incidence of death rate and adverse general behavior that did not show were dose-independent. The route of administration, acute intraperitoneal and oral doses, showed LD_{50} of 2.45 and 8.96 g/kg, respectively [51].

13.2.1. Animal toxicity

In the chronic studies, rats administered *A. afra* aqueous extract (0.1 or 1 g/kg/day) survived the 3 months of daily dosing with LD_{50} greater than 1 g/kg. No significant changes were observed in the general behavior, hematological and biochemical parameters except for a transient decrease in aspartate aminotransaminase (AST) activity. No significant changes were observed in the organ weights and histopathological results showed no morphological alterations. High doses of the extract were also shown to be hepatoprotective. The aqueous extract of *A. afra* has been shown to be nontoxic in acute use and low chronic toxicity potential in rodent models [51].

13.3. *C. occidentalis* L

C. occidentalis is an annual shrub found in many African and Asian countries. Its leaves and roots are used in some traditional herbal medicines, but its pods or beans are avoided or used sparingly [52]. In Ghana, however, the roasted seeds are used as a beverage in the treatment of hypertension [53]. Many popular herbal tonics and medicines for liver disorders contain the leaves or roots of the plant. *C. occidentalis* has also been used in the treatment of scabies, snake and scorpion bites, diabetes, edema, fever, inflammation, rheumatism and ringworm. It is widely used for the treatment of bacterial and fungal infections and to boost the immune system.

13.3.1. Animal toxicity

The fresh or dried/roasted seeds have demonstrated toxicity in several animal studies [54]. Toxicity in animals is usually seen on the kidney, liver, skeletal muscle and the heart. Grazing animals such as cattle, sheep, horses and goats have shown toxicity upon the ingestion of large amount of the seed pods, the most poisonous even though all parts of the plants have shown some level of toxicity [55, 56].

Although the toxicity of the plant has been demonstrated in different animal species, the toxicity of the pod and bean is dose-dependent: low doses result in mild liver damage and myodegeneration while higher doses cause fatal hepatic degeneration followed by myodegeneration [56]. As the amount of *Cassia* in the animal's diet increases, muscle degeneration becomes a predominant characteristic of the poisoning and cause of the clinical signs. Roasting the seeds from the pod has, however, been shown to reduce the toxicity. Studies in rats [57] and chicken [58] fed a ration with *C. occidentalis* seeds at different concentrations showed histopathological and biochemical changes in muscles, liver and central nervous system. Barbosa-Ferreira et al. [57] in a study involved Wistar rats in four groups of 10 animals each, three of them fed rations containing 1, 2 and 4%, respectively, of *C. occidentalis* seeds, and the control fed normal commercial ration for a period of 2 weeks; rats in the experimental groups showed lethargy, weakness, among other adverse reactions. Histopathological study showed fiber degenerations in the skeletal and cardiac muscles. In the liver parenchyma, vacuolar degeneration was observed and, in the kidney, mild necrosis in the proximal convoluted tubules. All the adverse effects occurred in a dose-dependent manner [57].

Haraguchi et al. [58] studied the chronic effect of varying concentrations of *C. occidentalis* seeds in broiler chicks. All birds were killed on day 49 of age. Low doses of seeds showed no significant variation in biochemical parameters compared to the control group. Degenerative changes in striated skeletal muscles particularly pectoral as well as the liver and myocardium were observed in chicks treated with 0.3 and 0.5% of *Cassia* beans.

13.3.2. Human toxicity

Studies have shown that the ingestion of *C. occidentalis* can cause severe purging possibly due to the anthracene glycoside content [59]. Whereas this may produce great discomfort and pain in adults, in a child, this can be fatal; thus, while few pods might not have any ill effect in an adult or an older child when eaten, it could cause death in a young child [60]. Other *Cassia* species products such as senna extract (*C. acutifolia*) consumed as health drink resulted in severe hepatotoxicity in an adult [61]. *C. senna* leaves and pods have been used in orthodox medicine and still form part of traditional pharmacopeia [53].

The clinical spectrum of *C. occidentalis* poisoning in children resembles the toxicity observed in animals. Most cases in children occur when they eat the beans. As with animals, the clinical toxic features depend upon the amount of beans eaten. While the consumption of two to three pods by a young child may not have any deleterious impact, a large quantity can lead to serious morbidity and even death [62, 63].

Since some children eat very few beans and remain asymptomatic, people tend to consider the beans as non-toxic. With a larger 'dose', such as the beans in six to seven pods, they develop a non-fatal illness with vomiting, diarrhea, malaise, giddiness, drowsiness, change in voice and general weakness among other effects. However, recovery occurs after about 3–4 days of illness. The fatal hepatomyoencephalopathy syndrome may occur with relatively larger amount of beans—such as the cupped hand of a child [63].

13.4. *Calotropis procera* (Aiton)

The plant is widely distributed in Asia, tropical and subtropical Africa [64]. In ancient Egypt, it was recommended for the treatment of nodular leprosy [64]. In Indian traditional medicine, the decoction is used for the treatment of asthma, dysentery, rheumatism, fever, painful muscular spasm and as a purgative and expectorant [65], and as a proteolytic enzyme for the coagulation of cow milk in Ghana [66]. The extract from the plant has been reported to possess antibacterial, nematocidal and larvicidal [67] and anticancer [68] properties. The flower of the plant has been shown to possess potent antimicrobial and anti-inflammatory activities [69].

13.4.1. Animal toxicity

C. procera has been shown to adversely affect early and late pregnancy in rats [70]. Acute toxicity studies in mice, however, showed no significant change in the hematological parameters. Behavioral changes, symptoms of toxicity and mortality were absent during the 24-h duration of the experiment. In the 3-month chronic toxicity study with 100 mg/kg, body weight per day, a 50% mortality of the animals was recorded. No significant changes in the hematological parameters were observed. This study suggested a safe use of the plant in single high dose but a serious health hazard may ensue with prolong use.

13.5. *Senna alata* (L.) Roxb

S. alata grows in several regions of Africa and in other parts of the world [71]. The leaves and stem bark of *S. alata* are widely used to treat hepatitis, skin diseases, jaundice, gastroenteritis, intestinal helminthiasis, eczema, tryphoenteritis and ringworm. The leaves of the plant have been shown to possess antibacterial activity on both Gram positive and negative bacteria, for example, *Bacillus megaterium, Streptococcus haemolyticus, Staphylococcus aureus, Salmonella typhi, Pseudomonas aeruginosa and Klebsiella pneumoniae* [71].

13.5.1. Animal toxicity

In acute toxicity studies, mice treated with the dose of 20 g/kg body weight showed some behavioral changes 120 min after oral administration. These changes included slow response to external stimuli, reduction of mobility and aggression, slight excitability sketching and sluggishness all of which disappeared after 24 h. On the contrary, no adverse changes were noted in mice treated with less than 12 g/kg body weight. Weight gain recorded was increased in both sexes 8 days after oral administration of *S. alata*.

In the sub-acute toxicity, the hydro-ethanolic extract of *S. alata* at doses of 500 and 1000 mg/kg given *per os* every 48 h for 26 days did not result in death of the animals. Also, there was no sign of toxicity *during* the experimental period. However, there was a progressive increase in body weight at the stated doses of 500 and 1000 mg/kg of the rats for 26 days of administration of the extract of *S. alata* which may indicate the improvement of the nutritional state of the animal. The relative weights of the control and treated animal groups showed variation from one organ to another: the hearts and livers from the control group had relative weights quite similar to those of the treated groups. Same observations were noted in the relative weights of the liver, lung and kidney [72].

The histopathological study of the liver of groups of rats showed a normal architecture but they showed slight abnormalities such as steatosis and ballooning of hepatocytes when treated orally with the extract of *S. alata* for 26 days at doses of 1000 mg/kg body weight. However, no necrosis, infiltration, edema and conjunction, which are the signs of hepatotoxicity, were found. The effect of *S. alata* seems to have a protective effect on hepatocytes and improves liver architecture, giving justification for the wide usage of the hydro-ethanolic extract of *S. alata* [72].

13.6. *Zanthoxylum xanthoxyloides* (lam.) Waterm

Z. xanthoxyloides (Lam.) is widely distributed in several African countries. It is known for varied uses in traditional medicine: the root-bark extract is used in treating elephantiasis, toothache, sexual impotence, gonorrhea, malaria, dysmenorrhea and abdominal pain [73]. Workers in West Africa have reported the anti-sickling and antimicrobial activity of the extracts of the plant [74]. In Nigeria, *Z. xanthoxyloides* is used as a chewing stick; water extracts from the plant showed activities against bacteria significant to periodontal disease [75]. It is a very popular anthelmintic among the various tribes in Uganda [76]. It has also been found that the alcoholic extracts of the root bark possess considerable antibacterial activity [77]. Its methanolic extract of the root bark has anthelmintic activity [76], anti-sickling [74] and is anti-inflammatory [78].

13.6.1. Animal toxicity

In a study of the acute toxicity of the methanol extract of *Z. xanthoxyloides*, mice were given 10.0 and 2.0 g/kg of extract. Animals that received 10.0 g/kg all died within 6 h of administration of the extract. However, those on 2.0 g/kg survived beyond the 24 h of observation.

No animals showed immediate behavioral changes on administration of the extract. Yet, mice on both doses showed piloerection and were restless for 24 h following extract administration. They, however, did not vomit nor was there ptosis. Those animals placed on higher doses went into convulsions and died in hyperextension. Post-mortem examination revealed no gross abnormality of the brain, the organs of the chest and abdominal cavities. On the other hand, histopathological examination showed congestion and focal necrosis in the liver and renal tubules [76].

13.7. *Vernonia amygdalina* del

V. amygdalina is a shrub which is widely found in West Africa. The leaves are very popular vegetables used for soup. The roots and the leaves are used in ethnomedicine to treat fever, hiccups, kidney problems and stomach discomfort among other uses [79]. Both aqueous and alcoholic extracts of the stem, bark, roots and leaves are used extensively as purgative, antimalarial and in the treatment of eczema [80]. The use of the plant has been validated in humans to possess potent antimalarial and antihelminthic properties [81], antitumorigenic properties [82] and antiparasitic activity. It has been found to be used for self-medication by parasitized chimpanzees [83]. It has also been shown that the leaf extract has both hypoglycemic and hypolipidemic properties in experimental animals [84].

13.7.1. Animal toxicity

Acute toxicity studies produced an LD_{50} of 500 mg/kg body weight in Wistar albino rats. Biochemical parameters such as total, conjugated and unconjugated bilirubin levels showed no significant increase. The levels of both alanine aminotransferase and alkaline phosphatase in the presence of *V. amygdalina* leaf extract increased slightly in a dose-dependent manner when compared with the control but none of the observed increases was statistically significant ($P > 0.05$) when compared to the control or when compared within doses. The processed extracts of the plant were able to reverse carbon tetrachloride-induced hepatotoxicity in rats [85].

13.8. Herbal mixtures containing *Alstonia congensis* Engler bark and *Xylopia aethiopica* fruits (Dunal) A. Rich

In Africa and other parts of the world, herbal medications are prepared mostly from a combination of two or more plant parts which contain many active constituents with multiple physiological activities and could be used in the treatment of various health conditions [72] and possibly to reduce toxicity. The herbal formulation prepared with *A. congensis* bark and *X. aethiopica* fruits in equal proportion is a popular local herbal product taken over a long time for the treatment of diabetes.

13.8.1. Animal toxicity

In the acute and sub-acute study of the mixture in Swiss albino mice and Wistar albino rats, respectively, no changes in the behavior and in the sensory nervous system responses were observed. Gastro-intestinal effects were not observed in either male or female mice used in the experiments. The median acute toxicity value (LD_{50}) of the extract was above 20.0 g/kg body weight [86]. There was no significant change observed in the protein levels of the rats treated with lower doses of the extract (50 and 100 mg/kg) compared with control, while an observed significant decrease in the protein levels of the rats treated with a high dose (500 mg/kg) may be a sign of impaired renal function. Also, there was a significant increase ($p < 0.05$) in the plasma creatinine levels of all the treated groups [86]. There was no significant increase in AST and alanine aminotransferase (ALT) in the animals treated with lower doses of the extract compared with control but a significant increase in ALT was observed in the group treated with a high dose of the extract (500 mg/kg). This implies that the extract at the doses used had no effects on the heart tissue but at a high dose could have some deleterious effects on the liver tissue. The extract did neither improve nor produced any deleterious effects on the hematological parameters [86].

13.9. *Aspalathus linearis* (Burm. F.) Dahlg

The popular herbal tea, rooibos, also known as the 'long-life tea' in South Africa [86], is produced from the plant *A. linearis*. It is endemic to the South Africa [87]. Rooibos tea is known to have several health benefits, including antispasmodic, antioxidant, antiaging and antieczema activities [87].

Rooibos is exported to the East and Europe [88] and is currently sold in several countries including The Netherlands, Japan, the United Kingdom, Germany and the United States of America. The tea is mainly patronized due to its health-promoting properties when compared to black tea (*Camellia sinensis*) [89]. Rooibos is used as a beverage by the Khoi-descended people of the Cape; pregnant women take it for the iron content, and to relieve nausea and heartburns associated with pregnancy. It also serves as a milk substitute for infants and as colic relief in babies. Rooibos is well known for its antioxidant activity which also relates to its hepatoprotective properties [87] and immune-modulating effect in stimulating antibody production [90].

13.9.1. Animal toxicity

The safety assessment of rooibos has been addressed by some studies [87, 89]. Although some compounds in rooibos have been shown to contain mutagenic properties [91], it is, however, very unlikely that the mutagenic effect of rooibos would be relevant to tea drinkers when considering the quantities consumed [87]. In a study in rats, chronic consumption of aqueous extracts of unfermented and fermented rooibos over a period of 10 weeks did not cause any adverse effects in the liver and kidney [87].

13.10. *Musanga cecropioides* R. Br. Ex Tedlie

This plant is widely found in the tropical rainforest, particularly in West Africa. In Nigeria, the boiled leaves are used by the Igbo tribe as a powerful oxytocic to induce or augment labor while others use the decoction as a remedy for hypertension [92]. Parts of the plant have been used by traditional healers in the treatment of an array of diseases including lumbago, rheumatism, leprosy, chest infections and trypanosomiasis [92].

13.10.1. Animal toxicity

Acute toxicity study of *M. cecropioides* aqueous stem bark extract showed no mortality in rats, at a limit dose of 3000 mg/kg body weight given orally. This is an indication that the extract has low acute toxicity when orally administered. Administration of the aqueous extract for 28 days in a chronic study did not affect most of the biochemical parameters except for creatinine which was significantly elevated. Hematological parameters were not significantly affected during the 28-day treatment. Liver enzymes, AST and ALT, were not affected in the treatment showing that the extract is non-toxic on the hepatocytes. The study concluded that the absence of clinical signs of acute toxicities in human when the extract was orally administered as an antihypertensive may reflect the oral route of administration, low dose administration as well as short duration of exposure when used as an antihypertensive agent [93].

14. Conclusion

There is an increasing use of medicinal plants and herbal medicines which contribute significantly to the health of humanity worldwide, especially in developing countries. The limited scientific knowledge among the general population has led to the general assumption that herbal medicines being natural are therefore safe. However, evidence is being adduced from toxicological studies that show plant products to be potentially toxic thus affecting their safe use.

The source of potential toxicity could be traced to a number of factors: the type of constituents some of which may be intrinsically toxic such as tropane alkaloids and cardiac glycosides though they had been used in traditional medicine. Also, it is noted that the route of administration and dose, of any chemical, are important regarding safety due to chemical or pharmacological interactions; this is undergirded by the need for a regulatory regime for quality.

Serious adverse effects of therapies involving aqueous traditional medicines are rare. However, efforts to investigate toxicity, organ toxicity and cytotoxicity, have involved the use of organic solvent plant extracts and routes of administration which constitute a drawback to the conclusions drawn from such studies.

Information on the traditional formulation and use of the herbal medicines should be satisfactory to avoid possible toxicity from the medicinal plants. Manufacturers of herbal medicines should consider standardization of the products while patrons of herbal medicines need to inform their health-care providers about any herbal products they use to ensure effective and safe care. This is to avoid interaction between herbal and allopathic medicines which could yield adverse reactions.

Author details

Merlin L.K. Mensah[1], Gustav Komlaga[2*], Arnold D. Forkuo[3], Caleb Firempong[4], Alexander K. Anning[5] and Rita A. Dickson[2]

*Address all correspondence to: gustkomla@yahoo.com

1 Department of Herbal Medicine, Faculty of Pharmacy and Pharmaceutical Sciences, Kwame Nkrumah University of Science and Technology, Kumasi, Ghana

2 Department of Pharmacognosy, Faculty of Pharmacy and Pharmaceutical Sciences, Kwame Nkrumah University of Science and Technology, Kumasi, Ghana

3 Department of Pharmacology, Faculty of Pharmacy and Pharmaceutical Sciences, Kwame Nkrumah University of Science and Technology, Kumasi, Ghana

4 Departments of Biochemistry and Biotechnology, Faculty of Science, Kwame Nkrumah University of Science and Technology, Kumasi, Ghana

5 Department of Theoretical and Applied Biology, Faculty of Science, Kwame Nkrumah University of Science and Technology, Kumasi, Ghana

References

[1] Langlois-Klassen D, Kipp W, Jhangri GS, Rubaale T. Use of traditional herbal medicine by AIDS patients in Kabarole District, western Uganda. The American Journal of Tropical Medicine and Hygiene. 2007;**77**(4):757-763

[2] Abdullahi AA. Trends and challenges of traditional medicine in Africa. African Journal of Traditional, Complementary, and Alternative Medicines. 2011;**8**(5 Suppl):115-123

[3] WHO, Fendall NR. Declaration of Alma-Ata. Lancet. Geneva: WHO Press; 1978. 1978;**2**;1308

[4] Mahomoodally MF. Traditional medicines in Africa: An appraisal of ten potent African medicinal plants. Evidence-based Complementary and Alternative Medicine. 2013; 2013:617459

[5] Kofi B, Mhame PP, Kasilo OM. Clinical practices of African traditional medicine. The African Health Monitor [Internet]. Special Issue 14; 2010:33-39. Available from: https://www.aho.afro.who.int/en/ahm/issue/13/reports/clinical-practices-african-traditional-medicine

[6] Petrovska B. Historical review of medicinal plants' usage. Pharmacognosy Reviews. 2012 Jan;**6**(11):1

[7] de Barros NF, Fiuza AR. Evidence-based medicine and prejudice-based medicine: The case of homeopathy. Cadernos de Saúde Pública. 2014;**30**(11):2368-2376

[8] WHO. WHO Guidelines on Safety Monitoring of Herbal Medicines in Pharmacovigilance Systems. Geneva: World Health Organization; 2004. 82 pp

[9] Amit Kumar Tyagi SP. Traditional medicine: The goldmine for modern drugs. Advanced Techniques in Biology & Medicine. 2015;**3**(1):1-2

[10] Komlaga G, Cojean S, Beniddir MA, Dickson RA, Champy P, Suyyagh-albouz S, et al. The antimalarial potential of three Ghanaian medicinal plants. Herbal Medicine Open Access. 2015;**1**(1):1-6

[11] Komlaga G, Cojean S, Dickson RA, Beniddir MA, Suyyagh-Albouz S, Mensah MLK, et al. Antiplasmodial activity of selected medicinal plants used to treat malaria in Ghana. Parasitology Research. 2016;**115**(8):3185-3195

[12] Tetteh AW, Mensah ML, Boadu KO, Thomford KP, Agyemang MO, Annan K, et al. Clinical evaluation of the safety and effectiveness of Adutwumwaa Malamix: A poly-herbal product for the treatment of uncomplicated malaria in Ghana. Journal of Applied Pharmaceutical Science. 2017;**7**(7):040-045

[13] UNL Environmental Health and Safety. Toxicology and Exposure Guidelines [Internet]. Lincoln: University of Nebrasha; 2002 [cited 2017 Sep 22]. p. 28. Available from: https://ehs.unl.edu/documents/tox_exposure_guidelines.pdf

[14] Denny KH, Stewart CW. Acute, sub-acute, sub-chronic and chronic general toxicity testing for preclinical drug development. In: A Comprehensive Guide to Toxicology in Preclinical Drug Development. Elsevier Inc.: London; 2013. pp. 87-105

[15] Herxheimer A. Basic information that prescribers are not getting about drugs. Lancet. 1987;**329**(8523):31-33

[16] WHO. The WHO Recommended Classification of Pesticides by Hazard, and Guidelines to Classification. Geneva: WHO Press; 2010. pp. 1-81

[17] Nasri H, Shirzad H. Toxicity and safety of medicinal plants. Journal of Herbmed Pharmacology. 2013;**2**(2):21-22

[18] Kuete V. Toxicological Survey of African Medicinal Plants. 1st ed. In: Kuete V, editor. London: Elsevier Inc.; 2014. pp. 1-742

[19] Fennell CW, Light ME, Sparg SG, Stafford GI, Van Staden J. Assessing African medicinal plants for efficacy and safety: Agricultural and storage practices. Journal of Ethnopharmacology. 2004;**95**(2-3):113-121

[20] Sharma OP, Sharma S, Pattabhi V, Mahato SB, Sharma PDA. Review of the hepatotoxic plant Lantana camara. Critical Reviews in Toxicology. 2007;**37**:313-352

[21] Komlaga G, Agyare C, Dickson RA, Mensah MLK, Annan K, Loiseau PM, et al. Medicinal plants and finished marketed herbal products used in the treatment of malaria in the Ashanti region, Ghana. Journal of Ethnopharmacology. 2015 Jul 4;**172**:333-346

[22] Van Andel T, Myren B, Van Onselen S. Ghana's herbal market. Journal of Ethnopharmacology. 2012;**140**(2):368-378

[23] Raman A, Lau C. Anti-diabetic properties and phytochemistry of Momordica charantia L. (Cucurbitaceae). Phytomedicine. 1996;**2**(4):349-362

[24] Dharmananda S. The Interactions of Herbs and Drugs [Internet]. [cited 2017 Sep 17]. Available from: https://www.itmonline.org/arts/herbdrug.htm

[25] Barbosa JD, de Oliveira CMC, Duarte MD, Riet-Correa G, Peixoto PV, Tokarnia CH. Poisoning of horses by bamboo, Bambusa vulgaris. Journal of Equine Veterinary Science 2006 Sep;**26**(9):393-398

[26] Deshpande SS. Handbook of Food Toxicology. Marcel Dekker. New York: Marcel Dekker. Inc.; 2002. pp. 1-5

[27] Hill MS. Understanding Environmental Pollution. 3rd ed. Cambridge: Cambridge University Press; 1997. 316 pp

[28] Lv L, Huang W, Yu X, Ren H, Sun R. Comparative research of different Bupleurum chinense composition to influence of hepatotoxicity of rats and oxidative damage mechanism. China Journal of Chinese Materia Medica. 2009;**34**(18):2364-2368

[29] Balammal G, Babu MS, Reddy PJ. Analysis of herbal medicines by modern chromatographic techniques. International Journal of Preclinical and Pharmaceutical Research. 2012;**3**(1):50-63

[30] Woolston MSC. Herb-drug interactions [Internet]. Health Day. 2017;**355**:134-138. Available from: https://consumer.healthday.com/encyclopedia/holistic-medicine-25/mis-alternative-medicine-news-19/herb-drug-interactions-646428.html

[31] Palombo EA. Phytochemicals from traditional medicinal plants used in the treatment of diarrhoea: Modes of action and effects on intestinal function. Phytotherapy Research. 2006;**20**(9):717-724

[32] Gurib-Fakim A. Medicinal plants: Traditions of yesterday and drugs of tomorrow. Molecular Aspects of Medicine. 2006:1-93

[33] WHO. General Guidelines for Methodologies on Research and Evaluation of Traditional Medicine. Vol. 1. Geneva: WHO Press; 2000

[34] Riss TL, Moravec RA, Niles AL. Cytotoxicity testing: Measuring viable cells, dead cells, and detecting mechanism of cell death. Methods in Molecular Biology. 2011;**740**:103-114

[35] Ricci SM, Zong W-X. Chemotherapeutic approaches for targeting cell death pathways. The Oncologist. 2006;**11**(4):342-357

[36] Blazka ME, Hayes W. Acute toxicity and eye irritancy. In: Principles and Methods of Toxicology. 5th ed. New York: CRC Press, Taylor and Francis Group, 2001. pp. 1131-1141

[37] McGaw LJ, Elgorashi EE, Eloff JN. Cytotoxicity of African medicinal plants against normal animal and human cells. In: Kuete V, editor. Toxicological Survey of African Medicinal Plants. 1st ed. London: Elsevier; 2014. pp. 181-233

[38] Schimmer O, Kruger A, Paulini H, Haefele F. An evaluation of 55 commercial plant extracts in the Ames mutagenicity test. Die Pharmazie. 1994;**49**(6):448-451

[39] Kassie F, Parzefall W, Musk S, Johnson I, Lamprecht G, Sontag G, et al. Genotoxic effects of crude juices from Brassica vegetables and juices and extracts from phytopharmaceutical preparations and spices of cruciferous plants origin in bacterial and mammalian cells. Chemico-Biological Interactions. 1996;**102**(1):1-16

[40] Fernandes De Sá Ferreira IC, Ferrão Vargas VM. Mutagenicity of medicinal plant extracts in salmonella/microsome assay. Phyther Res. 1999;**13**(5):397-400

[41] Muganza MD, Fruth BI, Nzunzu Lami J, Mesia GK, Kambu OK, Tona GL, et al. In vitro antiprotozoal and cytotoxic activity of 33 ethnopharmacologically selected medicinal plants from Democratic Republic of Congo. Journal of Ethnopharmacology [Internet]. 2012 May 7 [Cited 2014 Aug 6];**141**(1):301-308. Available from http://www.ncbi.nlm.nih.gov/pubmed/22394563

[42] Ansah C, Gooderham NJ. The popular herbal antimalarial, extract of Cryptolepis sanguinolenta, is potently cytotoxic. Toxicological Sciences. 2002 Dec 1;**70**(2):245-251

[43] Nazar H, Usmanghani K. Clinical evaluation to assess the safety and efficacy of coded herbal medicine "Dysmo-off" versus allopathic medicine "Diclofenac sodium" for the treatment of primary dysmenorrhea. Journal of Herbal Pharmacotherapy. 2006;**6**(1):89-126

[44] Ganesh S, Patki SP, Mitra S. Clinical evaluation of a herbal formulation in liver disorders. Aust J Med Herbal. 2009;**21**(1):10-14

[45] Turkson BK, Kofi PO, Achaab E, Woyome Y, MLK M, Sarpong K, et al. Clinical evaluation of the effectiveness and safety of mist amen Fevermix, a Ghanaian bi-herbal product, used in the management of uncomplicated malaria. Journal of Natural Science Research. 2015;**5**(10):28-33

[46] Bugyei KA, Boye GL, Addy ME. Clinical efficacy of a tea-bag formulation of Cryptolepis sanguinolenta root in the treatment of acute uncomplicated falciparum malaria. Ghana Medical Journal. 2010;**44**(1):3-9

[47] Ansah C, Khan A, Gooderham NJ. Vitro genotoxicity of the West African anti-malarial herbal Cryptolepis sanguinolenta and its major alkaloid cryptolepine. Toxicology. 2005 Mar 1;**208**(1):141-147

[48] Ajayi AF, Akhigbe RE, Adewumi OM, Olaleye SB. Haematological evaluation of Cryptolepis sanguinolenta stem ethanolic extract in rats plant material. Int J Med Biomedical Research. 2012;**1**(1):56-61

[49] Oliver-Bever BEP. Medicinal Plants in Tropical West Africa. Cambridge: Cambridge University Press; 1986. pp. 203-204

[50] Ansah C, Otsyina HR, Duwiejua M, Woode E, Aboagye FA, Aning KG. Toxicological assessment of Cryptolepis sanguinolenta for possible use in veterinary medicine. J Vet Med Anim Heal. 2009;**1**(1):11-16

[51] Mukinda JT, Syce JA. Acute and chronic toxicity of the aqueous extract of Artemisia afra in rodents. Journal of Ethnopharmacology. 2007 May 30;**112**(1):138-144

[52] Oudhia P. Major Cassia species of Chhattisgarh, India: Natural occurrence, traditional medicinal knowledge and trade. Available from: http://www.botanical.com/site/column_poudhia/108_cassia.html [Accessed: July 25, 2017]

[53] Ghana Herbal Pharmacopoeia. Accra, Ghana: Policy Research and Strategic Planning Institute (PORSPI); 1992

[54] Silva MGB, Aragao TP, Vasconcelos CFB, Ferreira PA, et al. Acute and subacute toxicity of Cassia occidentalis L. stem and leaf in Wistar rats. Journal of Ethnopharmacology. 2011;**136**:341-346

[55] Suliman HB, Shommein AM. Toxic effect of the roasted and unroasted beans of *Cassia occidentalis* in goats. Veterinary and Human Toxicology. 1986;**28**:6-11

[56] Nicholson SS, Thornton JT, Rimes AJ. Toxic myopathy in dairy cattle caused by *Cassia obtusifolia* in green-chop. Bovine Prac. 1977;**12**:120-123

[57] Barbosa-Ferreira M, Dagli ML, Maiorka PC, Gorniak SL. Sub-acute intoxication by *Senna occidentalis* seeds in rats. Food and Chemical Toxicology. 2005;**43**:497-503

[58] Haraguchi M, Dagli ML, Raspantini PC, Gorniak SL. The effects of low doses of *Senna occidentalis* seeds on broiler chickens. Veterinary Research Communications. 2003;**2**:321-328

[59] Fairbairn JW. The distribution of anthraquinone glycosides in Cassia senna L. Phytochemistry. 1987;**6**(9):1203-1207

[60] Vanderperren B, Rizzo M, Angenot L, Haufroid V, Jadoul M, Hantson P. Acute liver failure with renal impairment related to the abuse of senna anthraquinone glycosides. The Annals of Pharmacotherapy. 2005;**39**:1353-1357

[61] Wilson S. Cassia occidentalis. In: Some Plants are Poisonous. Victoria: Reed Books Australia; 1997. Available at: http://www.touchwoodbooks.co.nz/tsomeplants.html Accessed: February 24, 2006

[62] Vashishtha VM, Kumar A, John TJ, Nayak NC. *Cassia occidentalis* poisoning—As the probable cause of hepatomyoencephalopathy in children in western Uttar Pradesh. The Indian Journal of Medical Research. 2007;**125**:756-762

[63] Vashishtha VM, Kumar A, John TJ, Nayak NC. *Cassia occidentalis* poisoning causes fatal coma in children in western Uttar Pradesh. Indian Pediatrics. 2007;**44**:522-525

[64] Millar AG, Morris M. Plants of Dhofar; The Southern Region of Oman, Traditional, Economic and Medicinal Uses. Sultanate of Oman: The Office of the Advisor for Conservation of the Environment, Diwan of Royal Court; 1987. p. 42

[65] Quisumbing E. Medicinal Plants of Philippines. Quezon City, Philipines: The Katha Publishing Co., Inc.; 1978

[66] Chikpah SK, Teye M, Annor JAF, Teye GA. Elixir. Food Science. 2015;**79**:30166-30170

[67] Neal SN, Bhatti DS. Preliminary screening of some weeds and shrubs for their nematocidal activity against *Meloidogyne javanica*. Indian. Journal of Nematology. 1978;**13**:123-127

[68] Girdhar G, Deval K, Mittal PK, Vasudevan P. Mosquito control by Calotropis latex. Pesticides. 1984;**18**:82-87

[69] Ayoub SMH, Kingston DGI. Screening of plants used in Sudan folk medicine for anti-cancer activity. Fitoterapia. 1981;**52**:281-284

[70] Prakash AO, Gupta RB, Mathur R. Effect of oral administration of forty two indigenous plants extracts on early and late pregnancy in albino rats. Probe. 1978;**27**:315-323

[71] Awal MA, Ainu Nahar M, Shamim Hossain MA, Barri M, Rahman HME. Brine shrimp toxicity of leaf and seed extracts of Cassia alata Linn.and their antibacterial potency. Journal of Medical Sciences. 2004;**4**(3):188-193

[72] Pieme CA, Penlap VN, Nkegoum B, Taziebou CL, Tekwu EM, Etoa FX, Ngongang J. Evaluation of acute and subacute toxicities of aqueous ethanolic extract of leaves of *(L) Roxb(Ceasalpiniaceae)*. African Journal of Biotechnology. 2006;**5**(3):283-289

[73] Anokbonggo WW, Odoi-Adome R, Oluju PM. Traditional methods of diarrhoeal management in Uganda. Bulletin of the World Health Organisation. 1990;**68**:359-363

[74] Sofowora EA. Medicinal Plants and Traditional Medicine in Africa. Ibadan – Oweri – Kaduna – Lagos: Spectrum Books Limited; 1993. pp. 159-176; 179-189; 195-238

[75] Taiwo O, Xu HX, Lee SF. Antibacterial activities of extracts from Nigerian chewing sticks. Phytotherapy Research. 1999;**13**(8):675-679

[76] Ogwal-Okeng JW, Obua C, Anokbonggo WWW. Acute toxicity effects of the methanolic extract of Fagara zanthoxyloides (lam.) root-bark. African Health Sciences. 2003 Dec;**3**(3):124-126

[77] El-Said F, Fadulu SO, Kuye JO, Sofowora A. Native Cures in Nigeria; Part II: The antimicrobial properties of the buffered extracts of chewing sticks. Lloydia. 1971;**34**:172-175

[78] Oriowo MA. Anti-inflammatory activity of piperonyl-4-acrylic isobutyl amide, an extractive from *Zanthoxylum zanthoxyloides*. Planta Medica. 1982;**44**(1):54-56

[79] Hamowia AM, Saffaf AM. Pharmacological studies on *Vernonia amygdalina* (del) and *Tithonia diversifolia* (Gray). Veterinary Medical Journal Giza. 1994;**2**:91-97

[80] Kupcham SM. Drugs from natural products. Plant source in drugs discovery, science and development. American Chemical Society. 1971;**6**:311-318

[81] Abosi AO, Raseroka BH. *In vivo* antimalarial activity of *Vernonia amygdalina*. British Journal of Biomedical Science. 2003;**60**(2):89-91

[82] Izevbigie EB, Bryant JL, Walker A. A novel natural inhibitor of extracellular signal-regulated kinases and human breast cancer cell growth. Experimental Biol. Med. (Maywood). 2004;**229**(2):163-169

[83] Huffman MA. Animal self-medication and ethno-medicine: Exploration and exploitation of the medicinal properties of plants. The Proceedings of the Nutrition Society. 2003;**62**(2):371-381

[84] Akah PA, Okafor CI. Blood sugar lowering effect of Vernonia amygdalina Del, in an experimental rabbit model. Phytherapy Research. 1992;**6**(3):171-173

[85] Babalola OO, Anetor JI, Adeniyi FA. Amelioration of carbon tetrachloride-induced hepatotoxicity by terpenoid extract from leaves of *Vernonia amydgalina*. The African Journal of Medical Sciences. 2001;**30**(1-2):91-93

[86] Ogbonnia S, Adekunle AA, Bosa MK, Enwuru VN. Evaluation of acute and subacute toxicity of *Alstonia congensis* Engler (Apocynaceae) bark and *Xylopia aethiopica* (Dunal) a. rich (Annonaceae) fruits mixtures used in the treatment of diabetes. African Journal of Biotechnology. 2008;**7**(6):701-705

[87] Joubert E, De Beer D. Rooibos (*Aspalathus linearis*) beyond the farm gate: From herbal tea to potential phytopharmaceutical. South African Journal of Botany. 2011;**77**(4):869-886

[88] Mulholland DA, Drewes SE. Global phytochemistry: Indigenous medicinal chemistry on track in southern Africa. Phytochemistry. 2004;**65**(7):769-782

[89] Blommaert KLJ, Steenkamp J. Tannin and possible caffeine content of rooibos tea, *Aspalathus* (subgen. Nortiera) *linearis* (Burm. Fil) R. Dahlgr [Afrikaans]. Agroplantae. 1978;**10**:49

[90] Kunishiro K, Tai A, Yamamoto I. Effects of rooibos tea extract on antigen-specific antibody production and cytokine generation *in vitro* and *in vivo*. Bioscience, Biotechnology, and Biochemistry. 2001;**65**(10):2137-2145

[91] Snijman PW, Swanevelder S, Joubert E, Green IR, Gelderblom WCA. The antimutagenic activity of the major flavonoids of rooibos (*Aspalathus linearis*): Some dose-response effects on mutagen activation-flavonoid interactions. Mutation Research, Genetic Toxicology and Environmental Mutagenesis. 2007;**631**(2):111-123

[92] Burkill HM. In: Farinhes A-D, editor. The Useful Plants of West Tropical Africa. 2nd ed. Kew: Royal Botanical Gardens; 1985;**1**:346-349

[93] Adeneye AA, Ajagbonna OP, Adeleke TI, Bello SO. Preliminary toxicity and phytochemical studies of the stem bark aqueous extract of *Musanga cecropioides* in rats. Journal of Ethnopharmacology. 2006;**105**:374-379

4

Taraxacum Genus: Potential Antibacterial and Antifungal Activity

María Eugenia Martínez Valenzuela,
Katy Díaz Peralta, Lorena Jorquera Martínez and
Rolando Chamy Maggi

Abstract

Plants have been used in traditional medicine for centuries as antibacterial and antifungal agents. *Taraxacum* spp., commonly known as dandelion, is a well-known herbal remedy with a long history; however, limited scientific information is available to explain its traditional use. This review aims to provide current information and a general overview of the available literature concerning the antibacterial and antifungal properties of the *Taraxacum* genus to support its potential as a powerful herbal medicine. Though *Taraxacum* has demonstrated that it is capable of inhibiting the growth of a wide range of bacteria and fungi, the technical aspects of methodology lack standardization, and, therefore, the overall results of processing are difficult to compare between studies. Phytochemical composition and antimicrobial activity in *Taraxacum* are neither directly related, nor does the published data provide sufficient information for identifying the group of unique extraction conditions that are optimal against specific microorganisms. Antimicrobial research indicates that this plant is a promising species for treating several common infections in humans, animals, and plants.

Keywords: antimicrobial, antifungal, ethnopharmacology, extraction, *Taraxacum* species

1. Introduction

Plants have been used in traditional medicine for centuries due to the synthesis of several molecules that provide antibacterial and antifungal properties, the majority of which probably evolved as defenses against infection or predation [1]. The medicinal potential of many plants is still largely unexplored. Among the estimated 250,000–500,000 plant species, a relatively small percentage have been investigated phytochemically and the fraction submitted for biological or pharmacological screening is even smaller [2]; approximately 20% of the plant species in the world have been investigated for these properties [3]. In this context, dandelion serves as an interesting species with which to unify decades-old information regarding its biological potential against diverse microorganisms. This review gathers the existing results to advance the search for products that could strengthen the domestication and mass production of this plant.

The *Taraxacum* spp. commonly called dandelion is an herbaceous perennial plant of the *Asteraceae* (Compositae) family. This common weed is found worldwide, though originally introduced from Eurasia, and can be found growing in parks, gardens, pastures, orchards, roadsides, vegetable gardens, and among agricultural and horticultural crops [4]. Primarily used as food, the role of *Taraxacum* in traditional medicine was mentioned during ancient times by the Greek physician Dioscorides in the first century and during the renaissance by monks in Cyprus [5]. This plant has been used to treat cystitis, liver and gastric ailments, hepatic and renal detoxification, diabetes, as an anti-inflammatory and anticarcinogenic agent, and, to a lesser extent, as an antimicrobial and antiviral agent, as described in several reviews [6, 7]. Ethnopharmacologically, its use as an antimicrobial agent has been known worldwide among varying cultures, though it has always been administered as a cataplasm (poultice) or infusion. The traditional antimicrobial uses of *Taraxacum* worldwide are displayed in **Table 1**.

Asia and Europe have an important historical background regarding the traditional uses of *Taraxacum*, primarily *T. officinale*, *T. mongolicum*, and *T. coreanum*. This traditional knowledge has been the principal reason for studying the potential uses and crop requirements of *Taraxacum*; studies in America remain scarce [18]. Due to the unscientific approach often present in oral traditions, uncertainty surrounds whether *Taraxacum* use effectively treats microbial infection or, instead, treats only the symptoms. Therefore, scientific research is extremely important in avoiding misinterpretation and myths regarding *Taraxacum* or any other plant.

The first antibacterial scientific study for *Taraxacum* was reported a mere 35 years ago [19]. More than a decade later, studies related to *Taraxacum* antimicrobial activity gained significant

Species	Common use	Country	Part used	Consumption	References
T. cyprium	Catarrh and common cold, cough	Greece	Roots, leaves	—	[5]
T. mongolicum	Urinary tract infections	China	Leaf	Infusion	[8]
T. officinale	Malaria	Venezuela	Roots, leaves	Decoction	[9]
	Tuberculosis	Italy	—	—	[10]
	Cough	Italy	—	—	[11]
	Bacterial infection	Mexico	—	—	[12]
	Diuretic	Chikar	Roots	Tonico	[13]
T. panalpinum	Malaria	Portugal	Roots, leaves, juice	—	[14, 15]
T. platycarpum	Pleurodynia	Korea	Leaf, stem	Infusion Brewing	[16, 17]

Table 1. Ethnopharmacological information of *Taraxacum* genus used as an antimicrobial traditional medicine.

relevance as part of an Italian program between the University of Ferrara and the University of Naples for screening medicinal plants [20]. Nowadays, this plant is becoming a promising species in the treatment of several bacterial and fungal diseases due to the results of various antimicrobial-related studies. This chapter seeks to elucidate both the traditional uses and current state of *Taraxacum* in antimicrobial research to determine the potential that this genus has to become an industrial medicinal crop worldwide. Due to the high potential value that could be derived from the use of new technologies and industrial products developed from this type of plant species, the conservation and protection of the crop should be considered and sustainable global production strategies are developed in accordance with assessments of ecological, economic, and social factors.

2. Antimicrobial properties of the *Taraxacum* genus

Literature reviews providing information on the antimicrobial aspects of natural products, which had until now only been considered empirical, have been recently scientifically confirmed as a means of countering the increasing reports of pathogenic microorganisms resistant to synthetic antimicrobial agents. Some plant-derived compounds can control microbial growth, either separately or in association with conventional antimicrobials [21]. Currently, numerous studies seek to improve pathogen prevention by combining the application of medicinal herb extracts with an antibiotic or effective antipathogenic pesticide to reduce the active synthetic ingredient and resistant pathogenic strains.

2.1. *Taraxacum* species tested for antimicrobial properties

Among the *Taraxacum* genus, *T. officinale* is the most frequently reported species, with almost 80% of mentions in documents related to antimicrobial properties (see **Table 2**), followed by *T. mongolicum* and *T. coreanum*, though over 2500 *Taraxacum* species are currently identified [67]. Other, less studied species include *T. platycarpum*, *T. farinosum*, *T. ohwianum*, and *T. phaleratum*; however, the relevance of these species is confined to specific areas (mostly in Asia) in which they grow naturally since they are not deliberately cultivated for medicinal benefit. This indicates that the microbial properties of less than 1% of all *Taraxacum* species discovered have been studied, revealing the enormous research potential of this genus.

2.2. Bacterial and fungi strains tested

Taraxacum extracts have been tested on different bacterial and fungal strains affecting humans, animals, and plants to determine its antimicrobial profile, confirm its traditional usage, and expand its known uses. Antimicrobial agents are categorized based on the spectrum of action, namely "narrow" and "broad" spectrum, which indicates whether its use is specific for certain bacterial strains or active on a wider range. Bacterial infections can result in mild to life-threatening illnesses that require immediate antibiotic intervention. Alternatively, a superficial fungal infection is rarely life-threatening but can have debilitating effects and may spread to other people or become invasive or systemic, resulting in a life-threatening infection. The widespread, and sometimes inappropriate, use of chemical compounds can create antibiotic

Species	Autentification/ Voucher	C: Collected P: Purchase	Zone	Season	Plant part*	Sample manipulation	Ratio	Solvent	Extraction time	Temp.	Agitation	Inhibition activity**	Ref.
T. officinale Wigg.	No/No	NI	NI	NI	Flower	NI	1:10	Acetic acid 10%	1 h	RT	Homog.	+	[22]
T. officinale Wigg.	No/No	C	NI	Yes	Seeds	Grounded	1:10	Acetic acid 10%	1 h	RT	NI	+	[23]
T. officinale Weber	Yes/No	C	Yes	Yes	NI	Dried	NI	Water, ethanol and ethyl acetate	1 h	80°C	Maceration	+	[24]
T. officinale	Yes/Yes	C	Yes	NI	NI	Air-dried	1:14	Acetone	30 min	NI	NI	+	[25]
Taraxacum spp.	No/No	C	Yes	NI	NI	NI	1:10	Dichloromethane	3 h	20°C	Homog.	+	[26]
T. officinale	No/Yes	C	Yes	Yes	NI	NI	NI	Dichloromethane	3 days	NI	Homog.	+	[27]
T. coreanum	No/No	NI	NI	NI	NI	NI	1:3.3	Ethanol 75%	9 h	60°C	Reflux	+	[28]
T. mongolicum	No/No	C	NI	NI	Aerial	Frezee-dried and grounded 20-mesh	1:5	Ethanol 75%	2 days	NI	Soaked	+	[29]
T. officinale Weber	No/Yes	C	Yes	Yes	Root	Dried and grounded	NI	Ethanol 80%	NI	NI	Reflux	+	[20]
T. officinale F. H. Wigg	Yes/Yes	C	NI	NI	Aerial	Air-dried and crushed	1:1	Ethanol 90%	2 days	RT	Intermitent shaking	+	[30]
T. mongolicum H.					NI		1:10	Ethanol 95%	3 h	80°C		+	[31]
T. ohwianum	No/No	NI	NI	NI	NI	Freeze-dried, air-dried (40°C, 24 h), grounded 24-mesh	1:16	Ethanol 95%	24 h	RT (23°C)	Shaking	+	[32]
T. officinale	Yes/No	NI	NI	NI	Leaves	Air-dried	1:5	Ethylacetate	24 h	RT	150 rpm	+	[22]
T. officinale F.H. Wigg.	Yes/Yes	P	NI	NI	Root	Freeze-dried and blended	1:10	Hexane	Overnight	RT	70 rpm	+	[33]

Species	Autentification/ Voucher	C: Collected P: Purchase	Zone	Season	Plant part*	Sample manipulation	Ratio	Solvent	Extraction time	Temp.	Agitation	Inhibition activity**	Ref.
T. officinale	No/No	NI	NI	NI	Leaves	Air-dried 1 month and grounded	1:1.4	Methanol 75%	NI	NI	NI	+	[34]
T. officinale Weber	No/No	C	Yes	NI	Aerial	Air-dried a 40°C (36–48 h) and grounded	1:5	Methanol 80%	1 h	100°C	Reflux	+	[35]
T. officinale Weber ex. F. H. Wigg	No/Yes	NI	NI	NI	Leaves	NI	1:4	Methanol	5 days	RT	NI	+	[36]
T. officinale Weber	No/No	C	NI	NI	Aerial	Dry under shade and ground	1:10	Methanol	3 weeks	25°C	Homog.	+	[37]
T. platycarpum	No/No	NI	NI	NI	NI	Dried	NI	Methanol	3 h	80°C	NI	+	[38]
T. platycarpum	No/No	NI	NI	NI	NI	Dried	NI	Methanol	3 h	80°C	NI	+	[39]
T. officinale					NI		NI	Methanol	16 h	50°C		+	[40]
T. officinale	No/No	C	NI	NI	Leaves	Dried under shade and grounded	1:2.5	Methanol	24 h	37°C	120 rpm	+	[41]
T. mongolicum Hand-Mazz	Yes/Yes	C	Yes	Yes	NI	Air-dried and grounded	NI	Water	3 h	100°C	By boiling	+	[36]
T. officinale					NI		1:05	Water	NI	NI	Homog.	+	[42]
T. officinale	No/No	NI	NI	NI	NI	Dried at 25–30°C for 1 week., ground with a mortar	1:20	Water	24 h	35°C	Shaking	+	[43]
T. officinale F.H. (Webb)	No/No	C/P	NI	NI	Root	Cleaning prior freeze-dried, grounded	1:10	Water	3 h	RT	170 rpm	+	[44]

Species	Autentification/ Voucher	C: Collected P: Purchase	Zone	Season	Plant part*	Sample manipulation	Ratio	Solvent	Extraction time	Temp.	Agitation	Inhibition activity**	Ref.
T. officinale	No/No	NI	NI	NI	NI	NI	1:04	Water	45 min	100°C	NI	+	[45]
T. officinale Weber ex Wigger	No/No	NI	NI	NI	leaves	Grounded	1:01	Water	5 min	NI	NI	+	[46]
T. mongolicum	No/No	NI	NI	NI	NI	Grounded	NI	Water	1 h	100°C	By boiling	+	[47]
T. officinale	No/No	NI	NI	NI	NI	Dried at 60°C × 2 h and grounded 60-mesh	1:10	Water	NI	NI	NI	+	[48]
T. officinale H.	NI/NI	NI	NI	NI	NI	NI						+	[49]
T. officinale F.H. Wigg	NI/NI	C	Yes	Yes	Honey	NI	NI	NI	NI	NI	NI	+	[50]
T. farinosum Hausskn. & Bornm	NI/NI	C	NI	Yes	Root	NI	NI	NI	NI	NI	NI	+	[51]
T. officinale	Yes/No	C	Yes	Yes	NI	Dried 40°C × 5 days and grounded	NI	NI	NI	NI	Reflux	+	[52]
T. officinale	NI/NI	NI	NI	NI	NI	NI	NI	NI	NI	NI	NI	+W	[53]
T. officinale	No/No	P	NI	NI	NI	NI	NI	Ethanol 35%	NI	NI	NI	+W	[54]
T. platycarpum	No/No	P	NI	NI	NI	Grounded 50-mesh	1:10	Ethanol	24 h	RT	Homog.	+W	[55]
Taraxacum sp.	No/No	NI	NI	NI	Aerial	Grounded	1:10	Water	4 h	100°C	By boiling	+W	[56]
T. officinale F.H. Wigg.	No/No	C	Yes	Yes	Aerial	Frozen, cut and grounded	1:01	Ethanol 20%	24 h	RT	NI	–	[57]
T. officinale	No/No	NI	NI	NI	Leaves	Dried	NI	Ethanol 40%	NI	NI	NI	–	[58]

Species	Autentification/ Voucher	C: Collected P: Purchase	Zone	Season	Plant part*	Sample manipulation	Ratio	Solvent	Extraction time	Temp.	Agitation	Inhibition activity**	Ref.
T. officinale	No/No	Extract (P)	NI	NI	NI	Diluted	NI	ethanol 45%	NI	NI	NI	–	[59]
T. phaleratum G. Hagl et Rech	Yes/Yes	C	Yes	NI	Aerial	Air-dried and grounded	NI	Ethanol 70%	NI	RT	NI	–	[60]
T. officinale Cass.	No/No	P	NI	NI	Root	Dried	1:04	Ethanol	24 h	NI		–	[61]
T. officinale	No/No	C	Yes	NI	flower	Chopped and frozen	NI	Methanol 90%	30 min	4°C	Homog.	–	[62]
T. officinale Weber	Yes/Yes	NI	NI	NI	NI	Dried and grounded	1:40	Methanol	Overnight	RT	NI	–	[63]
T. mongolicum Hand-Mazz	No/Yes	C	NI	NI	Whole	NI	1:10	Water	Overnight	NI	Homog.	–	[64]
T. officinale	No/No	P	NI	NI	Root	Grounded	1:8.3	Water	30 min	100°C	By boiling	–	[65]
T. officinale	No/No	C	Yes	Yes	Leafs, roots	NI	1:03	Water		RT	Homog.	–	[66]

*NI, No indicated.

Table 2. Physical parameters on *Taraxacum* extracts for testing antimicrobial activity.

resistance. Due to this issue, the potential of *Taraxacum* as a useful, broad-spectrum antimicrobial and antifungal agent that can be "easily and worldwide grown," is highly valuable. A list of the strains against which *Taraxacum*'s antimicrobial activity has been tested is displayed in **Table 3**.

Bacterial strains	**Fungi strains**
Aeromonas hydrophila (−) [22]	*Alternaria alternata* (+) [46, 68]
Agrobacterium tumefaciens (+) [24]	*Aspergillus carbonarius* (+) [35]
Bacillus cereus (+) [22, 33, 36, 44] (−) [66]	*A. niger* (+) [23, 35, 37, 68, 69] (−) [27, 66]
B. pumilus (−) [66]	*A. flavus* (+) [37] (−) [66]
B. subtilis (+) [20, 24, 25, 27, 29, 34, 38, 39, 41, 48, 69] (−) [37, 64, 66]	*A. fumigatus* (+) [37](−) [66]
Campylobacter jejuni (+) [54, 59]	*Bipolaris sorokiniana* (+) [23, 67] (−) [68]
Chromobacterium violaceum (+) [66] (−) [65]	*Botrytis cinerea* (+) [23, 35, 67]
Clavibacter michiganense (+) [69]	*Candida albicans* (+) [27, 34, 36, 52] (−) [55, 57, 66]
Cupriavidus sp. (−) [66]	*C. glabrata* (−) [55, 66]
Enterobacter coccus (−) [37]	*C. krusei* (−) [66]
Enterococcus faecalis (+) [53] (−) [37, 66]	*C. parapsilesis* (−) [55, 66]
Erwinia carotovora (+) [24]	*C. utils* (−) [55]
Escherichia coli (+) [22, 24, 25, 27, 29, 34, 36, 38, 39, 41, 43, 45, 47, 48, 58, 70] (−) [20, 32, 33, 37, 44, 57, 62, 64, 66]	*C. tropicalis* (+) [55] *Cladosporium herbarum* (+) [71]
Helicobacter pylori (+) [31, 54]	*Cochliobolus sativus* (+) [68]
Klebsiella aerogenes (−) [66]	*Colletotrichium gloesporoides* (−) [68]
K. penumoniae (+) [29, 36] (−) [20, 37, 45, 66]	*C. lagenarium* (+) [42]
Listeria monocytogenes (+) [38, 39] (−) [66]	*Cryptococcus neoformans* (+) [36]
Micrococcus kristinae (+) [25]	*Exophiala (Wangiella) dermatitidis* (−) [66]
M. luteus (+) [37, 41]	*Fusarium avenaceum* (+) [68]
Mycobacterium aurum (−) [63]	*F. graminearum* (−) [69]
M. bovis (−) [63]	*F. oxysporum* (+) [23, 56, 69]
M. smegmatis (−) [63]	*Microsporum canis* (+) [51]
M. tuberculosis (−) [60]	*Monilinia laxa* (+) [35]
Propionihacterium acnes (+) [49]	*Mucor piriformis* (+) [46]
Proteus mirabilis (+) [43] (−) [20]	*Penicillium sp.* (−) [66]
P. vulgaris (+) [25, 29] (−) [70]	*P. digitatum* (+) [35]
Pseudomonas sp. (−) [50]	*P. expansum* (+) [26, 46] (−) [35]
P. aeruginosa (+) [24, 27, 29, 36, 41, 49, 70] (−) [20, 37, 57, 64, 66]	*P. italicum* (+) [35]

Bacterial strains	Fungi strains
P. fluorescens (+) [24]	*Ph. betae* (+) [23, 68]
P. syringae (+) [69]	*Phytophthora infestans* (+) [69]
Serratia/Rahnella sp. (−) [66]	*Pityrosporum ovale* (+) [49]
Salmonella typhimurium (+) [36] (−) [33, 44]	*Pythium debaryanum* (+) [69]
S. abony enterica (+) [58]	*Rhizoctonia solani* (+) [37, 56]
S. poona (−) [66]	*Saccharomyces cereviseae* (+) [34]
S. typhi (+) [44, 51] (−) [20]	*Saprolegnia australis* (−) [61]
Sarcina lutea (+) [24]	*Scedosporium apiospermum* (−) [66]
Serratia marcescens (+) [25] (−) [66]	*Trichophyton longifusus* (+) [51]
Shigella fiexeri (−) [70]	*T. mentagrophytes* (+) [27]
S. sonnei (+) [36]	*Verticillium albo-atrum* (+) [23] (−) [68]
Staphylococcus aureus (+) [22, 24, 25, 28, 29, 32–34, 36, 38, 39, 41, 43–45, 48–52, 70] (−) [20, 27, 37, 57, 58, 62, 64, 66]	
S. epidermidis (+) [28] (−) [66]	
Streptococcus haemolyticus (+) [20]	
S. agalactiae (+) [47]	
S. dysgalactiae (+) [47]	
Vibrio cholerae (+) [37]	
V. parahaemolyticus (+) [38, 39]	
Xanthomonas campestris (+) [69]	
(+) Extracts of *Taraxacum* active against the pathogen; (−) extracts of *Taraxacum* inactive against the pathogen.	

Table 3. Bacterial and fungal strains on which *Taraxacum* extracts have been tested.

2.2.1. Human pathogens

In the study of antibacterial properties of these plants, most attention has been focused on human pathogenic strains, including *S. aureus, E. faecalis, V. cholerae, B. subtilis, P. aeruginosa, K. pneumonia,* and *E. coli*. These are the pathogens commonly responsible for infections in gastrointestinal and massive organ systems such as the lungs and skin. *Taraxacum officinale* is the species generally studied to combat these pathogens, but it has demonstrated diverse results depending on the extraction characteristics or the bioassay performed. For instance, a methanolic extract of *T. officinale* at 0.2 mg/mL was as effective as an antibacterial agent against *M. luteus* and *V. cholera* with minimum inhibitory concentration (MIC) values of 1.0 and 12.5 mg/mL, respectively, but displayed no activity against *S. aureus, E. faecalis, E. bacter, V. cholerae, B. subtilis, P. aeruginosa, K. pneumonia, or E. coli* [37]. In the same study, the inhibition percentages achieved for mycelial growth of *A. niger, A. flavus, A. fumigatus,* and *R. solani* were 37, 71, 85, and 78%, respectively. Other works indicate that methanolic *T. officinale* leaf extracts ranging from 0.003 to 0.5 mg/mL were active against *S. aureus, P. aeruginosa, B. cereus, S. sonnei,*

S. enterica serovar *typhimurium, E. coli, K. pneumonia, C. albicans,* and *C. neoformans* with MIC values ranging from 0.04 to 5.0 mg/mL [36]. A similar extract at 10 mg/mL displayed moderate growth diameter inhibition for *S. typhi,* but was highly active for *S. aureus, B. cereus,* and *E. coli,* even when no activity was observed for *A. hydrophila* [22]. Ethanolic extracts of 2.0 mg/mL were active against *A. aureus, MRSA* clinical, and *B. cereus,* with MIC values between 0.38 and 0.5 mg/mL, but were not effective against *E. coli* or *S. typhi.* In the same work, a water extract at the same concentration showed no activity against any strain tested [33]. Moreover, 21 ethanolic extracts from various plants were tested against 20 *Salmonella* serovars. *Taraxacum* inhibited only 5% of these, and was therefore not considered for additional antimicrobial studies [72].

Recently, methanolic and chloroformic leaf extracts of *T. officinale* were found to be effective against *M. luteus, P. aeruginosa, B. subtilis, E. coli,* and *S. aureus* with MIC values of 0.3 mg/mL and no observable activity for water extracts [41]. In this study, the highest impact was noted with methanol and chloroform extracts against *S. aureus* and *E. coli,* respectively, and the lowest with both extracts against *P. aeruginosa.* Furthermore, an ethanolic extract was effective against *E. coli* and *S. aureus,* but no activity was observed for either extract against *K. pneumonia* and *P. aeruginosa* at 50, 100, and 200 mg/mL. Nevertheless, a water extract was effective only for *E. coli* at 100 and 200 mg/mL [45]. Water and ethanolic extracts at 1.0 mg/mL exhibit effective inhibition against *S. aureus* and fewer inhibitory effects were observed for *P. mirabilis;* against *S. aureus,* an ethanolic extract was active at 0.5 mg/mL, but a water extract was only active at 1.0 mg/mL; and inhibition was not achieved for either extracts at 0.1 mg/mL [73]. An ethanolic extract was slightly active against *B. subtilis* and *S. haemolyticus,* but was inactive against other Gram positive and Gram negative strains, resulting in no further studies with this extract [20]. Furthermore, only weak activity was achieved by methanolic extracts of this plant against *P. syringae* [74].

Both ethanolic and water extracts of *T. officinale* were active for *S. marcescens* and *M. kristinae.* The ethanolic extract alone was active on *P. vulgaris, E. coli, B. subtilis,* and *S. aureus* with MIC values ranging from 1.0 to 7.0 mg/mL for all strains tested [25]. Similar extracts had antimicrobial effects on four species that induce acne (*P. ovale, P. acnes, P. aeruginosa,* and *S. aureus*) in broth dilution tests with effects depending on the extract concentration, but no further information was available [49]. Moreover, a leaf extract (0.04 mg/well) was reported as a bactericidal agent against *S. aureus* and fungistatic against *C. albicans* [52]. Contrarily, extracts of 130 and 200 mg/mL from aerial parts were unable to prevent the growth of 34 microorganisms from genera *Bacillus, Enterobacter, Klebsiella, Listeria, Pseudomonas, Salmonella, Staphylococcus, Aspergillus,* and *Candida,* among others; therefore, it was considered inactive at these concentrations in a disc diffusion assay [66]. A methanolic *T. officinale* flower extract was not active against *E. coli* or *S. aureus* at 1.0 mg/mL in a diffusion agar assay [62] and no activity was found on *S. aureus, E. coli, P. aeruginosa,* or *C. albicans* using a leaf ethanolic extract when 0.05 mL were placed in sterile discs [57]. Furthermore, an ethanolic extract of leaves displayed no activity against *S. aureus, E. coli,* or *S. abony* by the serial dilution method [58], with the same results for root and leaf extracts on *M. aurum* and *M. smegmatis* at 0.5 mg/mL [63].

Raw extracts of *T. officinale* have been widely tested, as well as solvent fractions. In a study in which the methanolic leaf extract was fractioned by different solvents, the methyl chloride, ethyl acetate, and butanol fractions were active on *E. coli, S. aureus, B. subtilis, C. albicans,* and *S. cerevisiae* at 50 mg/mL, with inhibition percentages ranging from 13 to 76%. The water fraction showed moderate inhibition via the broth dilution method (10 and 14% for *E. coli* and *B. subtilis,* respectively) but no effect on the disc diffusion assay [34]. The only report in which a *Taraxacum* extract was compared to another natural antibacterial substance besides other plants extracts evaluated the use of *T. officinale* extract as an irrigation agent in endodontic treatments against *E. faecalis* in root canal infections. Leaf and root extracts at 0.7% were slightly active but propolis was more effective for this purpose [53]. In the case of commercial preparations, high activity has been reported for a commercial *T. officinale* ethanolic extract, showing antibacterial activity against *H. pylori* at 20 mg/mL with 26% inhibition but no observable activity for *C. jejuni* [54].

Considering other *Taraxacum* species, *T. platycarpum* anticandidal activity was determined against five different *Candida* sp. by agar diffusion assay. An ethanolic extract at 0.2 mg/mL weakly inhibited *C. tropicalis* but no other Candida strains [55]. A methanolic extract was active against *B. subtilis, S. aureus, L. monocytogenes, E. coli,* and *V. parahaemolyticus* at concentrations ranging from 0.5 to 2.0 mg/mL, with growth inhibition ranging from 5.1 to 100%, correlating to the concentration. In that study, chloroform, butanol, and ethyl acetate fractions were active in the disc diffusion assay for almost every strain tested, but an aqueous extract was inactive [38, 39].

An ethanolic extract of *T. mongolicum* at 0.2 mg/mL was not able to achieve growth inhibition in a microdilution assay for *B. subtilis, S. aureus, E. coli,* or *P. aeruginosa* [64]. In contrast, an ethanolic extract of this species was active for *E. coli, S. aureus,* and *P. aeruginosa* in the disc diffusion assay with MIC values between 0.05 and 0.1 mg/mL, which was three times higher than the values obtained for erythromycin. However, no activity was achieved for *S. fiexneri* or *P. vulgaris* [75]. Another report indicated that only the butanol fraction of an ethanolic extract of this plant was active on *H. pylori,* but water and methyl chloride fractions were inactive. Nevertheless, a different report indicated that a butanol fraction exerted higher inhibition (13%) than the aqueous fraction, possibly due to the flavonoid and luteolin content (28 and 1.1%, respectively) [31]. Against *S. aureus* and *S. epidermis,* an acetyl acetate fraction of an ethanolic *T. coreanum* extract was active at 0.5, 1.0, and 3.0 mg/disc, a chloroform fraction was active at 1.0 and 3.0 mg/disc, and a butanol fraction at 1.0 mg/mL, but displayed no activity against *MRSA* displayed [28]. An ethanolic *T. ohwianum* extract was active against *E. coli* at 240 and 320 mg/mL, but not against *S. aureus* [32]. These authors indicate that the pH and temperature of the bioassay were important parameters in the antimicrobial performance of the extract. An extract of the aerial parts of *T. phaleratum* was inactive at 0.2 mg/mL against *M. tuberculosis,* even when several solvent fractions were tested [60].

Limited studies have been conducted on humans establishing the antimicrobial potential of *Taraxacum* extracts. Chinese language studies have reported the effects of various formulas containing *T. mongolicum* for medical treatment. An herbal formula known as "fu zheng qu xie" was just as effective as the antibiotic gentamycin in 75 cases of gastric disease caused by *H. pylori.* Furthermore, an herbal formula called "jie du yang gan gao," which includes *T. mongolicum,* was significantly more effective than another botanical formulation in lowering elevated liver enzymes and curing patients with hepatitis B in a 96-person, double-blind trial [76].

2.2.2. *Plant pathogens*

Plant extracts have also been tested on bacteria and fungi that affect fruits and vegetables, causing rot diseases during postharvest handling, to find an alternative to chemical pesticides, which are harmful to the environment and human health. An aqueous *T. officinale* root extract (S) at different dilutions (S, S/2 to S/100) caused significant inhibition to mycelial growth in *A. alternata* (70% for S to 17% for S/100), *P. expansum* (67% for S to 5.3% for S/100), and *M. piriformis* (70% for S to 16% for S/100) [46]. In the case of *R. solani* and *C. sativus*, a *Taraxacum* acetyl acetate extract at a concentration of 100 mg/mL exhibited a weak effect on the growth of these plant pathogens and no inhibition of *F. oxysporum* [22]. A methanolic extract of *Taraxacum* at 0.2 mg/mL was not effective against *A. niger*, *A. flavus*, *A. fumigates*, or *R. solani* [37]. A methanolic extract of *Taraxacum* sp. displayed weak activity against *C. sativus*, *F. oxysporum*, and *R. solani* at 5 mg/disc and a water extract displayed no activity at all [56].

A *T. officinale* hydro-methanolic extract tested the inhibition of conidial germination and inhibition of germ tube elongation for several plant pathogens at several dilutions (0.25×, 0.5×, and 0.75×) using a microassay method on slides. Dilution at 0.75× showed inhibition of conidial germination values of 2, 3, 4, 9, 11, and 12% for *P. italicum*, *A. niger*, *A. carbonarius*, *B. cinerea*, *M. laxa*, and *P. digitatum*, respectively. For these same strains, excluding *A. carbonarius*, inhibition of germ tube elongation values were 56, 45, 38, 5 and 42%, respectively. For *P. expansum*, the plant extract did not show positive results for inhibition of conidial germination or inhibition of germ tube elongation. In artificially inoculated fruits, the extract applied to nectarines was not protective against brown rot development from *M. laxa*, while for apricots effects were similar to those of the negative control for *P. digitatum* [35]. Dichloromethane and diethyl ether *T. officinale* extracts were tested on *P. expansum* by applying either a solution or its vapor to paper discs. The dichloromethane extract was more active of the two models, though direct inoculation in apples offered no observable inhibition [26]. Water extracts of *T. officinale* and *T. platycarpum* were tested against *C. lagenarium* in cucumber, exhibiting inhibition rates of the anthracnose lesions of 1.9 and 13% in treated leaves, and 11 and 5.3% in untreated leaves, respectively. These results were not significant compared to other plant extracts [42]. *In vivo* evaluation of protective effects in plant tissue has not been as successful as the *in vitro* assays, which is typical in cases of inhibitory activity validation. To avoid these ineffective results, concentrations are increased to demonstrate the pathogen control effect.

2.2.3. *Animal pathogens*

Regarding animal pathogens, *Saprolegnia* infections can account for significant salmonid losses. Treatment is difficult and there are reservations regarding efficacy, prompting a search for suitable alternatives. A *T. officinale* root extract was not as effective as a fungistatic at 10, 100, 1000, or 10,000 mg/mL [61]. The effects of *Taraxacum* polysaccharides were studied on the preservation of white shrimp (*Penaeus vannamei*) during refrigerated storage (10 days at 4°C) by soaking the shrimps in aqueous extracts (1–3% w/v). Samples were periodically evaluated for total viable count, pH value, and total volatile basic nitrogen, which resulted in 2–3% of shrimp in fresh conditions (<30 mg/100 mg of total volatile basic nitrogen) and a total viable count that only increased slightly during storage. This indicated that the treatment effectively retarded bacterial growth during refrigerated storage, prolonging shrimp shelf life for up to 10 days [76].

In the case of the meat industry, an herb mixture including *T. officinale* as a substitute for fodder antibiotics in pig feeding revealed positive growth of the animal and no change in meat quality, confirming the possibility of using herbs as an antibiotic substitute in pig feed [77, 78]. Aqueous and ethanolic extracts of *T. mongolicum* could also inhibit four pathogenic bacteria responsible for cow mastitis, a serious disease in the cow industry, at concentrations of 0.13, 0.25, and 0.5 g/mL. In this case, the ethanolic extracts displayed slightly better antibacterial activities than aqueous extracts. For *E. coli, S. aureus, S. agalactiae,* and *S. dysgalactiae,* inhibition zone diameters were slightly larger for aqueous than for ethanolic extracts but showed between medium and high sensitivity [79]. Dandelion extract can not only be used to control pathogens but also to supplement the diet of animals, which could result in increased meat, milk, whey, and other yields, contributing to the food industry. Alternatively, the extracts could be utilized in the agricultural industry as biofertilizers to promote plant growth and strengthen the plant against biotic and abiotic stress.

2.3. *Taraxacum* antimicrobial action mechanisms

Innate plant immunity involves various defense responses, including cell wall reinforcements, lytic enzyme biosynthesis, secondary metabolite production, and pathogenesis-related proteins. To protect themselves from non-beneficial microorganisms, plants accumulate secondary metabolites that form chemical barriers to microbial attacks (phytoanticipins) and produce antimicrobials (phytoalexins) [80]. Phenolics and terpenoids are considered the primary mechanisms for plant defenses because these reduce microbial attacks by disrupting the cell membranes in microorganisms, bind to adhesins and cell wall compounds, and inactivate enzymes, among other roles [81]. The action mechanisms of natural compounds are related to the disintegration of the cytoplasmic membrane and destabilization of the proton motive force, electron flow, active transport, coagulation of the cell content, inhibition of protein synthesis, inhibition of DNA synthesis, and the synthesis of metabolites used for DNA synthesis [82]. Some action mechanisms are specific to certain targets and some targets may also be affected by more than one mechanism [83]. A general scheme of the action's sites and antimicrobial potential mechanism is presented in **Figure 1** of Supporting Information.

Even though *Taraxacum* is a plant with extremely high pathogen resistance, the underlying molecular mechanisms of antimicrobial activity are poorly studied [68]. Until now, most of the research on *Taraxacum* has focused on elucidating the compounds present in the extract, and, to a lesser extent, on the mechanism involved in the antimicrobial activity itself. One study specifically illustrated the effect of four proteins from *T. officinale* flowers on fungi by light microscopy and distinguished two modes of antimicrobial action, depending on the fungus tested. *Taraxacum* proteins completely blocked conidia germination or induced thickening of multiple local hyphae and irreversible cytoplasm plasmolysis [68, 69]. Different extracts from this genus showed positive inhibitory activity in controlled studies and were characterized by protein synthesis inhibition (e.g. chloramphenicol, tetracycline, gentamicin, and kanamycin) and cell wall synthesis (e.g. amphotericin, cefixime, cephalothin, and penicillin). These

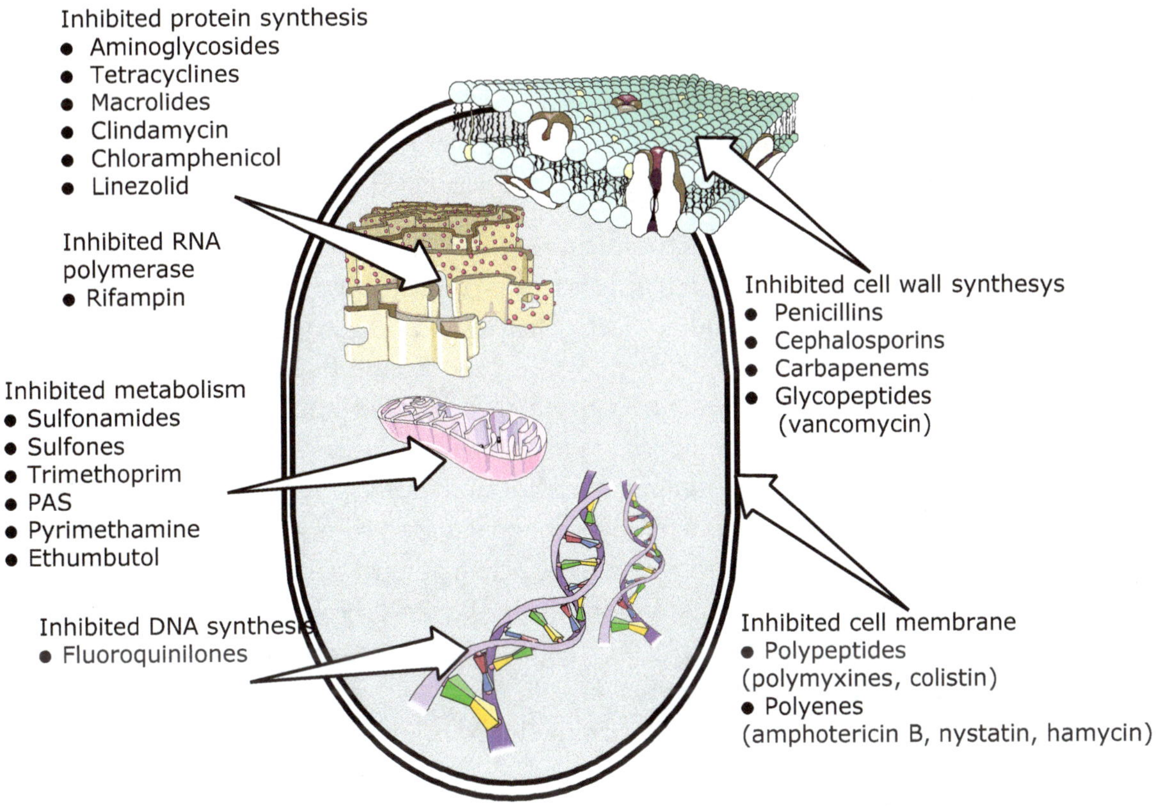

Figure 1. Main action mechanisms for antimicrobial agents (adapted from Mulvey and Simor [84]).

mechanisms need to be addressed to elucidate the *Taraxacum* active compound action mechanisms because a direct relation with the positive controls cannot be pursued.

Another response that has been studied is the modulation of microbe adherence to body tissues. Adhesion to epithelial cells has been represented as the first step in the subsequent bacterial invasion of host cells [59]. These authors reported the partial inhibition of intestinal adherence of *C. jejuni* HT-29 cells using a commercial ethanolic *Taraxacum* extract. Cytotoxic activity was less than 10%, but no antibacterial activity was observed. Moreover, *Taraxacum* has been tested with the aim of controlling bacterial diseases by inhibiting communication between bacteria. An ethanolic extract of *T. officinale* aerial parts disturbed bacterial communication systems (or quorum sensing) for *C. violaceum*, showing the moderately positive effect of the extract on the attenuation of microbial pathogenicity [30]. In contrast, an ethanolic and water extract of the rhizomes of the same plant showed no significant activity in the same assay [65].

2.4. *Taraxacum* compounds related to antimicrobial action

Several studies have named a wide range of compounds, including terpenes, flavonoids, and phenolic compounds, as responsible for the medicinal activity of different plants [85, 86]. For *Taraxacum*, only a few studies concerning its antimicrobial properties have considered chemical identification of the obtained extracts and this identification is chiefly qualitative (e.g. using colorimetric methods indicating presence or absence). Authors report the presence of terpenoids, triterpenoids, steroids, coumarins, phenols, saponins, flavonoids, flavones, flavonols, chalcones, phlobatannins, and cardiac glycosides in antimicrobial extracts [22, 27, 34, 36, 37, 43–45, 87, 88] but neither compound isolation nor further identification were performed.

Taraxasterol acetate, lupeol acetate, tranexamic acid, and squalene, among others, were identified in the dichloromethane extract of *T. officinale* leaves, which show low activity against *E. coli, P. aeruginosa, B. subtilis, C. albicans,* and *T. mentagrophytes* in an agar well assay at 30 μg but no observed activity against *S. aureus* or *A. niger* [27]. Terpenoids and flavonoids were identified in the ethanolic extracts of the *T. farinosum* root, which displayed antibacterial activity against *S. aureus, S. typhi, M. canis,* and *T. longifusus* in an agar well diffusion and agar tube dilution, while the herb extract was active only against the latter two strains [51]. Fractions of a methanolic root extract indicated the significant presence of phenolic-based compounds and hydroxyl-fatty acids with liquid and mass spectrometry, and were active against *S. aureus, MRSA* clinical, and *B. cereus* at 2 mg/mL, with MIC values ranging from 0.05 to 0.19 mg/mL, and crude extracts indicating values of 0.25–0.5 mg/mL [33]. An oligosaccharide extract (DOs) from this species exhibited high antibacterial activity against *E. coli, B. subtilis,* and *S. aureus* at 100 mg/mL, indicating that these oligosaccharides could potentially be used as antibacterial agents [48].

Concerning specific compounds, isolated *Taraxacum* peptides displayed antimicrobial activity at 6 μg/μL, corresponding to 52–79% of kanamycin activity against *P. syringae, B. subtilis,* and *X. campestris* at the same concentration [69], which is a promising value that warrants further experiments. These authors indicated that though *A. niger* appeared sensitive to four proteins (ToAMP1, ToAMP2, ToAMP3, and ToAMP4) from *T. officinale* flowers, *F. graminearum* was not susceptible to any of these proteins. All proteins displayed inhibition activity against *B. cinerea, B. sorokiniana, A. niger, P. debaryanum, F. oxysporum,* and *P. infestans,* with IC50 values ranging between 1.2 and 5.8 μM. The ToAMPs were also active against *P. syringae, B. subtilis,* and *X. campestris,* similar to a kanamycin control. Additionally, ToAMP2 was active against *C. michiganensis* at up to 0.5 μg/μL. The disease development of *P. infestans* was inhibited by ToAMP2 at 1.3 μM (20–40%) to 5.2 μM (10–20%). In further studies, *B. sorokiniana, C. gloeosporioides,* and *V. albo-atrum* were insensitive to ToAMP4, another peptide isolated from the seed extract of *T. officinale,* at concentrations below 15 mM. The IC50 values for the agent-sensitive fungi *A. alternata, A. niger, F. avenaceum,* and *P. betae* ranged from 2.9 to 13.1 mM, with MIC values from 1.0 to 8.0 mM; no activity was observed for *P. syringae, B. subtilis, E. coli,* or *C. michiganensis* [68, 69]. Peptides supposedly have broad-spectrum activity, lack of microbial resistance, and high efficacy [69], but some action mechanisms in these molecules are still poorly defined [89]. Peptides related to albumin 2S from *Taraxacum* seeds are active against phytopathogenic fungi and bacteria. Antifungal assays displayed different activities for the 2S isoforms (ToA1, ToA2, and ToA3). The spore germination of *B. cinerea, A. niger,* and *P. debaryanum* were the most tolerant, and *H. sativum, P. betae,* and *V. albo-atrum* were the most sensitive at concentrations ranging from 0.063 mg/mL to 0.25 mg/mL. *H. sativum* and *P. betae* were inhibited by ToA1, ToA2, and ToA3, but *F. oxysporum* and *V. albo-atrum* were only inhibited by ToA2 and ToA3, respectively. In potato tubers, *P. infestans* was inhibited by ToA3 at 0.06 mg/mL at 96 and 120 h, but at 144 h ToA2 inhibited better at 0.13 mg/mL [23].

Interestingly, an antimicrobial filtrate isolated from the fungal strains of *P. betae* (PG23) from *T. mongolicum* was proven active against *E. coli, S. aureus, A. hydrophila, E. tarda,* and *P. multocida,* and proposed as a potential antimicrobial product for poultry and aquatic disease control [88].

3. Driving forces and tendencies in *Taraxacum* antimicrobial research

Between 2000 and 2010, approximately 40 new drugs originating from terrestrial plants, terrestrial microorganisms, marine organisms, and terrestrial vertebrates and invertebrates against different bacteria, fungi, and viruses were launched on the market [90]. This follows distinct research tendencies. Studies related to antimicrobial and antifungal properties generally aim, in developing and developed countries, to respond to the necessity of finding new drugs or products based on traditional medicine at a low cost, confirming already established activity originating from oral tradition. The driving force behind studying new antimicrobial alternatives is the necessity of finding new drugs or natural products that act against diseases due to the increased drug resistance in the latter. Furthermore, the toxicity of synthetic compounds currently utilized in farming and agricultural industries has created a market for natural compounds that are safer, cheaper, and more effective against pathogens.

Modern phytochemistry, scientific equipment, and technology have had a significant impact on natural product chemistry, including isolation, extraction, purification, and structure determination. However, this discipline still demands that research investigators establish the clinical significance of natural compounds and recognize them as drugs or industrial products (pesticides, bactericides, pharmaceutical products, etc.) [91]. Bioactive compounds in botanical drugs are purportedly superior to monosubstances because of synergistic effects. Similarly, multidrug therapy is highly important against resistant microbial strains due to the enhanced efficacy, reduced toxicity, decreased adverse side effects, increased bioavailability, lowered dosage, and reduced evolution of antimicrobial resistance [92].

Even when antibiotics have been effective in treating infectious diseases, resistance to the action mechanisms has led to the emergence of new and the re-emergence of old infectious diseases. Several plant extracts exhibit synergistic activity against microorganisms, with natural products (including flavonoids and essential oils) and synthetic drugs effectively combating bacterial, fungal, and mycobacterial infections. The mode of action of combinations differs significantly from the individual use of the same drugs; hence, isolating a single component may not highlight its importance, simplifying the task of the pharmacological industries [93].

Acknowledgements

This work has been supported by Innova Chile CORFO Code FCR-CSB 09CEII-6991 and a doctoral fellowship awarded by the Pontifical Catholic University of Valparaíso, Chile Project DI Iniciación COD 039.454/2017 Pontificia Universidad Católica de Valparaíso.

Author details

María Eugenia Martínez Valenzuela[1], Katy Díaz Peralta[2], Lorena Jorquera Martínez[3] and Rolando Chamy Maggi[1]*

*Address all correspondence to: rolando.chamy@pucv.cl

1 Escuela de Ingeniería Bioquímica, Facultad de Ingeniería, Pontificia Universidad Católica de Valparaíso, Valparaíso, Chile

2 Departamento de Química, Universidad Técnico Federico Santa María, Valparaíso, Chile

3 Escuela de Ingeniería en Construcción, Facultad de Ingeniería, Pontificia Universidad Católica de Valparaíso, Valparaíso, Chile

References

[1] Modi C, Modi S, Patel H, Dudhatra G, Kumar A, Awale M. Herbal Antibacterials: A review. Journal Intercultural Ethnopharmacology. 2012;**1**:52-61. DOI: 10.5455/jice.20120207113423

[2] Mahesh B, Satish S. Antimicrobial activity of some important medicinal plant against plant and human pathogens. World Journal Agricola Science. 2008;**4**:839-843. DOI: 10.1556/EuJMI.3.2013.4.6

[3] Vashegyi I, Marozsán-Tóth Z, Galiba G, Dobrev P, Vankova R, Tóth B. Cold response of dedifferentiated barley cells at the gene expression, hormone composition, and freezing tolerance levels: Studies on callus cultures. Molecular Biotechnology. 2013;**54**:337-349. DOI: 10.1007/s12033-012-9569-9

[4] Stewart-Wade S, Neumann S, Collins L, Boland G. The biology of Canadian weeds. 117. *Taraxacum officinale* G.H. Weber ex Wiggers. Canadian Journal Plant Science. 2002;**82**:825-853. DOI: org/10.4141/P01-010

[5] Lardos A. The botanical materia medica of the Iatrosophikon – A collection of prescriptions from a monastery in *Cyprus*. Journal of Ethnopharmacology. 2006;**104**:387-406. DOI: 10.1016/j.jep.2005.12.035

[6] González-Castejón M, Visioli F, Rodríguez-Casado A. Diverse biological activities of dandelion. Nutrition Reviews. 2012;**70**:534-547. DOI: 10.1111/j.1753-4887.2012.00509.x

[7] Schütz K, Carle R, Schieber A. *Taraxacum* – A review on its phytochemical and pharmacological profile. Journal of Ethnopharmacology. 2006;**107**:313-323. DOI: 10.1016/j.jep.2006.07.021

[8] Li G.Pharmacology, toxicity and clinic of traditional Chinese medicine. In: Tianjin Science and Technique. Tianjin, China: Translation Publishing House; 1992. pp. 207-208

[9] Ou M, Li YW. The Traditional Chinese Drug and Its Usage. Hong Kong, China: Hai Feng Press; 1994. pp. 49-51

[10] Zhu M, Wong P, Li R. Effects of *Taraxacum mongolicum* on the bioavailability and disposition of ciprofloxacin in rats. Journal of Pharmaceutical Sciences. 1999;**88**:632-634. DOI: 10.1021/js980367q

[11] Caraballo A, Caraballo B, Rodríguez-Acosta A. Preliminary assessment of medicinal plants used as antimalarials, in the southeastern Venezuelan Amazon. Revista da Sociedade Brasileira de Medicina Tropical. 2004;**37**:186-188. DOI: 10.1590/S0037-86822004000200016

[12] Guarino C, De Simone L, Santoro S. Ethnobotanical study of the Sannio area, Campania, Southern Italy. Ethnobotany Research and Applications. 2008;**6**:255-317. DOI: 10.17348/era.6.0.255-317

[13] Saghir I, Awan A, Majid S, Khan M, Qureshi S, Bano S. Ethnobotanical studies of Chikar and its allied areas of district Muzaffarabad. Journal of Biological Sciences. 2001;**1**:1165-1170

[14] Guarrera P, Savo V. Perceived health properties of wild and cultivated food plants in local and popular traditions of Italy: A review. Journal of Ethnopharmacology. 2013;**146**:659-680. DOI: 10.1016/j.jep.2013.01.036

[15] Neves J, Matos C, Moutinho C, Queiroz G, Gomes L. Ethnopharmacological notes about ancient uses of medicinal plants in Trás-os-Montes (northern of Portugal). Journal of Ethnopharmacology. 2009;**124**:270-283. DOI: 10.1016/j.jep.2009.04.041

[16] Rodriguez-Fragoso L, Reyes-Esparza J, Burchiel S, Herrera-Ruiz D, Torres E. Risks and benefits of commonly used herbal medicines in Mexico. Toxicology and Applied Pharmacology. 2008;**227**:125-135. DOI: 10.1016/j.taap.2007.10.005

[17] Song M, Kim H. Ethnomedicinal application of plants in the western plain region of North Jeolla Province in Korea. Journal of Ethnopharmacology. 2011;**137**:167-175. DOI: 10.1016/j.jep.2011.05.001

[18] Martinez M, Poirrier P, Chamy R, Prüfer D, Schulze-Gronover C, Jorquera L, Ruiz G. *Taraxacum officinale* and related species – An ethnopharmacological review and its potential as a commercial medicinal plant. Journal of Ethnopharmacology. 2015;**169**:244-262. DOI: 10.1016/j.jep.2015.03.067

[19] Wat C, Johns T, Towers G. Phototoxic and antibiotic activities of plants of the Asteraceae used in folk medicine. Journal of Ethnopharmacology. 1980;**2**:279-290. DOI: 10.1016/S0378-8741(80)81006-3

[20] Izzo A, Di Carlo G, Biscardi D, De Fusco R, Mascolo N, Borrelli F, Capasso F, Fasulo M, Autore G. Biological screening of Italian medicinal plants for antibacterial activity. Phythotherapy Research. 1995;**9**:281-286. DOI: 10.1002/ptr.2650090410

[21] Silva N, Fernandes A. Biological properties of medicinal plants: A review of their antimicrobial activity. Journal of Venomous Animals and Toxins including Tropical Diseases. 2010;**16**:402-413. DOI: 10.1590/S1678-91992010000300006

[22] Ghaima K, Hashim N, Ali S. Antibacterial and antioxidant activities of ethyl acetate extract of nettle (*Urtica dioica*) and dandelion (*Taraxacum officinale*). Journal of Applied Pharmaceutical Science. 2013;**3**:96-99. DOI: 10.7324/JAPS.2013.3518

[23] Odintsova T, Rogozhin E, Sklyar I, Musolyamov A, Kudryavtsev A, Pukhalsky V, Smirnov A, Grishin E, Egorov T. Antifungal activity of storage 2S albumins from seeds of the invasive weed dandelion *Taraxacum officinale* Wigg. Protein and Peptide Letters. 2010;**17**:522-529. DOI: 10.2174/092986610790963591

[24] Stanojković A, Ceković J, Čomić L, Pivić R, Stanojković A. Antibacterial properties of some plants from the family *Asteraceae* growing wild in Serbia. Lekovite sirovine. 2008;**26/27**:11-20

[25] Jaca T, Kambizi L. Antibacterial properties of some wild leafy vegetables of the Eastern Cape Province, South Africa. Journal of Medicinal Plants.2011;**5**:2624-2628.DOI: http://www.academicjournals.org/journal/JMPR/article-abstract/3CA6E7916006

[26] Ikeura H, Somsak N, Kobayashi F, Kanlayanarat S, Hayata Y. Application of selected plant extracts to inhibit growth of *Penicillium expansum* on apple fruits. Plant Pathology Journal. 2011;**10**:79-84. DOI: 10.3923/ppj.2011.79.84

[27] Ragasa C, Apuada M, Rideout J. Terpenoids from *Taraxacum officinale*. NRCP Research Journal. 2009;**10**:17-26

[28] Im D, Lee K. Antioxidative and antibacterial activity and Tyrosinase inhibitory activity of the extract and fractions from *Taraxacum coreanum* Nakai. Korean Journal of Medicinal Crop Science. 2011;**19**:238-245. DOI: 10.7783/KJMCS.2011.19.4.238

[29] Qiao H, Sun T. Antibacterial activity of ethanol extract and fractions obtained from *Taraxacum mongolicum* flower. Research Journal of Pharmacognosy. 2014;**1**:35-39. Available from: http://rjpharmacognosy.ir/article_6336_609.html

[30] Zaki A, Shaaban M, Hashish N, Amer M, Lahloub M. Assessment of anti-quorum sensing activity for some ornamental and medicinal plants native to Egypt. Scientia Pharmaceutics. 2013;**81**:251-258. DOI: 10.3797/scipharm.1204-26

[31] Han S, Hwang J, Park S, Lee K, Ko K, Kim K, Kim K. Potential effect of solvent fractions of *Taraxacum mongolicum* H. on protection of gastric mucosa. Korean Journal of Medicinal Crop Science. 2005;**37**:84-89

[32] Sun H, Li Z, Liu W, Wang X, Zhang T, Feng Z. *In vitro* antibacterial activities of antibiotics and traditional chinese medicinal herb extracts on *Escherichia coli* and *Staphylococcus aureus*. Asian Journal of Chemistry. 2014;**26**:298-302. DOI: 10.14233/ajchem.2014.16174

[33] Kenny O, Brunton N, Walsh D, Hewage C, Mcloughlin P, Smyth T. Characterisation of antimicrobial extracts from dandelion root (*Taraxacum officinale*) using LC-SPE-NMR. Phytotherapy Research. 2015;**29**:526-532. DOI: 10.1002/ptr.5276

[34] Tettey C, Ocloo A, Nagajyothi P, Lee K. An *in vitro* analysis of antiproliferative and antimicrobial activities of solvent fractions of *Taraxacum officinale* (dandelion) leaf. Journal of Applied Pharmaceutical Science. 2014;**4**:41-45. DOI: 10.7324/JAPS.2014.40309

[35] Gatto M, Ippolito A, Linsalata V, Cascarano N, Nigro F, Vanadia S, Di Venere D. Activity of extracts from wild edible herbs against postharvest fungal diseases of fruit and vegetables. Postharvest Biology and Technology. 2011;**61**:72-82. DOI: 10.1016/j.postharvbio.2011.02.005

[36] Fabri R, Nogueira M, Dutra L, Bouzada M, Scio E. Potencial antioxidante e antimicrobiano de espécies da família Asteraceae. Revista Brasileira de Plantas Medicinais. 2011;**13**:183-189. DOI: 10.1590/S1516-05722011000200009

[37] Khan A, Qureshi R, Gillani S, Ullah F. Antimicrobial activity of selected medicinal plants of Margalla Hills, Islamabad, Pakistan. Journal of Medicinal Plants Research. 2011;**5**:4665-4670

[38] Kim K, Chun H, Han Y. Screening of antimicrobial activity of the dandelion (*Taraxacum platycarpum*) extract. Korean Society of Food Science and Nutrition. 1998;**14**:114-118

[39] Kim K, Min K, Lee S, Han Y. Isolation and identification of antimicrobial compound from dandelion (*Taraxacum platycarpum* D.). Journal of the Korean Society of Food Science and Nutrition. 1999;**28**:822-829

[40] Park J, Jang J, Lee M, Park E. Effect of dandelion (*Taraxacum officinale*) extracts on the intestinal microorganisms of streptozotocin-induced diabetic rats. Journal of the Korean Society of Food Science and Nutrition. 2002;**31**:1112-1118. DOI: 10.3746/jkfn.2002.31.6.1112

[41] Sohail Z, Afzal M, Afzal A, Rahman I, Shad S, Ahmed B, Anjum N, Qureshi K, Bibi A. *In vitro* antibacterial study of *Taraxacum officinale* leaves extracts against different bacterial pathogenic strains. Journal of Pharmacognosy and Phytochemistry. 2014;**3**:15-17

[42] Inagaki H, Yamaguchi A, Kato K, Kageyama C, Iyozumi H, Oki Y. Screening of weed extracts for antifungal properties against *Colletotrichum lagenarium*, the causal agent of anthracnose in cucumber. Weed Biology and Management. 2008;**8**:276-283. DOI: 10.1111/j.1445-6664.2008.00308.x

[43] Jassim A, Farhan S, Noori O. Identification of dandelion *Taraxacum officinale* leaves components and study its extracts effect on different microorganisms. Journal of Al-Nahrain University – Science. 2012;**15**:7-14

[44] Kenny O, Smyth T, Walsh D, Kelleher C, Hewage C, Brunton N. Investigating the potential of under-utilised plants from the Asteraceae Family as a source of natural antimicrobial and antioxidant extracts. Food Chemistry. 2014;**161**:79-86. DOI: 10.1016/j.foodchem.2014.03.126

[45] Lateef O, Issah Y. Screening ethanolic and aqueous leaf extracts of *Taraxacum offinale* for in vitro bacteria growth inhibition. Journal of Pharmaceutical and Biomedical Sciences. 2012;**20**:06

[46] Parveen S, Wani A, Ganie A, Pala S, Mir R. Antifungal activity of some plant extracts on some pathogenic fungi. Archives of Phytopathology and Plant Protection. 2013;**47**:279-284. DOI: 10.1080/03235408.2013.808857

[47] Peng S, Dai W, Yu H, Wang Y, Wang X, Sun S. Antibacterial activity of aqueous and ethanolic extracts of *Portulaca oleracea* L and *Taraxacum mongolicum* against pathogenic

bacteria of cow mastitis. International Journal of Applied Research in Veterinary Medicine. 2014;**12**:210-213. DOI: 10.18805/ijar.5960

[48] Qian Z, Jiang L. Preparation and antibacterial activity of the oligosaccharides derived from *Rhizoma phragmites*. Carbohydrate Polymers. 2014;**111**:356-358. DOI: 10.1016/j.carbpol.2014.04.043

[49] Chan G, Kim H. Antimicrobial effects of extracts of *Taraxacum officinale* H. on acnes strains. 국제통합보완대체의학회지 [International Journal of Integrated CAM]. 2011;**7**:3-16. DOI: 10.4172/1948-5948.1000287

[50] Redzic S, Kurtagic H, Prazina N, Tuka M, Avdagic T. The antimicrobial activity of honey in relation to the composition of pollen (Bosnia-Herzegovina, W. Balkan). Planta Medicinal. 2011;**77**:SL62. DOI: 10.1055/s-0031-1282185

[51] Sarer E, Sahin A, Gökbulut A. The investigation on the terpenoids and flavonoids of an endemic *Taraxacum* species from Turkey. Planta Medicinal. 2010;**76**:P303. DOI: 10.1055/s-0030-1264601

[52] Sharma V, Sharma H, Mehta D, Chhabra B, Thakur D, Sourirajan A, Dev K. Comparative analysis of antibacterial and antifungal properties of traditional medicinal plants of Shimla and Solan, Himachal Pradesh. International Journal of Pharmacy and Pharmaceutical Research. 2014;**6**:18-26. DOI: 10.1016/j.jtcme.2017.04.002

[53] Shafiq N, Al-Hashimi M. The antibacterial evaluation of dandelion extracts as root canal irrigating solutions (A comparative study). Journal of Bagdhdad College of Dentistry. 2014;**26**:35-40

[54] Cwikla C, Schmidt K, Matthias A, Bone K, Lehmann R, Tiralongo E. Investigations into the antibacterial activities of phytotherapeutics against *Helicobacter pylori* and *Campylobacter jejuni*. Phytotherapy Research. 2010;**24**:649-656. DOI: 10.1002/ptr.2933

[55] Kim J, Yi Y, Lim Y. Biological and antifungal activity of herbal plant extracts against *Candida* species. Korean Journal of Microbiology and Biotechnology. 2009;**37**:42-48

[56] Bahraminejad S, Abbasid S, Fazlali M. In vitro antifungal activity of 63 Iranian plant species against three different plant pathogenic fungi. African Journal of Biotechnology. 2011;**10**:16193-16201. DOI: 10.5897/AJB11.1203

[57] Borchardt J, Wyse D, Sheaffer C, Kauppi K, Fulcher R, Ehlke N, Biesboer D, Bey R. Antimicrobial activity of native and naturalized plants of Minnesota and Wisconsin. Journal of Medicinal Plants Research. 2008;**2**:98-110

[58] Ionescu D, Mihele D, Predan G, Rizea G, Dune A, Ivopol G. Antimicrobial activity of some hydroalcoholic extracts of artichoke (*Cynara scolymus*), burdock (*Arctium lappa*) and dandelion (*Taraxacum officinale*). Agricultural Food Engineering. 2013;**6**:113-120 Available from: http://webbut.unitbv.ro/Bulletin/Seri

[59] Bensch K, Tiralongo J, Schmidt K, Matthias A, Bone KM, Lehmann R, Tiralongo E. Investigations into the antiadhesive activity of herbal extracts against *Campylobacter jejuni*. Phytotherapy Research. 2011;**25**:1125-1132. DOI: 10.1002/ptr.3384

[60] Tosun F, Vural M, Palittapongarnpim P. Antimycobacterial screening of some Turkish plants. Journal of Ethnopharmacology. 2004;**95**:273-275. DOI: 10.1016/j.jep.2004.07.011

[61] Caruana S, Yoon G, Freeman M, Mackie J, Shinn A. The efficacy of selected plant extracts and bioflavonoids in controlling infections of *Saprolegnia australis* (Saprolegniales; Oomycetes). Aquaculture..2012;**358–359**:146-154. DOI: 10.1016/j.aquaculture.2012.06.035

[62] López-García J, Kuceková Z, Humpolícek P, Mlcek J, Sáha P, Humpolíček P, Mlček J, Sáha P. Polyphenolic extracts of edible flowers incorporated onto atelocollagen matrices and their effect on cell viability. Molecules. 2013;**18**:13435-13445. DOI: 10.3390/molecules181113435

[63] Newton S, Lau C, Gurcha S, Besra G, Wright C. The evaluation of forty-three plant species for *in vitro* antimycobacterial activities; isolation of active constituents from *Psoralea corylifolia* and *Sanguinaria canadensis*. Journal of Ethnopharmacology. 2002;**79**: 57-67. DOI: 10.1016/S0378-8741(01)00350-6

[64] Liu Y, Nielsen M, Staerk D, Jäger A. High-resolution bacterial growth inhibition profiling combined with HPLC-HRMS-SPE-NMR for identification of antibacterial constituents in Chinese plants used to treat snakebites. Journal of Ethnopharmacology. 2014;**155**: 1276-1283. DOI: 10.1016/j.jep.2014.07.019

[65] Tolmacheva A, Rogozhin E, Deryabin D. Antibacterial and quorum sensing regulatory activities of some traditional Eastern-European medicinal plants. Acta Pharmaceutica. 2014;**64**:173-186. DOI: 10.2478/acph-2014-0019

[66] Woods-Panzaru S, Nelson D, McCollum G, Ballard L, Millar B, Maeda Y, Goldsmith C, Rooney P, Loughrey A, Rao J, Moore J. An examination of antibacterial and antifungal properties of constituents described in traditional Ulster cures and remedies. Ulster Medical Journal. 2009;**78**:13-15. PMCID: PMC2629014

[67] The Plant List. Version 1.1. Published on the Internet. Available from: http://www.theplantlist.org/ [Accessed: May 2015]

[68] Astafieva A, Rogozhin E, Andreev Y, Odintsova T, Kozlov S, Grishin E, Egorov T. A novel cysteine-rich antifungal peptide ToAMP4 from *Taraxacum officinale* Wigg. flowers. Plant Physiology and Biochemistry. 2013;**70**:93-99. DOI: 10.1016/j.plaphy.2013.05.022

[69] Astafieva A, Rogozhin E, Odintsova T, Khadeeva N, Grishin E, Egorov T. Discovery of novel antimicrobial peptides with unusual cysteine motifs in dandelion *Taraxacum officinale* Wigg. flowers. Peptides. 2012;**36**:266-271. DOI: 10.1016/j.peptides.2012.05.009

[70] Gao D. Analysis of nutritional components of *Taraxacum mongolicum* and its antibacterial activity. Pharmacognosy Journal. 2010;**2**:502-505. DOI: 10.1016/S0975-3575(10)80039-2

[71] Hanawa F, Kanauchi M, Tahara S, Mizutani J. Lettucenin A as a phytoalexin of dandelion and its elicitation in dandelion cell cultures. Journal of the Faculty of Agriculture, Hokkaido University. 1995;**66**:151-162

[72] Voss-Rech D, Klein C, Techio V, Scheuermann G, Rech G, Fiorentin L. Antibacterial activity of vegetal extracts against serovars of *Salmonella*. Ciência Rural, Santa Maria. 2011;**41**:314-320. DOI: 10.1590/S0103-84782011000200022

[73] Al-kalby J, Alwan N. Effects of ethanolic extract of *Taraxacum officinale* leaves on some physiological and reproductive parameters of local adult male rabbits.Basrah Journal of Veterinary Research. 2007;**6**:42-55

[74] Elkhalfi B, Essari A, Serrano A, Soukri A. Antibacterial activity of plant methanolic extracts on a field isolate of *Pseudomonas syringae* pv tomato from the Casablanca region (Morocco). Advancesin Bioscience of Biotechnology. 2013;**4**:1-9. DOI: 10.4236/abb.2013.47A2001

[75] Chen Z. Clinical study of 96 cases with chronic hepatitis B treated with jiedu yanggan gao by a double-blind method. Zhong Xi Yi Jie He Za Zhi. 1990;**10**:71-74

[76] Wang H. Effect of dandelion polysaccharides on the retardation of the quality changes of white shrimp. International Journal of Biological Macromolecules. 2014;**68**:205-208. DOI: 10.1016/j.ijbiomac.2014.05.002

[77] Urbanczyk J, Hanczakowska E, Swiatkiewicz M. Herb mixture as an antibiotic substitute in pig feeding. Medycyna Weterynaryjna. 2002;**58**:887-889

[78] Yan L, Meng QW, Kim IM. The effects of dietary *Houttuynia cordata* and *Taraxacum officinale* extract powder on growth performance, nutrient digestibility, blood characteristics and meat quality in finishing pigs. Livestock Science. 2011;**141**:188-193. DOI: 10.1016/j.livsci.2011.05.017

[79] Yang L, Lü J, Feng Y. Partition and extraction of total flavonoids from *Taraxacum mongolicum* in PEG/$(NH_4)_2SO_4$ aqueous two-phase system. Chemical Industry and Engineering Progress. 2014;**33**:1992-1996

[80] González-Lamothe R, Mitchell G, Gattuso M, Diarra M, Malouin F, Bouarab K. Plant antimicrobial agents and their effects on plant and human pathogens. International Journal Molecular of Science. 2009;**10**:3400-3419. DOI: 10.3390/ijms10083400

[81] Cowan M. Plant products as antimicrobial agents. Clinical Microbiology Reviews. 1999;**12**:564-582. PMCID: PMC88925

[82] Singh S, Barrett J. Empirical antibacterial drμg discovery – Foundation in natural products. Biochemical Pharmacology. 2006;**71**:1006-1015. DOI: 10.1016/j.bcp.2005.12.016

[83] Burt S. Essential oils: Their antibacterial properties and potential applications in foods – A review. International Journal of Food Microbiology. 2004;**94**:223-253. DOI: 10.1016/j.ijfoodmicro.2004.03.022

[84] Mulvey M, Simor A. Antimicrobial resistance in hospitals: How concerned should we be? Canadian Medical Association Journal. 2009;**180**:408-415. DOI: 10.1503/cmaj.080239

[85] Chadwick M, Trewin H, Gawthrop F, Wagstaff C. Sesquiterpenoids lactones: Benefits to plants and people. International Journal of Molecular Science. 2013;**14**:12780-12805. DOI: 10.3390/ijms140612780

[86] Mir M, Sawhney S, Jassal M. Qualitative and quantitative analysis of phytochemicals of *Taraxacum officinale Wucpecker*. Journal of Pharmacy and Pharmacology. 2013;**2**:1-5

[87] Khan A, Qureshi R, Ullah F, Gilani S, Nosheen A, Sahreen S, Laghari M, Laghari M, Hussain I, Murad W. Phytochemical analysis of selected medicinal plants of Margalla Hills and surroundings. Journal of Medicinal Plants Research. 2011;**5**:6017-6023. DOI: 10.5897/JMPR11.869

[88] Zhang H, Xiong Y, Zhao H, Yi Y, Zhang C, Yu C, Xu C. An antimicrobial compound from the endophytic fungus *Phoma* sp. isolated from the medicinal plant *Taraxacum mongolicum*. Journal of the Taiwan Institute of Chemical Engineers. 2013;**44**:177-181. DOI: 10.1016/j.jtice.2012.11.013

[89] Barbosa P, Del Sarto R, Silva O, Franco O, Grossi-De-Sa M. Antibacterial peptides from plants: What they are and how they probably work. Biochemistry Research International. 2011. 9 pp. Article ID: 250349. DOI: 10.1155/2011/250349

[90] Brahmachari G. Natural products in drμg discovery: Impacts and opportunities – An assessment. Bioactive Natural Products: Opportunities and Challenges in Medicinal Chemistry. 2012;**1**:1-199

[91] Mahmood Z, Mahmood S. Antibiotic natural products: Opportunities and challanges. In: Microbial Pathogens and Strategies for Combating Them: Science, Technology and Education. Formatex Research Center. 2013;**2**:823-833

[92] Radulović N, Blagojević P, Stojanović-Radić Z, Stojanović N. Antimicrobial plant metabolites: Structural diversity and mechanism of action. Current Medicinal Chemistry. 2013;**20**:932-952. DOI: 10.2174/0929867313805219136

[93] Hemaiswarya S, Kruthiventi A, Doble M. Synergism between natural products and antibiotics against infectious diseases. Phytomedicine. 2008;**15**:639-652. DOI: 10.1016/j.phymed.2008.06.008

5

Application of Herbal Medicine as Proliferation and Differentiation Effectors of Human Stem Cells

Preethi Vidya Udagama and Vindya Udalamaththa

Abstract

One of the main streams of traditional medicine is herbal medicine; a wide range of medicinal plants and their individual parts are used for therapy. Though not scientifically validated, this traditional medicine practice is much popular in countries such as India, China and Sri Lanka and in many other countries in South, Southeast and Eastern Asia due mainly to its healing capabilities. More recently, scientists initiated the chemical analyses of these medicinal plants, obtaining invaluable results. The latest addition to such investigations is studies on effects of herbal extracts on different types of stem cells. An extensive summary of such reported studies is presented in this chapter, mainly categorizing these into proliferation stimulatory effects on stem cells and inhibitory effects on cancer stem cells (CSCs), where both properties are beneficial in cell therapy procedures. At present, standardizing the products and limited knowledge on the mechanisms of action and pathways of these have critically limited the use of herbal extracts in therapeutics. However, we believe that in the near future scientists would be focusing on herbal remedies to replace the use of synthetic stimulants and cancer drugs to overcome the disadvantages of these, such as toxicity, side effects and exorbitant costs.

Keywords: herbal extracts, stem cell therapy, cellular stimulants, proliferation and differentiation, cancer stem cells

1. Introduction

Traditional medicine is a popular treatment method for a wide range of diseases in many countries due to its claims of therapeutic activity by patients. The knowledge handed over from generation to generation since ancient ages is the foundation of traditional medicine; hence, the methods of treatment vary depending on the country and the region of origin.

In addition, a single region may use different types of traditional medicine due to different ethnic backgrounds of its citizens migrated from different regions of the world.

As the World Health Organization (WHO) defines 'Traditional medicine is the sum total of the knowledge, skills, and practices based on the theories, beliefs, and experiences indigenous to different cultures, whether explicable or not, used in the maintenance of health as well as in the prevention, diagnosis, improvement or treatment of physical and mental illness [1]'.

Herbal medicine is one of the main streams of every traditional medicine practice regardless of the different types such as Indian traditional medicine (ITM), Sri Lankan traditional medicine (SLTM), traditional Chinese medicine (TCM), Arabic traditional medicine (ATM), African traditional medicine and South American traditional medicine. According to the WHO, medicinal ingredients of herbal medicine include herbs, herbal materials, herbal preparations and finished herbal products that contain active ingredients as parts of plants or other plant materials or combinations; also, 75% of the world's population use herbs for their basic healthcare needs [2]. Archaeological proof of history in the use of herbal medicine dates back to more than 5000 years [3], along with evidence from ancient literature such as *Arkaprakasa* (pharmacology and pharmacy) and *Kumaratantra* (paediatric diseases and management) claimed to be written by the great king Ravana of Sri Lanka where different herbal preparations were introduced for treatment and management of different types of diseases [4]. An in-depth account of the historical events on the use of herbals is reviewed by Petrovska [5]. The same disease could be treated in different countries, with different types of plant-based remedies mainly depending on their indigenous plant varieties and traditional knowledge handed down to generations through thousands of years [6, 7].

Even though history strongly supports the use of herbal medicine, over the last century, traditional knowledge and its effective uses were challenged by Western medical practitioners due to lack of scientific validation of these claims and evidence [2]. However in the recent decades, perspectives on herbal medicine had been evolving into positive thoughts with the isolation of many different effective drugs from plant materials. Existing synthetic drugs are highly expensive, and most of these are required to be replaced due to their instability *in vivo* [8]. Continuous synthetic drug doses may cause side effects and toxicity [9]; hence, these disadvantages accelerated the search for alternatives derived from natural products. With the technological advances in health and basic sciences, multi screening drug facilities to investigate specific therapeutic activities was made possible. Isolated chemicals and bioactive compounds from plant materials are the main source of modern pharmaceutical drugs, which are either naturally derived or synthetic analogues of existing natural compounds [10]. Among the many different approved drugs derived from herbal material, anticancer drugs [11], antidiabetic drugs [12] and skin care products [13] have maintained topmost status in this long list. In cancer therapy, 25% of the drugs used in the last 20 years are directly derived from plant material [11], and 49% of the antidiabetic drugs approved in the last 10 years were plant derived [12]. Both in developing and developed countries, obesity is becoming a socio-economic burden rendering global populations unhealthy, leading to many non-communicable diseases [14]. There are many weight-reducing supplements prepared by herbal extracts selling in an increased rate in the local markets, even without clinical approval, due to the popularity of the products among the users. Hence, researches are in the timely search of antiobesity herbal preparations [14] as these would flourish as multimillion dollar businesses in the global market.

In order to investigate the different activities of plant-derived extracts, the use of experimental platforms is important prior to clinical trials. Human stem cells are one such experimental platform to investigate therapeutic activities of herbal extracts *in vitro*. Stem cells with the ability to self-renew and differentiate into many cell lineages have been accepted and extensively used by scientists globally as a reliable tool in their research. Of the many different sources of stem cells, bone marrow stem cells have been used widely in research due to their well-explained characteristics, but the usage paradigm is shifting towards umbilical cord- and cord blood-derived stem cells due to the advantages such as minimum ethical issues, high availability and easy isolation methods of the latter [15]. Since stem cells possess multi-lineage differentiation ability, stimulated differentiation of stem cells could be used to investigate on therapeutics applicable to different types of diseases. For example, human mesenchymal stem cells (hMSCs) could be differentiated into osteocytes, adipocytes and chondrocytes; hence, herbal extracts could be used to investigate the suppression or the stimulation of adipogenic, osteogenic and chondrogenic differentiation properties of stem cells and therefore used to investigate the therapeutic possibilities of diseases related to the above cell lineages *in vitro*. Human haematopoietic stem cells are the progenitors of cells of blood tissue; hence, those can be differentiated into different blood cell types, and herbal extracts could be used in the above manner to search for therapeutic agents for blood cell-related disorders. Induced pluripotent stem cells (iPSCs), a group of adult somatic cells which are genetically engineered to function as embryonic-like stem cells, are also widely used as disease model stem cell lines in investigations of therapeutic candidates for different disease targets [16]. iPSC-derived cardiomyocytes from patients with cardiovascular diseases and iPSC-derived neurons from patients with neurodegenerative disorders are currently used in high-throughput drug screening [17]. Undifferentiated stem cells are transplanted in order to regenerate tissue *in vivo*; hence, stimulation factors are important to increase the regeneration speed. The issues of synthetic growth factors and stimulants, i.e. possible side effects, high costs and low availability, remain unchanged; therefore, natural stimulants are preferred. Hence, research is ongoing in search of natural stimulants for stem cells [8]. Furthermore, growth factors, cytokines and vesicles secreted by hMSCs are known as the secretome of hMSCs, and these bioactive factors isolated singly or as a mixture are investigated as potential therapeutic agents, which could reduce the complexities of therapy using cell transplantations [18].

Although it is reported that over 53,000 plant species are used in herbal medicine globally [2], only a few are being tested and reported with scientific proof of their biological activities. The need for merging of traditional herbal medicine knowledge and cutting-edge scientific techniques is essential to produce novel drugs for the benefit of patients. Investigation of mechanisms of actions and pathways, stimulated by herbal extracts, is critical as this would support the scientific validation of such products prior to their market launch. Therefore, this chapter aims to elaborate such research published in the recent decade, in which herbal preparations, extracts and plant-derived bioactive compounds were utilized to produce scientific proof of anti-disease activity, proliferation stimulant activity and differentiation stimulation or suppression of stem cells and their related plausible mechanisms of action. Also, the chapter would identify research gaps related to effects of herbal extracts on stem cells for use in clinical therapy. This chapter harps on the potential of commercializing herbal-based stem cell therapy, which will also be affordable to the developing world.

2. Effects of herbal extracts on human stem cells

2.1. Stimulatory effects of herbal extracts on human stem cells

Our literature search for the use of herbal preparations to stimulate stem cell proliferation and differentiation in clinical trials resulted in no publications or records, explaining that this area of research is at its infancy harping on the vital necessity of this line of research. However, many studies have been reported on the use of animal models with end results of *in vitro* studies, cross-linking the above-mentioned research areas, suggesting that the impending phases of research would hopefully culminate in clinical trials, leading to natural products being marketed as commercial stem cell-stimulating agents.

There are several reviews published summarizing the effects of different herbal extracts and their isolated bioactive compounds on human and other mammalian stem cells isolated from different sources. Our review published in 2016 elaborates on osteogenic, anti-adipogenic, neurogenic, endothelial/vascular genesis, angiogenesis and proliferative effects of herbal extracts on human mesenchymal stem cells mostly confirmed by RNA expression studies [8]. Dried root of Korean herb *Dipsacus asper* had been used in Korean traditional medicine for the treatment of bone fracture and the crude extract, and an isolated compound from the herb hedraganin-3-O-(2-O-acetyl)-α-L-arabinopyranoside demonstrated the osteogenic differentiation ability on bone marrow-derived hMSCs via the upregulation of bone-specific proteins and alkaline phosphatase activity [19]. Aloe emodin, present in Aloe latex, showed anti-adipogenic activity on hMSCs by reducing expression levels of mRNAs (resistin, adiponectin, aP(2), lipoprotein lipase, PPARγ and tumour necrosis factor-α) involved in adipogenic pathways [20]. Treatment of adipose-derived hMSCs with dried root extract of *Angelica sinensis*, an herb used in traditional Chinese medicine, resulted in significantly higher differentiation of neural-like cells than a commonly used neural inducer, butylated hydroxyanisole [21]. The neuroprotective ability of the same extract was proven by decreased induced neurotoxicity in cultured cortical neurons, increasing the extract's value as a potential candidate in treating neurodegenerative disorders [22]. A patent was obtained for endothelial differentiation of hMSCs treated with olive leaf extract with overexpression of gene vascular endothelial growth factor, PCAM, platelet-derived growth factor receptor and vascular endothelial growth factor receptor (VEGFR)-1 [23]. An updated list of herbals and mechanism of actions on MSCs, as well as a list of phytochemicals (resveratrol, genistein, naringin, icariin) isolated from plant extracts, were presented in a similar review published in 2017 [24]. As elaborated here, all four isolated compounds had proven their ability to differentiate MSCs into osteoblasts and osteocytes, possibly through the Wnt signalling pathway, upregulating gene expression of RUNX2 and Sirt-1 genes [25–27]. Combined therapy of adipose-derived hMSCs with icariin showed significantly improved survival rates of hMSCs as well as increased expression of endothelial markers and smooth muscle markers in rat models with diabetes mellitus-induced erectile dysfunction (DMED) inhibiting oxidative stress via the regulation of PI3K/Akt-STAT3 signal pathway [28]. A previous review published in 2014 demonstrated the well-established link between herbal preparations used in Ayurveda for a wide array of disorders with their proliferation and differentiation effects which were utilized in similar capacities on stem cell differentiation and proliferation, providing scientific proof of thousands of years old Ayurvedic predictions and practices [29]. *Rasayana*, the branch of Ayurveda which explains rejuvenation and immunomodulation, has listed the use of approximately 200 herbs [28] which could be investigated for their regeneration capacities on stem cells. *Medhya Rasayana,* an intellectual/retention rejuvenation therapy method in Ayurveda that consists of four herbal plants, could be used individually or in combination [30]. Studies on stem cells treated with *Medhya Rasayana* extracts have shown the expression of nestin on stem cells, an early neural stem cell marker [29], confirming the ability of *Medhya* herbs to treat disorders related to the neural system by increasing the differentiation ability of stem cells.

A growing concern of ameliorating radiation-induced normal tissue injury is arising as it affects the well-being of cancer patients. Stem cell therapy is used to replace these cells and tissues, and many examples are elaborated in the review of Benderitter *et al.* [31]. Authors have reviewed a number of studies related to ameliorating radiation-induced myelopathy by transplanting neural stem cells to the spinal code [32], potential applications of transplanting salivary gland stem cells in patients with radiation-induced xerostomia [31], potential benefits of transplanting stem cells and biomaterial in animal models with osteoradionecrosis [33] and transplanting autologous fat drafts including adipose-derived stem cells to treat radiation-induced late skin complications [34]. As herbal extracts had proven their differentiation aiding capabilities in *in vitro* studies, they could act as stimulants to produce increased numbers of stem cells required for patient transplantations. The following figure illustrates the different sources of human mesenchymal stem cells (hMSCs) and their differentiation capabilities with advantages and disadvantages of herbal stimulants and synthetic stimulants (**Figure 1**) [8].

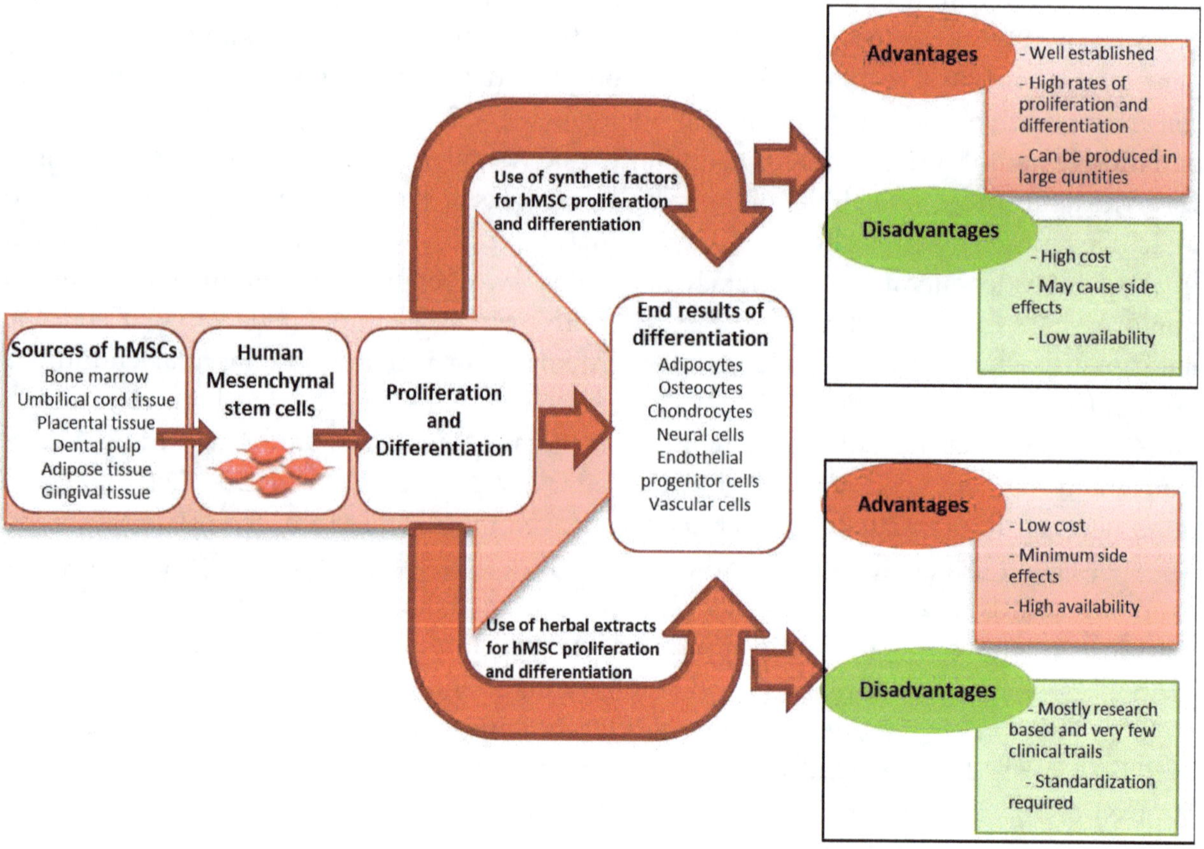

Figure 1. A glimpse of hMSC sources and their differentiation capabilities stimulated with herbal extracts or synthetic stimulants (Courtesy: Udalamaththa et al. [8]).

Although most of the reported research was on hMSCs, haematopoietic stem cells (HSCs) are also being investigated for their properties of proliferation and differentiation when treated with herbal extracts and their isolated compounds. Proliferation, differentiation and *in vitro* expansion of healthy hHSCs are important as many haematological malignancies disrupt the healthy hHSC populations. A review that summarizes a wide range of research publications on the use of Chinese herbal medicine (CHM) to promote recovery after HSC transplantation had elaborated the positive results of herbal extracts from plants such as Sheng Di Huang (*Rehmannia glutinosa*), Bai Zhu (*Atractylodes macrocephala*), Ren Shen (*Panax*), Dang Shen (*Codonopsis pilosula*), Mai Men Dong (*Ophiopogon japonicus*), Dang Gui (*Angelica sinensis*), Tai Zi Shen (*Pseudostellaria heterophylla*), Huang Qi (*Astragalus membranaceus*) and Ejiao (*Equus asinus*) [35]. A study on autologous and allogenic HSC transplanted in patients with chronic granulocytic leukaemia, acute non-lymphocytic leukaemia and lymphoma were treated with CHM concluded that treating with CHM reduces complications of transplantations and promotes recovery of haematopoietic functions [36]. More research on various other HSC transplantations against haematological malignancies such as severe aplastic anaemia patients [37], patients with myelodysplastic syndrome [38] and acute paediatric leukaemia [39] were cited herein [35], which had given positive results on patient survival rates, reduction of complications and increasing functional properties of haematopoietic cells. However, most of these studies were based on a low number of samples; hence, the need to perform such studies in large populations arises in order to validate and standardize the CHM procedures. *In vitro* studies and animal model studies had also been reported on HSC proliferation and differentiation to gather more scientific evidence to support small local clinical trials performed in isolation in individual countries. EMSA eritin, a polyherbal formulation had increased proliferation of HSC in irradiated BALB/c mice *in vivo* and triggered differentiation into the lymphopoiesis lineages [40]. Inducing of proliferation and attenuating of apoptosis were observed when an immune-mediated aplastic anaemia mouse model was treated with a modified Chinese herbal formula prepared with Radix astragali, Radix *Angelicae sinensis* and *Coptis chinensis Franch* [41].

Although stem cell therapy had boosted disease therapy into the next level of modern therapeutic medicine, a major limitation is their poor survival after transplantation into the host, which could be resolved by supplementing the microenvironment with vitamins and other antioxidants [29] and other preconditioning strategies such as exposure to hypoxic conditions, oxidative stress and heat shock treatments [42]. Scientists are studying natural plant extracts and their isolated compounds as alternatives to synthetic growth factors and other stimulants to precondition the microenvironment for the survival of stem cells *in vivo*, as there are many reports on the presence of a wide array of beneficial phytochemicals in plants. Pretreatment of adipose-derived hMSCs with *C. setidens* herbal extract had resulted in increased survival of hMSCs by inhibiting ROS-induced apoptosis, suggesting the suitability of the extract to prevent ROS-induced oxidative stress by regulating the oxidative stress-associated signalling pathway and suppressing the apoptosis-associated signal pathway [43]. Extract of *Origanum vulgare* had protected murine mesenchymal stem cells from oxidative stress when preconditioned with high doses via significantly decreasing caspase-3 activity [44]. *Tinospora cordifolia* and *Withania somnifera*, two widely used herbs used in Ayurveda for rejuvenating and anti-ageing treatment, had shown increase in proliferation and inhibition of senescence in WJ-MSCs *in vitro* [45], suggesting that pretreatment with these herbals would aid in *in vivo* transplantation procedures.

2.2. Inhibitory effects of herbal extracts on cancer stem cells

Cancer stem cells (CSCs), the cells which are capable of self-renewal and produce the heterogeneous lineage of cancer cells [46], has become the most complicated issue in cancer therapy. A number of studies were reported which resulted in the reduction of cancer cells with the treatment of isolated phytochemicals such as epigallocatechin-3-gallate (EGCG), curcumin, resveratrol, lycopene, pomegranate extracts, luteolin, genistein, piperin, β-carotene and sulforaphane [45]. Specifically, sulforaphane, a phytochemical isolated from broccoli, had apoptosis-inducing effects on pancreatic CSCs [47] and could target breast CSCs effectively [48].

However, in this scenario, scientists are changing their approach in the search for natural products by trying to select herbal extracts and preparations known to be effective against cancers in traditional medicine. This approach would be advantageous for both ends of traditional medicine and modern therapeutics, as traditional medicine will have a chance of proving the remedies in a scientific platform and also the modern therapeutics would have the benefit of using time tested anticancer remedies rather than screening thousands of plant extracts for this purpose without any clues. A review on targeting CSCs using TCM remedies and their active compounds had elaborated several approaches of herbal remedies acting on CSCs. Reversion of drug resistance of CSCs, inducing cell death and inhibiting cell proliferation, inhibiting metastasis and targeting CSCs-related miRNAs are the explained methods of TCM remedies targeting CSCs [49]. Berberine liposomes, isolated from rhizome of *Coptis chinensis*, showed anticancer effects on human breast CSCs transplanted in nude mice by penetrating the cell membrane, accumulating in mitochondria of CSCs and resulting in reversion of drug resistance and apoptotic pathway inducing cell death and inhibiting cell proliferation [50]. Curcumin and epigallocatechin gallate (EGCG) had synergistically targeted breast CSCs by downregulating stemness genes and inducing differentiation of these into non-stem cells [51]. Prostate cancer metastasis had been reduced by a combination of quercetin, extracted from *Dysosma veitchii* and EGCG by reducing activity of LEF-1/TCF responsive receptor [52]. Honokiol, a lignan isolated from *Magnolia officinalis*, had inhibited renal cancer metastasis by regulating miR-141/ZEB2 signalling [53]. Triphala, a widely used formulation in Ayurveda, had shown anticancer properties on human colon cancer stem cells by p53-independent proliferation inhibition and apoptosis inducing [54]. Also, a Sri Lankan group of scientists had investigated on anticancer properties of gedunin, a major compound found in *Azadirachta indica*, which confirmed its apoptotic-inducing properties against human embryonal carcinoma cells—a cancer stem cell model [55].

2.3. Commercial herbal products with claims of stem cell rejuvenation

Many herbal products are commercialized with claims to be rejuvenating adult stem cells which are considered as stem cell supplements. The first stem cell enhancer was developed and patented by Dr. Sahelian of Stemtech HealthSciences, Inc. in 2005 [56] which included extracts of freshwater microalgae and marine macroalgae [57]. Stem Cell 100® is a patent pending product prepared from bioactive compounds of herbal plants *Astragalus membranaceus, Vaccinium,* Pine bark, *Camellia sinensis, Pterocarpus marsupium, Polygonum multiflorum, Schisandra,* Fo-Ti root and *Drynaria* rhizome mainly derived from TCM [58]. ProxyStem is another patent pending nutraceutical stem cell supplement with claims to be working on pro-inflammatory pathways, endothelial cell health, oxidative stress protection, mitochondrial function and artery support [59].

Another product, NutraStem Active, was awarded a patent for claims of its ability to promote adult stem cells with its four ingredients—blueberry extract, green tea extract, L-carnosine and vitamin D3 [60]. Stem-Kine, a clinically proven stem cell supplement, includes ellagic acid which protects stem cells from free radicals [61]; it is a polyphenol compound extracted from mainly a plant of the berry family [62].

3. Pros and cons of using herbal remedies to stimulate stem cells

Traditional herbal treatment provides a straightforward method to identify the link between plant/herbal remedies and their use in curing different diseases. Modern scientists now use the same strategy to identify herbal plants and their isolated compounds which could be used as stem cell stimulants for much needed stem cell therapeutic procedures. Studies were initiated in this line of research in developed countries as well as in the developing countries acquiring their own traditional herbal treatment knowledge. China seems to be much ahead in this hybrid system of research using Chinese traditional herbs/isolated compounds and cutting-edge screening technologies. Although there is a plethora of internationally published research by research groups from China, many clinical trials and small population studies seem to be concealed from the rest of the world as these reports are published in local journals in their native language [35]. China is not alone in this exercise. Other countries such as Iran and Pakistan too with rich traditional medicine cultures and also into stem cell research are posing the same issue, as the data they produce are not communicated to the international scientific community. This is an unfortunate situation which could be rectified to be more productive through collaborative research with the rest of the world.

In certain instances, developing countries offer their knowledge of traditional herbal medicine together with their rich local plant diversity to collaborate with developed countries to obtain cutting-edge technologies to achieve high potential results in their research. However, the strict local regulations and policies on shipping indigenous plant material or their compounds in developing countries, in order to protect their own plant species, had restricted this productive collaborative research frame work, as this process is lengthy which would lead to late initiation of laboratory investigations.

Another concern is that of the withdrawal of traditional herbal practitioners from providing information on their herbal remedies to the scientists for investigations; it is the latter who have the ability to scientifically prove that these remedies are actually therapeutically potent. Traditional practices are said to be handed down from generation to generation within families, and most of these practitioners treat patients *pro bono*, as a social service. Since these practitioners claim to have satisfactory results from providing such treatment, they have no reason to give away their herbal remedies, which had been a family secret for over hundreds of years. However, the modern graduates of traditional medicine are more into scientifically validating their treatment methods, as it is beneficial for their practice to have scientifically proven results to compete with Western medicine practitioners. Most traditional medicine practitioners vary the constituents of herbal preparations and the ratios used in their prescriptions even for the same disease depending on the patient's individual constitution, indicative of the practise of 'personalized/precision medicine'. 'Ayugenomics' irrevocably established that a genetic basis did indeed exist to the said individual constitutions [63]; differential DNA methylation signatures in the three distinct 'prakriti' phenotypes (based on distinctly descriptive physiological, psychological and anatomical features of different individuals) demonstrated the epigenetic basis of traditional human classification in Ayurveda with relevance to personalized medicine [64]. Yet, allopathic medicine strongly believes in standard preparations where only the dose is varied among individual patients. Hence, there arises the question whether modern standardized herbal preparations would be universally effective on every patient.

Nevertheless, herbal remedies that were scientifically investigated for their properties with elucidated mechanisms and pathways of action too may face further obstacles prior to their market launch. As mentioned in the review of Udalamaththa *et al.*, a large-scale manufacturing process may reduce the crude properties of herbal remedies, solvents used to prepare extracts may produce adverse effects when used in therapy, complexity and variability of bioactive compounds may make clinical applications challenging [8]. As standardization of herbal products is a must prior to the market launch, similar and stringent regulations will be applied to herbal stem cell stimulants which are to be used in therapy.

Yet, despite all issues involved, pharmaceutical companies are competing for patents and commercializing herbal stimulants, supplements and many more drugs which could be used in stem cell therapy.

4. Conclusion

Herbal medicine has at all times been a trusted treatment method from ancient eras. The paucity of the use of herbal medicine or related treatment methods in allopathic medicine practices or other types of therapy using cutting-edge technology may pose the 'missing part of the puzzle' which scientists and clinicians have strived to solve. However, in recent years, both traditional medicine and novel technologies in synergy have resulted in beneficial outcomes advantageous to the patients. Examples presented in this chapter provide a glimpse of recent studies where herbal medicine and stem cells have been amalgamated in search of treatment against 'incurable diseases'. Although the use of medicinal plants in stem cell research is in its infancy, with small population studies within local communities, with low numbers of related patents and many complexities in application in a clinical setting, the attraction of this area of research has never ebbed due to the promising results emerging from basic scientific research. Preliminary trials leading to the initiation of in-depth studies may well result in inexpensive, available, nontoxic drugs, stimulants and supplements useful in stem cell therapy.

Acknowledgements

The authors gratefully acknowledge funding by the National Science Foundation, Sri Lanka (RG/2015/HS/01).

Author details

Preethi Vidya Udagama* and Vindya Udalamaththa

*Address all correspondence to: preethi@zoology.cmb.ac.lk

Department of Zoology and Environment Sciences, Faculty of Science, University of Colombo, Colombo, Sri Lanka

References

[1] World Health Organization, [Internet]. 2017. Available from: http://who.int/medicines/areas/traditional/definitions/en/ [Accessed: August 25, 2017]

[2] Pan SY, Litscher G, Gao SH, Zhou SF, Yu ZL, Chen HQ, Zhang SF, Tang MK, Sun JN, Ko KM. Historical perspective of traditional indigenous medical practices: The current renaissance and conservation of herbal resources. Evidence-Based Complementary and Alternative Medicine. Apr 27, 2014;**2014**:525340

[3] Edwards E, Da-Costa-Rocha I, Lawrence MJ, Cable C, Heinrich M. Use and efficacy of herbal medicines: Part 1—Historical and traditional use. The Pharmaceutical Journal. Aug 11, 2012;**288**:685-686

[4] Sharma CP. *Ravana:* A great scholar and scientist. Journal of Gampaha Wickramarachchi Ayurveda Institute. 2000;**2**(1):19-20

[5] Petrovska BB. Historical review of medicinal plants' usage. Pharmacognosy Reviews. Jan 2012;**6**(11):1

[6] Andrade-Cetto A, Heinrich M. Mexican plants with hypoglycaemic effect used in the treatment of diabetes. Journal of Ethnopharmacology. Jul 14, 2005;**99**(3):325-348

[7] Parikh NH, Parikh PK, Kothari C. Indigenous plant medicines for health care: Treatment of Diabetes mellitus and hyperlipidemia. Chinese Journal of Natural Medicines. May 1, 2014;**12**(5):335-344

[8] Udalamaththa VL, Jayasinghe CD, Udagama PV. Potential role of herbal remedies in stem cell therapy: Proliferation and differentiation of human mesenchymal stromal cells. Stem Cell Research & Therapy. Aug 11, 2016;**7**(1):110

[9] Ali TF, Hasan T. Phlorotannin-incorporated mesenchymal stem cells and their promising role in osteogenesis imperfecta. Journal of Medical Hypotheses and Ideas. Jul 31, 2012;**6**(2):85-89

[10] Newman DJ, Cragg GM. Natural products as sources of new drugs over the last 25 years. Journal of Natural Products. Mar 23, 2007;**70**(3):461-477

[11] Amin A, Gali-Muhtasib H, Ocker M, Schneider-Stock R. Overview of major classes of plant-derived anticancer drugs. International Journal of Biomedical Science: IJBS. Mar 2009;**5**(1):1

[12] Gothai S, Ganesan P, Park SY, Fakurazi S, Choi DK, Arulselvan P. Natural phyto-bioactive compounds for the treatment of type 2 diabetes: Inflammation as a target. Nutrients. Aug 4, 2016;**8**(8):461

[13] Stallings AF, Lupo MP. Practical uses of botanicals in skin care. The Journal of Clinical and Aesthetic Dermatology. Jan 2009;**2**(1):36

[14] Mohamed GA, Ibrahim SR, Elkhayat ES, El Dine RS. Natural anti-obesity agents. Bulletin of Faculty of Pharmacy, Cairo University. Dec 31, 2014;**52**(2):269-284

[15] Hass R, Kasper C, Böhm S, Jacobs R. Different populations and sources of human mesenchymal stem cells (MSC): A comparison of adult and neonatal tissue-derived MSC. Cell Communication and Signaling. May 14, 2011;**9**(1):12

[16] Wilson KD, Wu JC. Induced pluripotent stem cells. Journal of American Medical Association. Apr 28, 2015;**313**(16):1613-1614

[17] Kim C. iPSC technology-powerful hand for disease modeling and therapeutic screen. BMB Reports. May 2015;**48**(5):256

[18] Pires AO, Mendes-Pinheiro B, Teixeira FG, Anjo SI, Ribeiro-Samy S, Gomes ED, Serra SC, Silva NA, Manadas B, Sousa N, Salgado AJ. Unveiling the differences of secretome of human bone marrow mesenchymal stem cells, adipose tissue-derived stem cells, and human umbilical cord perivascular cells: A proteomic analysis. Stem Cells and Development. May 25, 2016;**25**(14):1073-1083

[19] Kim BS, Kim YC, Zadeh H, Park YJ, Pi SH, Shin HS, You HK. Effects of the dichloromethane fraction of Dipsaci Radix on the osteoblastic differentiation of human alveolar bone marrow-derived mesenchymal stem cells. Bioscience, Biotechnology, and Biochemistry. Jan 23, 2011;**75**(1):13-19

[20] Subash-Babu P, Alshatwi AA. Aloe-emodin inhibits adipocyte differentiation and maturation during in vitro human mesenchymal stem cell adipogenesis. Journal of Biochemical and Molecular Toxicology. Aug 1, 2012;**26**(8):291-300

[21] Wang Q, Zhou L, Guo Y, Liu G, Cheng J, Yu H. Differentiation of human adipose-derived stem cells into neuron-like cells by Radix Angelicae Sinensis. Neural Regeneration Research. Dec 15, 2013;**8**(35):3353

[22] Huang SH, Lin CM, Chiang BH. Protective effects of Angelica Sinensis extract on amyloid beta-peptide-induced neurotoxicity. Phytomedicine. 2008;**15**(9):710-721

[23] Use of olive leaf extracts in a pharmaceutical composition for inducing angiogenesis and vasculogenesis US 20120141435 A1. In: Patents. 2012. Available from: https://www.google.com/patents/US20120141435. [Accessed: November 18, 2015]

[24] Kornicka K, Kocherova I, Marycz K. The effects of chosen plant extracts and compounds on mesenchymal stem cells—A bridge between molecular nutrition and regenerative medicine-concise review. Phytotherapy Research. Jan 1, 2017;**31**(7):947-958

[25] Tseng PC, Hou SM, Chen RJ, Peng HW, Hsieh CF, Kuo ML, Yen ML. Resveratrol promotes osteogenesis of human mesenchymal stem cells by upregulating RUNX2 gene expression via the SIRT1/FOXO3A axis. Journal of Bone and Mineral Research. Oct 1, 2011;**26**(10):2552-2563

[26] Zhou H, Shang L, Li X, Zhang X, Gao G, Guo C, Chen B, Liu Q, Gong Y, Shao C. Resveratrol augments the canonical Wnt signaling pathway in promoting osteoblastic differentiation of multipotent mesenchymal cells. Experimental Cell Research. Oct 15, 2009;**315**(17):2953-2962

[27] Beher D, Wu J, Cumine S, Kim KW, Lu SC, Atangan L, Wang M. Resveratrol is not a direct activator of SIRT1 enzyme activity. Chemical Biology & Drug Design. Dec 1, 2009;**74**(6):619-624

[28] Wang X, Liu C, Xu Y, Chen P, Shen Y, Xu Y, Zhao Y, Chen W, Zhang X, Ouyang Y, Wang Y. Combination of mesenchymal stem cell injection with icariin for the treatment of diabetes-associated erectile dysfunction. PLoS One. Mar 28, 2017;**12**(3):e0174145

[29] Joshi KS, Bhonde R. Insights from Ayurveda for translational stem cell research. Journal of Ayurveda and Integrative Medicine. Jan 2014;**5**(1):4

[30] Gomathi M, Balachandar V. Novel therapeutic approaches: Rett syndrome and human induced pluripotent stem cell technology. Stem Cell Investigation. 2017;**4**:20

[31] Benderitter M, Caviggioli F, Chapel A, Coppes RP, Guha C, Klinger M, Malard O, Stewart F, Tamarat R, Van Luijk P, Limoli CL. Stem cell therapies for the treatment of radiation-induced normal tissue side effects. Antioxidants & Redox Signaling. Jul 10, 2014;**21**(2):338-355

[32] Rezvani M, Birds DA, Hodges H, Hopewell JW, Milledew K, Wilkinson JH. Modification of radiation myelopathy by the transplantation of neural stem cells in the rat. Radiation Research. Oct 2001;**156**(4):408-412

[33] Espitalier F, Vinatier C, Lerouxel E, Guicheux J, Pilet P, Moreau F, Daculsi G, Weiss P, Malard OA. Comparison between bone reconstruction following the use of mesenchymal stem cells and total bone marrow in association with calcium phosphate scaffold in irradiated bone. Biomaterials. Feb 28, 2009;**30**(5):763-769

[34] Akita S, Akino K, Hirano A, Ohtsuru A, Yamashita S. Noncultured autologous adipose-derived stem cells therapy for chronic radiation injury. Stem Cells International. Dec 1, 2010;**2010**:532704-532712

[35] Fleischer T, Chang TT, Yen HR. Post-hematopoietic stem cell transplantation in patients with hematologic disorders: Chinese herbal medicine for an unmet need. Journal of Integrative Medicine. Sep 30, 2016;**14**(5):322-335

[36] Yu RX, Zhou YH, Zhu NX. Twelve cases of malignant hematopathy treated by combined therapy of hematopoietic stem cell transplantation and Chinese herbal medicine. ZhongguoZhong Xi Yi Jie He ZaZhi. 2001;**21**(2):90-93

[37] Ye BD, Zhang X, Shao KD, Chen D, Zhang Y, DJ W, QH Y, Shen JP, Shen YP, Zhou YH. Combined use of Chinese medicine with allogeneic hematopoietic stem cell transplantation for severe aplastic anemia patients. Chinese Journal of Integrative Medicine. Dec 1, 2014;**20**(12):903-909

[38] Zhang Y, Ye BD, Qian LL, Gao YT, Wen XW, Shen JP, Zhou YH. Treatment of myelodysplastic syndrome by hematopoietic stem cell transplantation combined with Chinese medical syndrome typing: A clinical study. ZhongguoZhong Xi Yi Jie He ZaZhi. 2015;**35**(1):53-56. Chinese with abstract in English

[39] Shi L, Cheng Z, Chen SM, Qin XL, Wang H. Autologous peripheral blood stem cell transplantation combined with traditional Chinese medicine therapy on acute leukemia inchildren. Shi Yong ErKe Lin Chuang ZaZhi. 2010;**25**(3):209-210. Chinese with abstract in English

[40] Ibrahim M, Widjajanto E, Widodo MA, Sumitro SB. Adequate stimulation of hematopoietic stem cell proliferation by a polyherbal formulation (EMSA eritin) leading to lymphocyte differentiation in BALB/c mice after radiation. Biomarkers and Genomic Medicine. Sep 30, 2015;**7**(3):110-115

[41] Zhou J, Li X, Deng P, Wei Y, Liu J, Chen M, Xu Y, Zhang D, Zhu L, Lou L, Dong B. Chinese herbal formula, modified Danggui Buxue tang, attenuates apoptosis of hematopoietic stem cells in immune-mediated aplastic Anemia mouse model. Journal of Immunology Research. 2017;**2017**:9786972

[42] Haider HK, Ashraf M. Preconditioning and stem cell survival. Journal of Cardiovascular Translational Research. Apr 1, 2010;**3**(2):89-102

[43] Lee JH, Jung HK, Han YS, Yoon YM, Yun CW, Sun HY, Cho HW, Lee SH. Antioxidant effects of *Cirsium setidens* extract on oxidative stress in human mesenchymal stem cells. Molecular Medicine Reports. Oct 1, 2016;**14**(4):3777-3784

[44] Mohammadzadeh-Vardin M, Sagha M. Using herbal preconditioning, extract of *Origanum vulgare* protects the mesenchymal stem cells from the oxidative stress. In: Abstracts of the 12th Royan International Congress on Stem Cell Biology & Technology; Iran. Cell Journal. 2016;**18**(Suppl 1):50

[45] Sanap A, Chandravanshi B, Shah T, Tillu G, Dhanushkodi A, Bhonde R, Joshi K. Herbal pre-conditioning induces proliferation and delays senescence in Wharton's jelly mesenchymal stem cells. Biomedicine & Pharmacotherapy. Sep 1, 2017;**93**:772-778

[46] Scarpa ES, Ninfali P. Phytochemicals as innovative therapeutic tools against cancer stem cells. International Journal of Molecular Sciences. Jul 10, 2015;**16**(7):15727-15742

[47] Kallifatidis G, Rausch V, Baumann B, Apel A, Beckermann BM, Groth A, Mattern J, Li Z, Kolb A, Moldenhauer G, Altevogt P. Sulforaphane targets pancreatic tumour-initiating cells by NF-κB-induced antiapoptotic signalling. Gut. Jul 1, 2009;**58**(7):949-963

[48] Li Y, Zhang T, Korkaya H, Liu S, Lee HF, Newman B, Yu Y, Clouthier SG, Schwartz SJ, Wicha MS, Sun D. Sulforaphane, a dietary component of broccoli/broccoli sprouts, inhibits breast cancer stem cells. Clinical Cancer Research. May 1, 2010;**16**(9):2580-2590

[49] Hong M, Tan HY, Li S, Cheung F, Wang N, Nagamatsu T, Feng Y. Cancer stem cells: The potential targets of Chinese medicines and their active compounds. International Journal of Molecular Sciences. Jun 7, 2016;**17**(6):893

[50] Ma X, Zhou J, Zhang CX, Li XY, Li N, RJ J, Shi JF, Sun MG, Zhao WY, LM M, Yan Y. Modulation of drug-resistant membrane and apoptosis proteins of breast cancer stem cells by targeting berberine liposomes. Biomaterials. Jun 30, 2013;**34**(18):4452-4465

[51] Chung SS, Vadgama JV. Curcumin and epigallocatechin gallate inhibit the cancer stem cell phenotype via down-regulation of STAT3–NFκB signaling. Anticancer Research. Jan 1, 2015;**35**(1):39-46

[52] Tang SN, Singh C, Nall D, Meeker D, Shankar S, Srivastava RK. The dietary bioflavonoid quercetin synergizes with epigallocatechingallate (EGCG) to inhibit prostate cancer stem cell characteristics, invasion, migration and epithelial-mesenchymal transition. Journal of Molecular Signaling. Aug 18, 2010;**5**(1):14

[53] Li W, Wang Q, Su Q, Ma D, An C, Ma L, Liang H. Honokiol suppresses renal cancer cells' metastasis via dual-blocking epithelial-mesenchymal transition and cancer stem cell properties through modulating miR-141/ZEB2 signaling. Molecules and Cells. May 2014;**37**(5):383

[54] Vadde R, Radhakrishnan S, Reddivari L, Vanamala JK. Triphala extract suppresses proliferation and induces apoptosis in human colon cancer stem cells via suppressing c-Myc/Cyclin D1 and elevation of Bax/Bcl-2 ratio. BioMed Research International. Jun 17, 2015;**2015**:649263

[55] Tharmarajah L, Samarakoon SR, Ediriweera MK, Piyathilaka P, Tennekoon KH, Senathilake KS, Rajagopalan U, Galhena PB, Thabrew I. In vitro anticancer effect

of Gedunin on human Teratocarcinomal (NTERA-2) cancer stem-like cells. BioMed Research International. Jun 7, 2017;**2017**:2413197

[56] Ray Sahelian. Stem Cell Enhancers and Natural Medicine Information [Internet]. 2016. Available from: http://www.raysahelian.com/stemcellenhancers.html [Accessed: September 3, 2017]

[57] Cerule [Internet]. 2016. Available from: http://www.cerule.com/stemenhance-ultra-en/ [Accessed: September 3, 2017]

[58] Stem Cell 100 [Internet]. 2011. Available from: http://www.stemcell100.com/ [Accessed: September 2, 2017]

[59] RevGenetics [Internet]. 2017. Available from: https://store.revgenetics.com/products/proxystem-stem-cell-pro-supplement [Accessed: September 2, 2017]

[60] Natura Therapeutics, Inc. [Internet]. 2007-2014. Available from: http://www.naturath-erapeutics.com/nutrastem_sport [Accessed: September 3, 2017]

[61] Stem-Kine [Internet]. 2017. Available from: https://www.stem-kine.com/order/ [Accessed: September 3, 2017]

[62] PubChem, Open Chemistry Data Base [Internet]. 2004. Available from: https://pubchem.ncbi.nlm.nih.gov/compound/ellagic_acid#section=Top [Accessed: September 3, 2017]

[63] Patwardhan B, Bodeker G. Ayurvedic genomics: Establishing a genetic basis for mind-body typologies. Journal of Alternative Complementary Medicine. Jun 2008;**14**(5):571

[64] Rotti H, Mallya S, Kabekkodu SP, Chakrabarty S, Bhale S, Bharadwaj R, Bhat BK, Dedge AP, Dhumal VR, Gangadharan GG, Gopinath PM, Govindaraj P, Joshi KS, Kondaiah P, Nair S, Nair SN, Nayak J, Prasanna BV, Shintre P, Sule M, Thangaraj K, Patwardhan B, Valiathan MV, Satyamoorthy KDNA. Methylation analysis of phenotype specific stratified Indian population. Journal of Translational Medicine. May 8, 2015;**13**:151

6

Herbal Medicine Use during Pregnancy: Benefits and Untoward Effects

Tariku Laelago

Abstract

The use of herbal medicine has been on an increase over time. The most commonly used herbs are ginger, cranberry, valerian, raspberry leaf, chamomile, peppermint, thyme, fenugreek, green tea, sage, anise, garlic and bitter kola. The use of herbal medicine during pregnancy is associated with educational status of women, income level of household and age of women. Herbal medicines were used during pregnancy to treat nausea and vomiting, reduce the risk of preeclampsia, shorten labour and treat common cold and urinary tract infection. Using herbal medicine occasionally causes trouble. Heartburn, pre-mature labour, miscarriage, increase in blood flow, abortion and allergic reactions are the common troubles of herbal medicine use during pregnancy. Using herbal medicine during the first trimester and the third trimester is unsafe for the foetus. Pregnant women should talk to health professionals before consuming any herbal medicines. The unfortunate consequences of using herbal medicine during pregnancy need further study for various herbs. Therefore, clinical trial research should be done to identify unfortunate consequences of herbal medicine use during pregnancy.

Keywords: benefits, herbal medicine, pregnancy, safety, untoward effect

1. Introduction

Herbal medicine has been used for disease prevention and treating ailments worldwide. It is known that between 65 and 85% of the world population used herbal medicine as their primary form of health care [1]. The prevalence of herbal medicine use during pregnancy ranges from 12 to 82.3% [2, 3]. Ginger, garlic, raspberry, cranberry, valerian, chamomile, peppermint and fenugreek are frequently used herbal medicines during pregnancy [2, 4–11]. Using herbal medicine during pregnancy has controversial issues. Even though, herbal medicine is easily available as compared to other medicines, the safety issue during pregnancy is a concern. Using herbal medicine in first 3 months and late in third trimester is dangerous for the foetus. Before using any herbal medicine, it is better to consult the doctor and the pharmacist to ensure that the herbs are appropriate and safe to use during pregnancy [12]. In pregnancy, mothers are concerned about all medications that may affect their health, the health of the foetus, and the pregnancy outcomes. Availing evidence-based information about benefits and untoward effects of herbal medicine use during pregnancy is important for safer pregnancy and healthy foetus. The aim of this chapter is to provide the best available information on benefits and untoward effects of herbal medicine use during pregnancy. This chapter identified the prevalence of herbal medicine use during pregnancy across regions and countries. The chapter also identified the commonly used herbs and described the character of women who used herbs during pregnancy. The benefits and untoward effects of commonly used herbal medicine during pregnancy are reviewed based on scientific findings.

2. Herbal medicine use during pregnancy: benefits and untoward effects

Herbal medicine use during pregnancy is common across regions and countries. The prevalence of herbal medicine use during pregnancy is varied across regions and countries. Multinational study conducted in different countries showed that 28.9% of pregnant women used herbal medicine during pregnancy [2, 4]. A literature review from the Middle East revealed that up to 82.2% of the women used herbal medicine at some point during pregnancy. The study also identified that many women used herbal medicine during the first trimester [5]. An observational cohort study done in South West England found that 26.7% of the women used a complementary or alternative medicine at least once during pregnancy. The use of herbs rose from 6% in the first trimester to 12.4% in the second trimester and to 26.3% in third trimester [13]. In Australia, 36% of the women took at least one herbal medicine during pregnancy [14]. Studies done in Africa showed the prevalence of herbal medicine use during pregnancy was between 12 and 73.1% [3, 6–9, 15–19].

The most commonly consumed herbal medicines during pregnancy include; ginger [2, 4–11], cranberry [2, 4, 10–11], valerian [2, 4, 10], raspberry leaf [2, 4, 10–11, 13], chamomile [13–14], peppermint [5, 13], rosehip [13], thyme [5], fenugreek [5, 9], green tea, sage, and aniseed [5]. Eucalyptus, tenaadam (*Ruta chalepensis*), damakess (*Ocimum lamiifolium*), feto, omore are also other herbal medicines used during pregnancy [6–8]. Garlic [6–8, 15–18], palm kernel oil, bitter kola and dogonyaro (*Azadirachta indica*) are other herbs that are used during pregnancy [15–18].

Being students, having no education, having low income and having tertiary education level make women more likely to use herbal medicine during pregnancy [2, 4, 6–8, 15–18]. The other factors that make women more likely to consume herbal medicines are being primiparas [2, 4, 9], non-smoking [2, 9] and old age women [13–14].

Based on the available researches and literature reviews, the most commonly used herbal medicines during pregnancy are identified. The benefits and untoward effects of the herbs are also reviewed.

2.1. Ginger (*Zingiber officinale*)

Common names of ginger is African ginger, black ginger, Cochin ginger, gingembre, ginger root, imber, and Jamaica ginger [20].

2.1.1. *Benefits of ginger*

Ginger is used as anti-nauseant and anti-emetic for nausea and for hyperemesis gravidarum. The recommended daily dose of ginger is up to 1g dried powder [21]. A single blind clinical trial showed ginger as an effective herbal medicine for decreasing nausea and vomiting during pregnancy. This study also suggested a daily total of 100 mg ginger in a capsule [22].

A randomized controlled clinical trial conducted on 120 women over 20 weeks of gestation with symptoms of morning sickness showed consumption of 1500 mg of dried ginger for 4 days improves nausea and vomiting. The study also revealed that newborns whose mothers consumed ginger during pregnancy had normal birth weights and normal APGAR score [23]. Consumption of ginger in amounts used in food preparation is likely to be safe. Taking 1–2 g dried ginger over the course of a day has been shown to relive symptoms of minor disorder of pregnancy [24–26]. Using higher doses of ginger is not safe for pregnant women. Thus, pregnant women should not use higher dose of ginger.

2.1.2. *Untoward effects of ginger*

A literature review reported that ginger is not a safe herb. It is a potential abortifacient with high doses (>1000 mg daily consumption). Higher doses of ginger can cause thinning of blood, stomach discomfort and heartburn [24–27].

2.2. Garlic (*Allium sativa*)

Garlic is a perennial herb cultivated in different countries. It is commonly used as a food ingredient and as a spice in different countries [28].

2.2.1. *Benefits of garlic*

Study conducted on antimicrobial and antifungal activity of garlic showed antibacterial and antifungal features of garlic make it nutritious to consume during pregnancy [29]. Garlic enhances a woman's immune system; this in turn helps women to have healthy pregnancy and healthy babies. Eating garlic during pregnancy is important to reduce the risk of preeclampsia and protein retention in urine [30]. A randomized controlled study was conducted where 100 primigravida were treated with either garlic tablets (800 mg/day) or placebo during the third trimester of pregnancy to determine the effect of garlic tablets supplementation on preeclampsia. With the exception of a garlic odour, the few side effects like nausea were reported because of garlic consumption during the third trimester of pregnancy. Pregnancy outcomes were comparable in both treated with garlic and the placebo group. The study did not report any incidence of major or minor malformations in newborn infants and there were no spontaneous abortions of the foetuses [31].

2.2.2. *Untoward effects of garlic*

Excessive use of garlic should be avoided in early pregnancy. Pregnant women with thyroid disorders should avoid its use. Pregnant women should also avoid using garlic prior to surgery including caesarean as it may interfere with blood clotting. Another untoward effect of using garlic during pregnancy is that it may aggravate heartburn [32].

2.3. Cranberry (*Vaccinium macrocarpon*)

There are different types of cranberries: American cranberry, Arandano Americano, Arandano Trepador, Cranberries, European cranberry, Grosse Moosbeere, kranbeere, large cranberry, Moosebeere, Mossberry [20].

2.3.1. *Benefits of cranberry*

Using cranberry during pregnancy is important to prevent urinary tract infection [33], stomach ulcer [34–35], periodontal diseases [36–38] and influenza [39]. A survey conducted on 400 Norwegian postpartum women reported that cranberry was one of the most commonly used herbs during pregnancy, mostly for urinary tract infection [40].

2.3.2. *Untoward effects of cranberry*

The untoward effects of cranberry use during pregnancy needs further investigations.

2.4. Valerian (*Valeriana officinalis*)

Valerian is native to Europe and Asia and has naturalized in Eastern North America. It has been extensively cultivated in Northern Europe [41].

2.4.1. *Benefits of valerian*

Valerian is used as a mild sedative to help patients fall asleep and relieve stress and anxiety. There is a lack of safety information on consumption of valerian during pregnancy. It is highly recommended that pregnant women talk to the doctor before taking valerian during pregnancy [24, 26, 42]. Study conducted on effect of valerian consumption during pregnancy on cortical volume and the levels of zinc and copper in brain tissue of mouse foetus showed valerian consumption in pregnancy had no significant effect on brain weight and cerebral cortex volume and copper level in foetal brain [43].

2.4.2. *Untoward effects of valerian*

Studies conducted on mouse foetus presented that consumption of valerian during pregnancy had significant decrease in the level of zinc in the brain [43]. This finding suggests that valerian use during pregnancy should be limited.

2.5. Bitter kola

Bitter kola is a plant that comes from Africa. Africans have been using bitter kola for pregnant women since ages. Nowadays, bitter kola popularity has spread worldwide [44].

2.5.1. Benefits of bitter kola

Drinking bitter kola is good for pregnancy. Bitter kola contains nutrients and vitamins good for pregnancy. For Africans, bitter kola is the best supplement for pregnant women. Health benefits of bitter kola include treating nausea and vomiting, making uterus healthier, strengthening pregnant women and normalizing blood circulation in pregnant women. Bitter kola contains very strong caffeine. One bean of bitter kola contains the same amount of caffeine as two glasses of coffee. Thus, pregnant women have to drink the recommended dose (one small cup of bitter kola in a day) [44].

2.5.2. Untoward effects of bitter kola

Using very high doses of bitter kola is not recommended. A very high dose of bitter kola is not good for the uterus of the woman [45].

2.6. Fenugreek (*Trigonella foenum-graecum*)

Fenugreek is an annual leguminous herb that belongs to the family fabaceae, which is found as a wild plant and cultivated in Northern India. It is a galactagogue [46].

2.6.1. Benefits of fenugreek

Consumption of fenugreek during pregnancy increases milk production in pregnant women. The exact mechanism of fenugreek consumption and increasing milk production is not well understood. However, it is believed that seeds of fenugreek contain the precursor of a hormone that increases milk production [45, 46].

2.6.2. Untoward effect of fenugreek

Large amounts of fenugreek may cause uterine contractions, miscarriage or premature labour. It could affect blood sugar levels, so pregnant women with insulin-dependent diabetes mellitus should avoid it. It can also cause heartburn [47].

2.7. Red raspberry leaf (*Rubus idaeus*)

Red raspberry leaf is known as garden raspberry leaf. The deciduous raspberry plant produces it [48].

2.7.1. Benefits of red raspberry

Red raspberry leaf has mineral rich nutritive and uterine tonic to promote an expedient labour with minimal bleeding. It can also be used as an astringent to diarrhoea. In a study based on two clinical trials, there was positive association with red raspberry use and astringency in the case of diarrhoea. Daily recommended dose is 1.5–5 g [23–24]. Traditionally, red raspberry leaf has been used in late pregnancy to shorten the duration of labour and to reduce complications of pregnancy. Pregnant women should consult a doctor or a pharmacist for advice before using red raspberry leaf in pregnancy in a tea or infusion [49]. Red raspberry fruit is not believed to pose risk to the mother or to the baby during pregnancy. Some women take it as a labour aid during the last 2 months before delivery, whereas others take it throughout the pregnancy. In a randomized clinical trial, 192 women at 32 weeks of gestation received 1.2 g of raspberry leaf tablets twice daily. The study reported no adverse effects to mothers or infants. The active treatment with raspberry leaf shortened the second stage of labour and lowered the rate of forceps delivery. A retrospective observational study conducted on 108 pregnant women showed that 57 women who ingested raspberry leaves were less likely to have an artificial rupture of membranes or to require caesarean section, forceps or vacuum birth than 51 controls [50–51]. Women have used red raspberry leaves for painful periods in pregnancy, morning sickness, to prevent miscarriage, easing labour and delivery and enriching breast milk [52].

2.7.2. *Untoward effects of red raspberry*

The untoward effect of red raspberry needs further investigations.

2.8. Chamomile (*Matricaria recutita*)

There are two types of chamomile: German and Roman. The common German variety comes from the flower *Matricaria recutita*, and the less common Roman variety comes from the flower *Chamaemelum nobile*. German chamomile is used in teas and other supplements such as capsule and oils [53].

2.8.1. *Benefits of chamomile*

Chamomile is used as a mild sedative and to aid digestion [32]. It has been used for the treatment of morning sickness [54]. German chamomile is the type used most often as a medicinal herb, extracts of which have been reported to increase the tone of uterus muscle [53]. Chamomile does not contain caffeine, which makes it safer for pregnant women, but there is some controversy over the safety of certain herbs not fully described by the Food and Drug Administration. There is insufficient information to say for sure whether chamomile can cause harm during pregnancy. As with many other herbs, the full effect of chamomile, especially in association with other medicines and herbs, has not been studied conclusively [55].

2.8.2. *Untoward effect of chamomile*

Chamomile may cause increased blood flow, contractions, miscarriage or premature labour. It can also cause allergic reactions [47].

2.9. Clary sage (*Salvia officinale*)

Clary sage is a plant native to Italy, Syria and Southern France and grows in dry soil. The essential oil is distilled from the flowers and flowering tips [56].

2.9.1. Benefits of clary sage

It is recommended that clary sage only be used from 37 weeks onwards. It may be used to induce labour if the body is ready to go into labour. It may stimulate the release of oxytocin in pregnant women [56]. Using clary sage is highly recommended during labour to help contractions to intensify and become more effective in pulling up the horizontal uterine muscles to open the cervix and move the baby down into the pelvis and into the birth canal. The simplest and most common way to use clary sage during labour is to put a few drops on to dry cloth; the mother will inhale the aroma when she needs it to help herself become more calm and relaxed during contractions [56–57].

2.9.2. Untoward effects of clary sage

Large doses best avoided for concern of potential miscarriage and abortifacient effect [47].

2.10. Anise (*Pimpinella anisum*)

Anise is known as aniseed. There are two types of anise: anise (*Pimpinella anisum*) and star anise (*Illicium verum*) Chinese star anise [58].

2.10.1. Benefits of anise

Orally, anise is used for dyspepsia, flatulence, rhinorrhoea (runny nose) and as an expectorant, diuretic, and appetite stimulant. Anise is also used to increase lactation and facilitate birth. Topically, anise is used for lice, scabies and psoriasis treatment. Using anise during pregnancy is likely safe when used orally in amounts commonly found in food. There is insufficient reliable information available about safety of anise when taken orally in medicinal amounts during pregnancy [59]. Anise used in small amounts in herbal tea is safer in pregnancy because exposure is relatively low [58].

2.10.2. Untoward effects of anise

When used topically, anise in combination with other herbs can cause localized pruritis. In allergic patients, inhaled or ingested anise can cause rhino conjunctivitis, occupational asthma and anaphylaxis [59]. Essential oil and concentrated anise should be avoided in pregnancy for the concern that they might trigger early labour [58].

2.11. Green tea (*Camellia sinensis*)

Green tea is mostly consumed in Middle East.

2.11.1. Benefits of green tea

Green tea is important to regulate blood sugar, cholesterol and blood pressure levels. It also speeds up the body's metabolic rate and provides a natural source of energy. It can help stabilize a pregnant mother's mood [60]. However, drinking too high a dose of green tea is not recommended. The recommended dose of caffeine per day is 300 mg [61].

2.11.2. Untoward effect of green tea

Pregnant women who consumed green tea are at risk of spontaneous abortion as shown by the following two studies. A case control study conducted on 3149 pregnant women showed that serum paraxanthine (caffeine metabolite) was higher in women who had spontaneous abortions than in controls [62]. Another case control study conducted on 1498 pregnant women also showed that consumption of 375 mg or more caffeine per day during pregnancy might increase the risk of spontaneous abortion [63]. Pregnant women who consumed high caffeine during pregnancy have a chance to deliver low birth weight infants. This is supported by the following studies. A prospective study conducted on 2291 pregnant women reported that women who consumed more than 600 mg of caffeine per day are at greater risk for having low birth weight infants [64]. A prospective study conducted on 63 women also reported that pregnant women who consumed more than 300 mg/day of caffeine had low birth weight newborns [65]. Studies showed consumption of high doses of caffeine had increased risk of stillbirth. A prospective follow-up conducted on 18,478 singleton pregnancies showed that the consumption of eight or more cups of coffee in a day doubled the risk of having stillbirth compared with women who did not consume coffee [66].

Even though the above studies are conducted on coffee consumption, consumption of high doses of green tea can have adverse effects on mothers and their infants. Caffeine found in coffee and green tea is not very different. Consumption of too much caffeine (more than 300 mg per day or more than eight cups per day) can cause miscarriage as seen by the above research findings. Consumption of too much caffeine can also cause trouble of sleeping.

2.12. Thyme (*Thymus vulgaris*)

It is known as common thyme, French thyme, garden thyme, oil thyme, red thyme oil, rubbed thyme, Spanish thyme, thyme aetheroleum, thyme essential oil, thyme oil, thyme herbal, van ajwain, vanya yavani, white thyme oil [67].

2.12.1. Benefits of thyme

A literature review conducted on herbal medicine use during pregnancy showed thyme is used to manage bloating and stomach aches. It is also used for treatment of common cold and urinary tract infection [2]. When used in amounts commonly found in food, thyme has a generally recognized safe status in the US. There is insufficient reliable information available about the safety of thyme when used in medicinal amounts during pregnancy [67]. Therefore, pregnant women should avoid using thyme in medicinal amount.

2.12.2. Untoward effects of thyme

Consumption of a large dose of thyme has an emmenagogue effect. Therefore, it is better to avoid it, especially in early pregnancy, because of concern of potential miscarriage [47].

2.13. Coconut

Countries within the Southeast Asian region are rich in coconut oil and other coconut by-products [67–69].

2.13.1. Benefits of coconut

Studies reported that coconut oil has been used to facilitate labour, delivery and prevent congenital malformation [70–72]. Coconut oil during pregnancy can be used as part of a healthy nutrient-dense whole food diet. Coconut oil supplies rich amounts of saturated fat with high amounts of lauric acid. The saturated fat content helps to build up adequate fat stores in pregnancy and in preparation for breast-feeding [73].

2.13.2. Untoward effects of coconut

The study conducted to investigate the effect of virgin coconut oil on mice showed that virgin coconut oil could affect infant growth and appearance via maternal intake. The study also suggests the use of virgin coconut oil as herbal medicine to be treated with caution [74].

2.14. Echinacea (Echinacea spp)

Echinacea species came from North America and were traditionally used by the Indians for a variety of diseases, including mouth sores, colds, injuries, tooth pain and insect bites [75].

2.14.1. Benefits of Echinacea

One clinical trial study shows positive association of echinacea consumption in reducing duration and recurrence of cold and urinary tract infection [76]. The recommended dose is 5–20 ml tincture.

2.14.2. Untoward effects of Echinacea

The untoward effect of using echinacea during pregnancy needs further study.

2.15. Peppermint (*Mentha piperita*)

Peppermint is one of the world's oldest medicinal herbs and is used in both Eastern and Western traditions. Ancient Greek, Roman and Egyptian cultures used the herbs in cooking and medicine. Peppermint is currently one of the most economically important aromatic and medicinal crops produced in the US [77].

2.15.1. Benefits of peppermint

Several clinical trials have shown that peppermint essential oil, a super concentrated form of herbs, can help relive irritable bowel syndrome [78]. Natural medicine's comprehensive database showed there are no reports in the scientific literature of peppermint being either safe or contra-indicated during pregnancy. Peppermint leaves and oil are believed to be safe during pregnancy when consumed in food amounts [79]. Study conducted on use of antiemetic herbs in pregnancy indicated that peppermint is used for treatment of pregnancy-induced nausea [80].

2.15.2. Untoward effects of peppermint

The untoward effect of peppermint consumption during pregnancy needs further investigation.

3. Conclusion

The use of herbal medicine during pregnancy is a common phenomenon. Different studies have shown that many women used one or more herbal medicines during pregnancy. Some women used herbal medicine in first trimester while others used it in second or third trimester or throughout pregnancy.

The common benefits of using herbal medicine during pregnancy include managing vomiting and nausea, reducing the risk of preeclampsia, managing urinary tract infection and common cold, and shortening of duration of labour.

The common untoward effects of using herbal medicine in pregnancy are heartburn, premature labour, miscarriage, increase blood flow, abortion and allergic reactions.

Different studies revealed that using herbal medicine during the first 12 weeks and the last 12 weeks of gestation is dangerous for the foetus. Pregnant women should consult doctors or pharmacists before using any herbal medicines.

The untoward effects of using herbal medicine during pregnancy need further investigation for many herbs. Thus, researches, especially a clinical trial study should be conducted to identify untoward effect of herbal medicine use during pregnancy.

Terminologies

Antiemetic	a drug that prevents or alleviates nausea and vomiting.
Astringent	a substance that contracts the tissues or canals of the body, thereby diminishing discharges, as of mucus or blood.
Emmenagogue	increases blood flow.
Abortifacient	cause a miscarriage "from Latin: abortus "miscarriage" and faciens 'making' is a substance that induce abortion.

Miscarriage	a term used for a pregnancy that ends on its own, within the first 20 weeks of gestation.
APGAR	referred to as an acronym for: appearance, pulse, grimace, activity and respiration.
Pruritis	itchy skin that makes one scratch.
Anaphylaxis	serious life threatening allergic reaction.
Galactagogue	milk-producing agent.
Tinctures	liquid extracts made from herbs that are taken orally (by mouth).

Author details

Tariku Laelago

Address all correspondence to: tarikulalago@gmail.com

Hossana College of Health Sciences, Hossana, Ethiopia

References

[1] World Health Organization. Traditional medicine. Fact sheet Number 134. Available form: http://www.who.int/mediacentre/factsheets/fs134/en/ [Accessed: December 01, 2017]

[2] Lisha J, Shantakumar N. Herbal medicines use during pregnancy: A review from the Middle East. Oman Medical Journal. 2015;**30**(4):229-236

[3] Mothupi Mc. Use of herbal medicine during pregnancy among women with access to public healthcare in Nairobi, Kenya: A cross-sectional survey. BMC Complementary and Alternative Medicine. 2014;**14**:432. Available form: http://www.biomedcentral.com/1472-6882/14/432

[4] Kennedy D, Lupattelli A, Koren G, Nordeng H. Safety classification of herbal medicines used in pregnancy in a multinational study. BMC Complementary and Alternative Medicine. 2016;**16**:102. DOI: 10.1186/s12906-016-1079-z

[5] Kennedy D, Lupattelli A, Koren G and Nordeng H. Herbal medicine use in pregnancy: Results of a multinational study. BMC Complementary and Alternative Medicine. 2013, 13:355. Available form: http://www.biomedcentral.com/1472-6882/13/355

[6] Mekuria A, Erku D, Gebresillassie B, Birru E, Tizazu A, Ahmedin A. Prevalence and associated factors of herbal medicine use among pregnant women on antenatal care follow-up at University of Gondar Referral and Teaching Hospital, Ethiopia: A cross-sectional study. BMC Complementary and Alternative Medicine. 2017;**17**:86. DOI: 10.1186/s12906-017-1608-4

[7] Bayisa B, Tatiparthi R, Mulisa E. Use of herbal medicine among pregnant women on antenatal care at Nekemte Hospital Western Ethiopia. Natural Pharmaceutical Products. 2014;**9**(4):e17368

[8] Laelago T, Yohannes T, Lemango F. Prevalence of herbal medicine use and associated factor among women aattending antenatal care in public health facilities of Hossana Town. Achieves of Public Health. 2016;**173**:1-8

[9] Orief Y, Farghaly N, Ibrahim M. Use of herbal medicines among pregnant women attending family health centers in Alexandria. Middle East Fertility Society Journal. 2014;**19**:42-50

[10] Pregnant women use herbal medicine. Science Nordic. Available form: http://sciencenordic.com [Accessed: October 28, 2017]

[11] Holst L, Wright D, Haavik S, Nordeng H. The use and user of herbal medicines during pregnancy. Journal of Alternative and Complementary Medicine. 2009;**15**:787-792

[12] Herbal and Traditional Medicines in Pregnancy. The Royal Women's Hospital Fact Sheet. Available from: www.thewomens.org.au. [Accessed: October 28, 2017]

[13] Bishop JL, Northstone K, Green JR, Thompson EA. The use of complementary and alternative medicine in pregnancy: Data from the avon longitudinal study of parents and children (ALSPAC). Complementary Therapies in Medicine. 2011;**19**:303-310

[14] Forster D, Denning A, Wills G, Bolger M, McCarthy E. Herbal medicine use during pregnancy in a group of Australian women. BMC Pregnancy and Childbirth. 2006;**6**:21

[15] Fakeye T, Adisa R, Mus I. Attitude and use of herbal medicines among pregnant women in Nigeria. BMC Complementary and Alternative Medicine. 2009;**9**:53. DOI: 10.1186/1472-6882-9-53

[16] Duru CB, Nnebue CC, Uwakwe KA, Diwe KC, Agunwa CC, Achigbu KI, et al. Prevalence and pattern of herbal medicine use in pregnancy among women attending clinics in a tertiary hospital in Imo State, South East Nigeria. International Journal of Current Research in Biosciences and Plant Biology. 2016;**3**(2):5-14. DOI: 10.20546/ijcrbp.2016.302.002

[17] Duru CB, Uwakwe AK, Chinomnso CN, Mbachi II, Diwe CK, Chuka C, et al. Socio-demographic determinants of herbal medicine use in pregnancy among Nigerian women attending clinics in a tertiary Hospital in Imo State, south-east, Nigeria. American Journal of Medicine Studies. 2016;**4**(1):1-10

[18] Tamuno A, Ohonsi O, Fadare J. Use of Herbal Medicine Among Pregnant Women Attending A Tertiary Hospital In Northern Nigeria. The Internet Journal of Gynecology and Obstetrics. 2010;**15**(2)

[19] Nyeko R, Tumwesigye NM, Halage AA. Prevalence and factors associated with use of herbal medicines during pregnancy among women attending postnatal clinics in Gulu district, Northern Uganda. BMC Pregnancy and Childbirth. 2016;**16**:296. DOI: 10.1186/s12884-016-1095-5

[20] Jellin JM, Batz F, Hitchens K. Natural Medicines Comprehensive Database. Vol. 1530. Stockton CA: Therapeutic Research Faculty; 2002

[21] Low Dog T. Women's Health in Complementary and Integrative Medicine: A Clinical Guide. St Louis, MO: Elsevier; 2004

[22] Ozgoli G, Goli M, Simbar M. Effect of ginger capsule on pregnancy, effects of ginger capsules on pregnancy, nausea, and vomiting. Journal of Alternative and Complementary Medicine. 2009;**15**(3):243-246

[23] Willetts KE, Ekangaki A, Eden JA. Effect of a ginger extract on pregnancy-induced nausea: A randomised controlled trial. The Australian & New Zealand Journal of Obstetrics & Gynaecology. 2003;**43**:139-144

[24] Loke Y, editor. Pregnancy and Breastfeeding Medicines Guide. 1st ed. Melbourne: The Royal Women's Hospital, Pharmacy Department; 2010

[25] Braun L, Cohen M. Herbs and Natural Supplements. 3rd ed. Churchill Livingstone, Australia: Elsevier; 2010

[26] Australian Pharmaceutical Formulary and Handbook. 22nd ed. Canberra: Pharmaceutical Society of Australia; 2012

[27] Wilkinson JM. What do we know about herbal morning sickness treatments? A literature survey. Midwifery. 2000;**16**:224-228

[28] Bayan L, Koulivand PH, Gorji A. Garlic: A review of potential therapeutic effects. Avicenna Journal of Phytomedicine. 2014;**4**:1-14

[29] Groppo F, Ramacciato J, Motta R, Ferraresi P, Sartoratto A. Antimicrobial and antifungal activity of garlic. International Journal of Dental Hygiene. 2007;**5**(2):109-115. DOI: 10.1111/j.16015037.2007.00230

[30] Charlson M, McFerren M. Garlic: what we know and what we don't know. Archives of Internal Medicine. 2007;**167**(4):325-326. DOI: 10.1001/archinte.167.4.325

[31] Ziaei S, Hantoshzadeh S, Rezasoltani P, Lamyian M. The effect of garlic tablet on plasma lipids and platelet aggregation in nulliparous pregnant at high risk of pre-eclampsia. European Journal of Obstetrics and Gynecology and Reproductive Biology. 2001;**99**:201-206

[32] Parle M, Bansal N. Herbal medicine: are they safe? Natural Product Radiance. 2005;**5**(1): 6-14

[33] Jepson RG, Mihaljevic L, Craig J. Cranberries for preventing urinary tract infections. Cochrane Database of Systematic Reviews. 2004;**2**:CD001321

[34] Shmuely H, Burger O, Neeman I, Yahav J, Samra Z, Niv Y, et al. Susceptibility of helicobacter pylori isolates to the anti-adhesion activity of a high-molecular-weight constituent of cranberry. Diagnostic Microbiology and Infectious Disease. 2004;**50**(4):231-235

[35] Burger O, Ofek I, Tabak M, Weiss EI, Sharon N, Neeman I. A high molecular mass constituent of cranberry juice inhibits helicobacter pylori adhesion to human gastric mucus. FEMS Immunology and Medical Microbiology. 2000;**29**(4):295-301

[36] Weiss EL, Lev-Dor R, Sharon N, Ofek I. Inhibitory effect of a high molecular-weight constituent of cranberry on adhesion of oral bacteria. Critical Reviews in Food Science and Nutrition. 2002;**42**(3):285-292

[37] Koo H, Nino de Guzman P, Schobel BD, Vacca Smith AV, Bowen WH. Influence of cranberry juice on e85 glucan-mediated processes involved in *Streptococcus mutans* biofilm development. Caries Research. 2006;**40**(1):20-27

[38] Labrecque J, Bodet C, Chandad F Grenier D. Effects of a high-molecular- weight cranberry fraction on growth, iofilm formation and adherence of Porphyromonas gingivalis. Journal of Antimicrobial Chemotherapy. 2006;**58**(2):439-443

[39] Weiss EI, Houri-Haddad Y, Greenbaum E, Hochman N, Ofek I, Zakay-Rones Z. Cranberry juice constituents affect influenza virus adhesion and infectivity. Antiviral Research. 2005;**66**(1):9-12

[40] Nordeng H, Havnen GC. Use of herbal medicine in pregnancy: A survey among 400 Norwegian women. Pharmacoepidemiology and Drug Safety. 2004;**13**:371-338

[41] Valerian Longwood Herbal Task Force. Available from: http://www.mcp.edu/herbal/default.htm [Accessed: November 12, 2017]

[42] The Royal women's hospital. Herbal and traditional medicines in pregnancy. www.thewomens.org.au [Accessed: October 29, 2017]

[43] Mohamoudin A, Rajei Z, Haghir H, Banihashemia S, Hami J. Effect of valerian consumption during pregnancy on cortical volume of and the level of zinc and copper in brain tissue of mouse foetus. Journal of Chiness Integrated Medicines. 2012;**10**:1

[44] Amazing Benefits of Bitter Kola. Available form: https://drhealthbenefits.com/pregnancy/-pregnant-nutrition/health-benefits-of-bitter-kola-in-pregnancy

[45] Thomas JE, Bandara M, Lee EL, Driedger D, Acharya S. Biochemical monitoring in fenugreek to develop functional food and medicinal variants. New Biotechnology. 2011;**28**:110-117

[46] Shinde P, Patil P, Bairagi V. Herbs in pregnancy and lactation: A review. Appraisal International Journal of Pharmaceutical Sciences Research. 2012;**3**:3001-3006

[47] Herbs Remedies to Avoid in Pregnancy. Available from: https://www.babycentre.co.uk/a536346/herbal-remedies-in-pregnancy [Accessed: November 10, 2017]

[48] Red Rasberry Leaf. Available from: https://en.m.wikipedia.org [Accessed: October 29, 2017]

[49] Holst L, Haavik S, Nordeng H. Raspberry leaf-should it be recommended to pregnant women? Complementary Therapies in Clinical Practice. 2009;**15**:204-208

[50] Simpson M, Parsons M, Greenwood J, Wade K. Raspberry leaf in pregnancy: Its safety and efficacy in labor. Journal of Midwifery and Women's Health. 2001;**46**(2):51-59

[51] Parsons M, Simpson M, Ponton T. Raspberry leaf and its effect on labour: Safety and efficacy. Australian College of Midwives Incorporated Journal. 1999;**12**(3):20-25

[52] Red Rasberry Leaf. Available from: www.highlandmidwife.com [Accessed: November 1, 2017]

[53] Barnes J, Anderson LA, Phillipson JD, editors. Herbal Medicines. Available form: http://www.medicinescomplete.com [Accessed: November 02, 2017]

[54] Briggs GG, Freeman RK. Drugs in Pregnancy and Lactation. 10th ed. Philadelphia: Wolters Kluwer Health; 2015

[55] Dilthey MR. Is chamomile tea safe during early pregnancy? Available from: LIVESTRON.COM.html [Accessed: November 20, 2017]

[56] Vicki Hobbs Phoenix Therapies Pregnancy Centre. Aromatherapy in Pregnancy. phoenixtherapies.au/wp-content [Accessed: October 27, 2017]

[57] Kassem N. Use of Early Sage Oil in Pregnancy. Available from: https.www.livesrtong.com/article/37143 [Accessed October 26, 2017]

[58] How Safe is Anise in Pregnancy. Available from: www.wise qeek.orq/what is star anise aniso.htm [Accessed: November 28, 2017]

[59] The Natural Medicine Comprehensive Database. Available from: www.naturaldatabase [Accessed: November 10, 2017]

[60] Keating A, Chez RA. Effect of green tea on pregnant women health. Alternative Therapies in Health and Medicine. 2002;**8**:89-91

[61] Health Beginning. Herbs and Herbal Teas: Safety during Pregnancy or While Breast Feeding. Available from: https://www.york.ca/wps/wcm/connect/yorkpublic/759e421145ae-4aa680eb-a5801db09903/herbs+and+herbal+teas+safety+during+pregnancy+or+while+breastfeeding.pdf?MOD=AJPERES [Accessed: November10, 2017]

[62] Klebanoff MA, Levine RJ, DerSimonian R, Clemens JD, Wilkins DG. Maternal serum paraxanthine, a caffeine metabolite, and the risk of spontaneous abortion. The New England Journal of Medicine. 1999;**341**:1639-1644

[63] Rasch V. Cigarette, alcohol, and caffeine consumption: Risk factors for spontaneous abortion. Acta Obstetricia et Gynecologica Scandinavica. 2003;**82**:182-188

[64] Balat O, Balat A, Ugur M, Pence S. The effect of smoking and caffeine on the fetus and placenta in pregnancy. Clinical and Experimental Obstetrics & Gynecology. 2003;**30**:57-59

[65] Wisborg K, Kesmodel U, Bech B, Hedegaard M, Henriksen TB. Maternal consumption of coffee during pregnancy and stillbirth and infant death in first year of life: Prospective study. British Medical Journal. 2003;**326**:420

[66] Bracken MB, Triche EW, Belanger K, Hellenbrand K, Leaderer BP. Association of maternal caffeine consumption with decrements in fetal growth. American Journal of Epidemiology. 2003;**157**:456-466

[67] Natural Medicine Comprehensive Database. Available from: http://naturaldatabase.therapeuticresearch.com/home.aspx?cs=&s=ND&AspxAutoDetectCookieSupport [Accessed: November 6, 2017]

[68] Rahman AA, Sulaiman SA, Ahmad Z, Daud WNW, Hamid AM. Prevalence and pattern of use of herbal medicine during pregnancy in Tumpat district, kelanta. Malaysian Journal of Medical Sciences. 2008;**15**:40-48

[69] Fife B. Coconut Cure: Preventing and Treating Common Health Problems with Coconut. USA: Piccadilly Books, Ltd; 2005

[70] Fife B. Procedure formulas and recipes. In: Coconut Cure: Preventing and Treating Common Health Problems with Cocont. USA: Piccadilly Books, Ltd; 2005. pp. 184-185

[71] Rahman AA, Ahmad Z, Naing L, Sulaiman SA, Hamid AM, Daud WN. The use of herbal medicines during pregnancy and perinatal mortality in Tumpat district, Kelantan, Malaysia. The Southeast Asian Journal of Tropical Medicine and Public Health. 2007;**38**:1150-1157

[72] Liau KM, Lee YY, Chen CK, Rasool AHG. An open label pilot study to assess the efficacy and safety of virgin coconut oil in reducing visceral adiposity. ISRN Pharmacology. 2011. DOI: 10.5402/2011/949686

[73] Rahman AA, Sulaiman SA, Ahmad Z, Nudri W, Daud W, Hamid AM. Prevalence and pattern of use of herbal medicines using pregnancy in tumpat district, kelantan. Malaysian Journal of Medical Sciences. 2008;**15**(3):40-48

[74] Coconut Oil Necessary for Building Hormones and a Healthy Baby. Available from: http://natural-fertility-info.com/coconut-oil-necessary-for-buildinghormones-and-a-healthy-baby.htm [Accessed: November 10, 2017]

[75] Gunasekaran A, Shaker MR, Mohd-Zin SW, Abdullah A, Ahmad-Annuarand A, Abdul-Aziz NM. Maternal intake of dietary virgin coconut oil modifies essential fatty acids and causes low body weight and spiky fur in mice. BMC Complementary and Alternative Medicine. 2017;**17**:79. DOI: 10.1186/s12906-017-1600-z

[76] Skopinska-Ruewska E, Wojtasik E. Immunotropowe diazaena jeuwek (echinacea purpurea, Echinacea pallida, Echinacea angustifolia). In: Skopinska-Ruewska E, editor. Wpae substancji naturalnych na ukaed odpornoOciowy. Warszawa: fundacja Promocy Zdrowiu-Medycna naturalna; 2002. pp. 32-42

[77] Holst L, Wright D, Haavik S, Nordeng H. Safety and efficacy of herbal remedies in obstetrics-review and clinical implications. Midwifery. 2011;**27**:80-86

[78] Peppermint. Available from: http://www.mcp.edu/herbal/default.htm and the center for holistic pediatrics education and research. Available form: http://www.childrenshospital.org/holistic. [Accessed: October 23, 2017]

[79] Shahin M, Shadi K, Pardise M, Anahita G, Reza A, Reza M. The effect of entericcoated, delayed-release peppermint oil on irritable bowel syndrome. Digestive Diseases and Sciences. 2010;**55**(5):1385-1390

[80] Westfall RE. Use of anti-emetic herbs in pregnancy: women's choices, and the question of safety and efficacy. Complementary Therapies in Nursing & Midwifery. 2004;**10**:30-36

7

Herbal Medicine

Nontokozo Z. Msomi and Mthokozisi B.C. Simelane

Abstract

Herbal medicine has gained cumulative popularity in today's medical practice. These treatments are the synthesis of therapeutic experiences of generations of traditional physicians for over hundreds of years. However, most of these applications are unorthodox, with over 80% of the world's population depending on some form of traditional medicine. The increase in the use of herbal products is due to their cultural acceptability, availability, affordability, efficacy and safety claims. This upsurge has led to the improvements in the quality and analysis of herbal products to be made with clinical research advancements in their safety and efficacy. The World Health Organization has recognized the importance of herbal medicine to the health of many people. Therefore, developing guidelines to evaluate herbal medicine by using modern control procedures and applying suitable standards. The current review aims to describe the present state and the projected future of herbal medicine.

Keywords: herbal medicine, safety and toxicity, regulations

1. Introduction

The practice of herbal medicine is the oldest form of healthcare which has been used for decades in developing and developed countries. Primitive people have depended on nature for food, shelter, clothing and medicine to cure ailments. These humans distinguished useful herbs with beneficial effects from those that were inactive or toxic [1]. According to literature approximately 50,000 plant species are stated to have medicinal properties [2]. Thus, the basis of modern medicinal drugs such as aspirin, morphine, digitoxin and quinine were synthesized through scientific validation of herbal medicine [3, 4]. Plant based drugs awareness advanced gradually and has been passed on, therefore setting a foundation for many traditional medicine systems around the globe [1].

Today herbal medicine is still the primary healthcare system for about 80% of the world's population, especially in the developing countries [1, 5, 6]. There has been also a sudden increase in the utilization of herbs as prescription drugs in developed countries such as France and Germany [3, 7]. However, there is a concern that not all herbal medicines are safe as reported [8]. Over the years the use of traditional medicine has provided us with valuable formulas on the selection, preparation and application of herbal remedies. The same vigorous method clinically and scientifically must be implemented to verify the effectiveness and safety of curative products, to be viable alternative to western medicine [4].

2. Herbal medicine

The World Health Organization (WHO) defines herbal medicine as a practice which includes herbs, herbal materials, herbal preparations and finished herbal products, that contain as active ingredients parts of plants, or other plant materials, or combinations [9]. These herbs are derived from plant parts such as leaves, stems, flowers, roots, and seeds [10].

Herbal drugs contain active ingredients, plant parts or plant materials in the processed or crude state with certain excipients, i.e., dilutions, solvents or preservatives [10, 11]. These active ingredients protect plants from damage and diseases and contribute to the plants aroma, flavor and color. Scientifically, they are known as phytochemicals which include several classes such as saponins, flavonoids, glycosides, tannins, alkaloids and terpenoids [12]. Phytochemicals have been scientifically validated over the years to provide health benefits for humans [13]. For example herbal remedies used as sedative and stomachic mixtures contain mainly aromatic plant species which have therapeutic essential oils, possessing antibacterial, stomach-soothing and antispasmodic properties. Plant species which have a high tannin content are used in mixtures for diarrhea and stomach ulcers; generally showing antimicrobials, astringents and anti-inflammatory activities [14, 15]. Bioactive and disease preventing phytochemicals present in medicinal plants are shown in **Table 1**.

Class	Characteristic	Use	Pharmacological activity	Reference
Alkaloids	Organic nitrogenous bases, bitter taste, colorless/yellow, crystalline solids, liquids	Biosynthesis of pharmaceuticals	Anticancer, antimicrobial, amoebicidal, anti-inflammatory,	[16, 17]
Saponins	Soap-like forming property, bitter taste,	Detergent, wetting and emulsifying agent	Antifeedant, antifungal, antiobesity, antioxidant	[18]
Tannins	Water-soluble, leather hides,	Used for cationic dyes, production of ink,	Antimutagens, anticarcinogens, antimicrobial,	[12, 19]
Flavonoids	Free radical scavenger	Prevents microbial infection,	Anti-inflammatory, antimicrobial, antibacterial, antioxidant	[20]

Table 1. Properties of some major constituents of medicinal plants.

3. Historical perspective of herbal medicine

The use of plants as medicines dates 60,000 years ago according to ancient Babylon reports. In Egypt and China written material on herbal medicine dates approximately 5000 years back, in Asia Minor and Greece it dates 2500 years ago [21]. There are various herbal medicinal systems, the practices and philosophy of each are influenced by the region within which it first evolved [22]. In China, they have their own system known as the Traditional Chinese medicine which has been used throughout history [23]. The oldest known herbal book in the world *The Devine Farmer's Classic of Herbalism* was compiled in China about 2000 years ago, numerous herbal pharmacopeias and various monographs on specific herbs exist through the composed information on herbs [3]. Ayurveda, a healthcare system that has been used in India for over 5000 years, that was founded by ancient Hindu healers and saints. Its *materia medica* provides a comprehensive description of over 1500 herbs and 10,000 formulations. The Indian government has recognized Ayurveda to be a complete healthcare system in comparison to western medicine [24]. Kampo medicine, the Japanese herbal medicine dates back over 1500 years with approximately 148 formulations [25].

4. Common herbal medicines

4.1. *Echinacea purpurea*

Echinacea has an extensive history on the use as medicines, mainly for infections such as septic wounds and syphilis, also as an anti-toxin for snakebites [26]. The species *Echinacea purpurea* from this genus is a well-known medicinal plant used in treating snake bites, toothache, skin disorders, bowel pain, chronic arthritis, seizure and cancer, traditionally [27]. *E. purpurea* possesses secondary metabolites including caffeic acid derivatives, alkamides, glycoproteins and polysaccharides alleged to be biologically and pharmacologically active [26, 27]. Allergic reactions can occur and are usually mild, but individuals with a history of asthma, atopy, or allergic rhinitis may experience severe allergic reactions that include dyspnea and anaphylaxis [26, 28]. Other adverse effects include abdominal pain, urticarial, nausea, erythematous, rash and pruritus [26].

4.2. Garlic

Traditionally, garlic (*Allium sativum*) has been used to treat colds, chronic bronchitis, coughs, respiratory catarrh, bronchitic asthma and influenza [26]. Additionally it is used mainly to manage hypertension and hypercholesterolemia. It contains alliin, which upon chopping or crushing is activated by alliinase in the absence of acid or heat [8, 28]. Allicin produces both hydrophilic (cysteine) and lipophilic (sulfides, ajoene) sulfur compounds which are accountable for pharmacologic effects. Garlic is administered via oil-filled capsules, condensed dried powder, and enteric-coated tablets and capsules; it is also aged in aqueous alcohol [28]. Adverse effects of garlic extract include burning sensation in the gastrointestinal tract, diaphoresis, nausea, and light headedness. The extract may also cause contact dermatitis and excessive ingestion may cause morbid spontaneous spinal epidural hematoma [8, 28].

4.3. Ginkgo

Ginkgo (*Ginkgo biloba*) and its leaf extracts contain active compounds which have been found to improve circulation and cognition. The extracts are sold in both solid and liquid forms and appear to be relatively safe [28]. Medicinal use of ginkgo dates back 2800 BC, the seeds are used as an expectorant, antitussive and anti-asthmatic, and the leaves aid in asthma and cardiovascular disorders [26]. The most common side effects are dizziness, headache, restlessness, vomiting, nausea, diarrhea and dermal sensitivity. Cross-allergenicity with poison ivy has been reported. Ginkgo as an inhibitor of platelet-activating factor may alter bleeding times, therefore it may cause an upsurge of the anticoagulant effect of aspirin and warfarin [28].

4.4. Ginseng

Ginseng (*Eleutherococcus senticosus*) is the fourth most extensively used Chinese medicinal herb, treating a variety of conditions. It is used as a general tonic and is claimed to increase the body's resistance against stress and builds up general vitality besides treating diabetes, depression and hypertension [29]. Products are made from dehydrated roots, such as extracts, elixirs and tea, also tablets and capsules. Numerous active constituents, ginsenosides, respectively have specific pharmacologic effects that sometimes compete with each other, thus the whole root is used in preparations [28]. Excessive doses of ginseng have been reported to cause insomnia, agitation and elevation of blood pressure, mastalgia and vaginal bleeding have been detected at acclaimed doses [8].

4.5. Kava

Kava (*Piper methysticum*) is believed to be beneficial for health by soothing nervous illnesses, inducing sleep and relaxation, reducing weight and counteracting fatigue. It is often used to treat asthma, urinary infections, fever, headaches, syphilis, rheumatism and gonorrhea, it is also used as a stomachic and diuretic [26]. Kava is commonly known as an anxiolytic agent. Reported side effects include dizziness, gastrointestinal discomfort, headaches and localized numbness after oral ingestion. Long term use at high doses may cause scaly, dry skin and discoloration of nails and the skin, eye redness and photosensitivity. Diplopia and photophobia may also occur after excessive consumption. Interaction of central nervous system depressants and kava may lead to a comatose state [8, 28].

4.6. St John's wort

St John's wort (*Hypericum perforation*) is specified to possess astringent and sedative properties. It has been used for neuralgia, excitability, fibrositis, menopausal neurosis, sciatica, wounds, depression and anxiety. Modern interest is focused on its antidepressant use [26]. St John's wort possesses active compounds such as hyperforin, hypericin and melatonin. It is reported to have side effects which include fatigue, constipation, nausea, vomiting, dry mouth, headaches, dizziness and photosensitivity [8].

4.7. Ma huang

Ma huang (*Ephedra sinica*) is a medicinal plant traditionally used to treat hay fever, bronchial asthma, colds, coughs, enuresis, myasthenia gravis, narcolepsy, rheumatism and chronic postural hypotension. It contains a number of alkaloids including ephedrine and pseudoephedrine [26]. Ma huang is not considered as a safe herb, with adverse effects including insomnia, dizziness, headaches, nervousness, stroke, seizures, hypertension, psychosis, irritability, myocardial infarction, premature ventricular contraction and death [28].

4.8. Valerian

Valerian (*Valeriana officinalis*) is a medicinal plant commonly used as a mild sedative and anxiolytic. Numerous constituents are found in the root of this plant, valerenic acid (C15 sesquiterpenoid) and valerena-4,7(11)-diene have been suggested to possess the active ingredients accountable for the sedative effect [30]. Valerian has been reported to cause excitability, headache, gastrointestinal complaints and ataxia. An oral overdose may result in abdominal cramps, onset of fatigue, light headedness, chest tightness, and tremors of feet and hands [28].

5. Why people use herbal medicine?

5.1. Accessibility and affordability

The documentation of medicinal plants of numerous cultures is extensive, these plants have been used in treating various diseases even without the knowledge of their constituents and accurate functions [31]. The high practice of herbal medicine is due to cultural acceptability, as plant remedies have been around for centuries [32]. In countries such as Zambia, Tanzania and Uganda the ratio of herbal medicine practitioners to the population was found to be 1:200–1:400. However, the ratio of western medicine practitioners is 1:20,000 or less [33]. A survey conducted in 1991 revealed that traditional practitioners in sub-Saharan Africa out number western practitioners by 100 to 1 [34]. Herbal medicine has remained affordable in comparison to high cost western medicine [35]. In over populated countries such as India, the rural population has almost no access to modern medicine, therefore, they are compelled to rely on herbal medicine for their basic healthcare needs [36].

5.2. An alternative approach to healthcare

Plants are perceived to be healthier than conventional biosynthetic drugs. Reports on conventional drugs adverse effects has been found to be much higher compared to herbal toxicity reports [4]. Other reasons for the use of herbal medicine include: (i) several claims on the efficacy and safety of plant medicines [11], (ii) improvements in the quality of herbal medicines with the development of scientific evaluation [21], (iii) to relieve symptoms related to chronic or terminal illnesses [37], such as HIV/AIDS, malaria, diabetes and sickle-cell anemia [38]. A survey conducted in the USA showed that 78% of patients living with HIV/AIDS use some form of herbal medicine. In such cases, western medicine is perceived to have failed the public [4].

6. Challenges facing the use of herbal medicine

6.1. Safety and toxicological concerns of herbal medicine

The products of herbal medicine have a long history of being safe [39], however the misuse of these medicines may have side effects due to toxic constituents [29]. In some countries, toxicological assessment of herbal medicine and associated products are not employed before placing them in the market [8]. Herbal medicine of a single plant may contain hundreds of constituents and mixed products may contain numerous times that number. The time required to isolate every single active ingredient from every herb would be tremendous [22]. Moreover, these countries lack operative machinery to legalize manufacturing quality standards and practices. Thus making hazardous herbal products continually available to consumers [8]. A study related on the use of traditional eye medicine reported that it caused 26% of childhood blindness in Malawi and Nigeria, and 25% of corneal ulcer in Tanzania [4]. Pyrrolizidine alkaloids have been reported to be fatal, these are molecules within certain plants causing hepatotoxicity through a veno-occlusion illness [10]. Nausea and probably vomiting can occur with some herbs such as ephedra and echinacea. Herbs consumed as teas have been reported to cause diarrhea and hematologic, cardiac and gastrointestinal effects [40]. Herbal products from Asia have been reported to be problematic since it contains numerous contaminants. A study on the assessment of 260 Asian patent medications reported that 25% of these products contained high levels of heavy metals and 7% contained undeclared drugs, decisively and unlawfully added to produce desired effects [41].

6.2. Challenges of quality control

Quality control of herbal drugs and their formulations is of vital importance in order to justifying their acceptability in modern system of medicine. A major concern facing the herbal drug market is the unavailability of the source and quality of herbal materials and their formulations [42]. Other factors such as the temperature, use of fresh plants, light exposure, nutrients, water availability, period and time of harvest, method of harvesting, drying, packing, storage and transportation of raw herbal material, etc., can critically affect the beneficial value of medicinal plants and quality. Some plant elements are heat labile and the plants containing them need to be dried at low temperatures [11].

6.3. Lack of knowledge about herbal medicine within government regulations

Herbal remedies can be sold as supplements, for supporting, maintaining, stimulating and promoting health in many countries. These supplements require a label that defines the ingredients are intended to affect the functions within humans in line with Act 101 of 1965 and amendments (2002) [14]. The evidence on the efficacy, safety and quality of such herbal products is unknown, therefore, raising a concern on the safety of these herbal medicines [8].

6.4. Need for scientific and clinical evaluation of herbal medicine

The concern surrounding safety of herbal medicinal products is increasing [8]. In order to allay these concerns and achieve public reliance on herbal medicine, manufacturers, researchers and regulatory authorities must follow inclusive clinical trials and vigorous scientific methodologies to ensure the quality and safety of herbal products [41]. The safety evaluation of any herbal drug considers two important factors; the nature and significance of the adversarial effect. Toxicity screening can disclose some of the risks related to the use of herbal medicine [43]. In 1991, WHO issued guidelines for the assessment of herbal medicine which include: (i) Quality assessment: crude plant material; plant preparation; finished product. (ii) Stability: shelf life. (iii) Safety assessment: documentation of safety based on experience or toxicology studies. (iv) Assessment of efficacy: documented evidence of traditional use or activity determination (animals, human) [6].The US Food and Drug Administration (FDA), the International Conference on Harmonization (ICH) and the United States Pharmacopeia (USPC, 1994–2001) follow these guidelines to validate herbal products [1].

7. National policies of herbal medicine

A national policy on herbal medicine may include the following: a defining role of herbal medicine in the health care system, provision for the necessary regulations and laws, contemplation of intellectual property concerns [22]. National policies vary from country to country regarding herbal medicine. Herbal medicines are classified as either prescription or non-prescription medicines. The Working Party on Natural and Nutritional Supplements was established by the Australian Parliament to evaluate the safety, efficacy, quality and labeling of herbal products (Therapeutic Good Act, 1990). The act states "that traditional claims for herbal remedies be allowed, providing general advertising requirements are complied with and providing such claims are justified by literature references" [11]. Herbal medicine in Canada must meet the terms of the National Health Products Regulations. In accordance to these regulations, a product license is required for all herbal products to be sold in Canada. The recommended use, potency, comprehensive information on the medicinal constituents, source and nonmedicinal constituents need to be provided in order for a license to be granted. The companies that manufacture, pack, label and import herbal medicine also need a site license [3].

The Dietary Supplement Health and Education Act (DSHEA) of 1994, states that any herb, natural and botanical concentrate, constituent and metabolite of extract, is categorized as a dietary supplement. These supplementations do not need any sanction from the FDA. Herbal medicine which is categorized as dietary supplements under DSHEA, are alleged to be safe and the FDA does not have the authority to require them to be approved for efficacy and safety before they enter the market. However, manufacturers of these herbal products are required to provide purity and identification standards, and confirm that claims made concerning their products are precise [39, 44].

In Chile the Unidad de Medicina Tradicional was established in 1992, with the aim of incorporating herbal medicine with established efficacy into health programs (Law No. 19.253,

October 1993). Directive No. 435/81 defines herbal drugs with therapeutic proposed claims and/or dosage recommendations as being medications, restricted from being sold in drugstores and pharmacies. Registration for marketing authorization is required for herbal products. These products are lawfully distinguished as follows: (1) drugs intended to alleviate, cure or prevent disease; (2) food products with therapeutic properties and for medicinal use, and (3) food products with nutritious purposes [11].

In Europe, the European Directive 2004/24/EC released in 2004 by the European Parliament and by the Council of Europe provides the guidelines for the use of herbal medicines. The guidelines state that for herbal medicine to be released in the market, it needs authorization from the national regulatory authorities of each country in Europe and the herbal products must have a standard level of efficacy and safety. The registration of herbal products from outside the European Union (EU) require substantial evidence of their medicinal use, at most a period of 15 years within EU and 15 years elsewhere [3]. In Germany, more than 300 monographs on medicinal plants have been regulatory evaluated, and in France more than 200 herbs have been recorded as acceptable ingredients of herbal medicine [4].

The widespread use of herbal medicine in Brazil is favored by two present public policies i.e. the National Policy on Integrative and Complementary Practices in the Public Health System (PNPIC) and the National Policy on Medicinal Plants and Herbal Medicines (PNPMF), through the Law 971/2006 and the Declaration 5813/2006, respectively. Currently, 382 herbal medicines are registered in Brazil, 357 of these are single medicines and the other 25 are composed of more than one medicinal plant [45].

8. The market for herbal medicine in the developed world

Herbal medicine has gained increasing popularity in the last two decades in industrialized countries. The congress of the United States of America (USA) established the Office of Alternative Medicine in the year 1989 within the National Institute of Health (NIH). This was formed to interest scientists in the field of medicinal plants [3]. According to the 2007 NIH survey, 4 out of 10 adults (38.8%) and 1 out of 9 children (11.8%) used some form of herbal medicine [37]. In USA, presently about 25% of prescription drugs contain at least one plant derived ingredient [21], the herbal market in this country has doubled from $4 billion since 1996 [6]. In 1989, the European Scientific Cooperative on Phytotherapy was formed with an aim to advance herbal medicine [3]. The herbal medicine market in European countries has been growing steadily from $6 billion in 1991 to over $20 billion currently, particularly in Germany, France and Italy [4, 6]. In Germany, herbal medicine is identified as one of the elements of naturopathy [46], approximately 600–700 plant derived medicines are accessible and prescribed by approximately 70% of German physicians [47]. In 2011, 20% of herbal drugs were sold as prescriptions and 80% over the counter in Germany [46]. In the year 2005, The National Centre for Complementary and Alternative Medicine at the National Institutes of Health in the USA spent about US$ 33 million on herbal medicine, the National Canadian Institutes disbursed approximately US$ 89 million for research in traditional therapies in 2004. These scientific evaluations have led to an upsurge in the investment of herbal medicine [3].

9. Future prospects of herbal medicine

In the past decade, about 121 pharmaceutical products have been formulated based on herbal medicine knowledge [42]. According to literature at least 25% of modern medicines are derived from plants, such as aspirin, picrotoxin and numerous others are synthetic analogues built on prototype compounds isolated from plants [48]. Because of the increase in the acceptance of plant derived drugs, the use of plants in medicine as a source of therapeutic agents will expand rapidly in the future [42]. This has extremely increased international trade of herbal medicine, attracting a number of pharmaceutical companies, including the multinationals [11]. The interest of WHO by documenting the use of medicinal plants used by ethnic groups, has increased scientific validation of the use of these plants. This will make people better informed concerning the effectiveness and safety of the treatment [21]. The regulation of herbs has assisted in improving herbal products, however additional changes need to be applied to advance and indorse high quality research [10].

10. Conclusion

The use of herbal medicine is not restricted to developing countries. Over the years, there has been an escalating interest in the use of herbal medicine worldwide. This has greatly expanded the demand for plant products, since herbal medicine has an advantage of being inexpensive with minimal side effects compared to synthetic medicines. The growth of the herbal drug market has attracted pharmaceutical companies which in turn have driven scientific validation and clinical studies on herbal medicines. Thus far, few programs have been established to study the safety and efficacy of herbal medicines as originally proposed by the WHO Guidelines for the assessment of herbal medicines. These guidelines have been helpful in establishing the role of herbal medicine in the health care industry. However, the data to provide a precise assessment on the safety, quality and efficacy of herbal medicine is inadequate generating concerns regarding the use of herbal products.

Author details

Nontokozo Z. Msomi and Mthokozisi B.C. Simelane*

*Address all correspondence to: simelanem2@ukzn.ac.za

Department of Biochemistry, School of Life Science, University of KwaZulu-Natal, Pietermaritzburg, South Africa

References

[1] Kunle OF, Egharevba HO, Ahmadu PO. Standardization of herbal medicines –A review. Journal of Biodiversity and Conservation. 2012;**4**(3):101-112. DOI: 10.5897/IJBC11.163

[2] Barboza GE, Cantero JJ, Núñez C, Pacciaroni A, Espinar LA. Medicinal plants: A general review and a phytochemical and ethnopharmacological screening of the native Argentine Flora. Kurtziana. 2009;**34**:7-365. ISSN:1852-5962

[3] Wachtel-Galor S, Benzie IFF. Herbal medicine. In: Benzie I, Wachtel-Galor S, editors. Herbal Medicine: Biomolecular and Clinical Aspects. 2nd ed. Boca Raton: CRC Press/ Taylor & Francis; 2011. ISBN: 13: 978-1-4398-0713-2

[4] Pal SK, Shukla Y. Herbal medicine: Current status and the future. Asian Pacific Journal of Cancer Prevention. 2003;**4**:281-288

[5] Okigbo RN, Anuagasi CL, Amadi JE. Advances in selected medicinal and aromatic plants indigenous to Africa. Journal of Medicinal Plants Research. 2009;**3**(2):86-95. ISSN: 1996-0875©2009

[6] Kamboj VP. Herbal medicine. Current Reviews. 2000;**78**(1):35-39

[7] Edzard E. The efficacy of herbal medicine – An overview. Fundamental & Clinical Pharmacology. 2005;**19**:405-409. DOI: 10.1111/j.1472-8206.2005.00335.x

[8] Ekor M. The growing use of herbal medicines: Issues relating to adverse reactions and challenges in monitoring safety. Frontiers in Pharmacology. 2014;**4**:1-10. DOI: 10.3389/ fphar.2013.00177

[9] Organization WH. General guidelines for methodologies on research and evaluation of traditional medicine 2000. Geneva: World Health Organization

[10] Bent S. Herbal medicine in the United States: Review of efficacy, safety, and regulation. Journal of General Internal Medicine. 2008;**23**(6):854-859. DOI: 10.1007/s11606-008-0632-y

[11] Calixto JB. Efficacy, safety, quality control, marketing and regulatory guidelines for herbal medicines (phytotherapeutic agents). Brazilian Journal of Medical and Biological Research. 2000;**33**:179-189. ISSN: 0100-879X

[12] Saxena M, Saxena J, Nema R, Singh D, Gupta A. Phytochemistry of medicinal plants. Journal of Pharmacognosy and Phytochemistry. 2013;**1**(6):168-182. ISSN: 2278-4136

[13] Hasler CM, Blumberg JB. Symposium on phytochemicals: Biochemistry and physiology. Journal of Nutrition. 1999;**129**:756-757. ISSN: 756S–757S

[14] Ndhlala AR, Stafford GI, Finnie JF, Staden JV. Commercial herbal preparations in KwaZulu-Natal, South Africa: The urban face of traditional medicine. South African Journal of Botany. 2011;**77**:830-843. DOI: 10.1016/j.sajb.2011.09.002

[15] Cano JH, Volpato G. Herbal mixtures in the traditional medicine of Eastern Cuba. Journal of Ethnopharmacology. 2004;**90**(2-3):293-316. DOI: 10.1016/j.jep.2003.10.012

[16] Harborne JB. Phytochemical Methods a Guide to Modern Techniques of Plant Analysis. London: Chapman and Hall Ltd; 1973. ISBN: 13: 978-0-412-23050-9

[17] Kauri R, Arora S. Alkaloids-important therapeutic secondary metabolites of plant origin. Journal of Critical Reviews. 2015;**2**(3):1-8. ISSN: 2394-5125

[18] Guclu-Ustundag O, Mazza G. Saponins: Properties, applications and processing. Critical Reviews in Food Science and Nutrition. 2007;**47**:231-258. DOI: 10.1080/10408390600698197 ISSN: 1040-8398

[19] Chung K-T, Wong TY, Wei C-I, Huang Y-W, Lin Y. Tannins and human health: A review. Critical Reviews in Food Science and Nutrition. 1998;**38**(6):421-464. DOI: 10.1080/10408699891274273

[20] Kumar S, Pandey AK. Chemistry and biological activities of flavonoids: An overview. The ScientificWorld Journal. 2013;**2013**:1-16. DOI: 10.1155/2013/162750

[21] Qazi MA, Molvi K. Herbal medicine: A comprehensive review. Journal of Pharmaceutical Research. 2016;**8**(2):1-5

[22] WHO. National Policy on Traditional Medicine and Regulation of Herbal Medicines. Geneva: World Health Organization; 2005

[23] Wnag S, Li Y. Trdaitiional Chinese medicine. In: Devinsky O, Schachter S, Pacia S, editors. Complementary and Alternative Therapies for Epilepsy. New York: Demos Medical Publishing; 2005. pp. 177-182. ISBN: 1-888799-89-7

[24] Goyal M, Sasmal D, Nagori BP. Ayurveda the ancient science of healing: An insight. In: Vallisuta O, Olimat SM, editors. Drug Discovery Research in Pharmacognosy. Croatia: InTech; 2012. pp. 1-10. ISBN: 978-953-51-0213-7

[25] Watanabe K, Matsuura K, Gao P, Hottenbacher L, Tokunaga H, Nishimura K, et al. Traditional Japanese Kampo medicine: Clinical research between modernity and traditional medicine–The state of research and methodological suggestions for the future. Evidence-Based Complementary and Alternative Medicine. 2011;**2011**:1-19. DOI: 10.1093/ecam/neq067

[26] Barnes J, Anderson LA, Phillipson JD. Herbal Medicine. 3rd ed. Pharmaceutical Press; 2007. ISBN: 978 0 85369 623 0

[27] Manayi A, Vazirian M, Saeidnia S. *Echinacea purpurea*: Pharmacology, phytochemistry and analysis methods. Pharmacognosy Reviews. 2015;**9**(17):63-72. DOI: 10.4103/0973-7847.156353

[28] Boullata JI, Nace AM. Safety issues with herbal medicine. Pharmacotherapy. 2000;**20**(3):257-269. DOI: 10.1592/phco.20.4.257.34886

[29] George P. Concerns regarding the safety and toxicity of medicinal plants –An overview. Journal of Applied Pharmaceutical Science. 2011;**1**(6):40-44. ISSN: 2231-3354

[30] Pyle BW, Tran HT, Pickel B, Haslam TM, Gao Z, MacNevin G, et al. Enzymatic synthesis of valerena-4,7(11)-diene by a unique sesquiterpene synthase from the Valerian plant (*Valeriana officinalis*). The FEBS Journal. 2012;**279**:3136-3146. DOI: 10.1111/j.1742-4658.2012.08692.x

[31] Patel D, Kumar R, Laloo D, Hemalatha S. Natural medicines from plant source used for therapy of diabetes mellitus: An overview of its pharmacological aspects. Asian Pacific Journal of Tropical Disease. 2012:239-250. DOI: 10.1016/S2222-1808(12)60054-1

[32] Wassie SM, Aragie LL, Taye BW, Mekonnen LB. Knowledge, attitude, and utilization of traditional medicine among the communities of Merawi town, Northwest Ethiopia: A cross-sectional study. Evidence-Based Complementary and Alternative Medicine. 2015;**2015**:1-7. DOI: 10.1155/2015/138073

[33] Mhame P. the role of traditional knowledge (TK) in the National Economy: the importance and scope of TK, particularly traditional medicine in Tanzania. In: UNCTAD Expert Meeting on Systems and National Experiences for Protecting Traditional Knowledge, Innovations and Practices, Geneva; October 30–November 1, 2000;**2000**

[34] WHO. WHO Traditional Medicine Strategy 2002-2005. Geneva: 2002

[35] Maroyi A. Traditional use of medicinal plants in South-Central Zimbabwe: Review and perspectives. Journal of Ethnobiology and Ethnomedicine. 2013;**9**(31):1-18. DOI: 10.1186/1746-4269-9-31

[36] Pandey M, Rastogi S, Rawat A. Indian traditional ayurvedic system of medicine and nutritional supplementation. Evidence-Based Complementary and Alternative Medicine. 2013;**2013**:1-12. DOI: 10.1155/2013/376327

[37] Barnes PM, Bloom B. Complementary and alternative medicine use among adults and children: United States, 2007. National Health Statistics Reports, 2008 Contract No.: 12

[38] Borokini TI, Omotayo FO. Phytochemical and ethnobotanical study of some selected medicinal plants from Nigeria. Journal of Medicinal Plants Research. 2010;**6**(7):1106-1118. DOI: 10.5897/JMPR09.430

[39] Moreira DL, Teixeira SS, Monteiro MHD, De-Oliveira ACAX, Paumgartten FJR. Traditional use and safety of herbal medicines. Revista Brasileira de Farmacognosia. 2014;**24**:248-257. DOI: 10.1016/j.bjp.2014.03.006

[40] Cui L, Liuc M, Chang X, Sunb K. The inhibiting effect of the *Coptis chinensis* polysaccharide on the type II diabetic mice. Biomedicine & Pharmacotherapy. 2016;**81**:111-119. DOI: 10.1016/j.biopha.2016.03.038

[41] Rana KK, Rana S. Review on present status and future of herbal medicine. The beats of natural. Sciences. 2014;**1**(2):1-8

[42] Verma S, Singh SP. Current and future status of herbal medicines. Veterinary World. 2008;**1**(11):347-350

[43] Ifeoma O, Oluwakanyinsola S. Screening of herbal medicines for potential toxicities. In: Gowder S, editor. New Insights into Toxicity and Drug Testing. Croatia: InTech; 2013. pp. 63-88

[44] Li W. Botanical drugs: A future for herbal medicines. Journal of Contemporary Health Law & Policy. 2002;**19**(1):117-149

[45] Carvalho ACB, Ramalho LS, Marques RFO, Perfeito JP. Regulation of herbal medicines in Brazil. Journal of Ethnopharmacology. 2014;**158**:503-506. DOI: 10.1016/j.jep.2014.08.019

[46] Joos S, Glassen K, Musselmann B. Herbal medicine in primary healthcare in Germany: The patient's perspective. Evidence-Based Complementary and Alternative Medicine. 2012;**2012**:1-10. DOI: 10.1155/2012/294638

[47] Das A, Prasad R, Bhatnagar K, Lavekar GS, Verma A. Synergism between medicinal plants and microbes. In: Chauhan AK, Varma A, editors. Microbes Health and Environment New Delhi: I.K International Publishing House Pvt. Ltd.; 2006. ISBN: 81-88237-79-5

[48] Msomi NZ, Simelane MBC. Olea europaea subsp. africana (Oleaceae). In: El-Shemy HA, editor. Active Ingredients from Aromatic and Medicinal Plants. Croatia: InTech; 2017. pp. 159-174

8

Plant-Derived Medicines with Potential Use in Wound Treatment

Tina Maver, Manja Kurečič, Dragica Maja Smrke,
Karin Stana Kleinschek and Uroš Maver

Abstract

The skin is among the largest and one of the most important organs in the human body. It represents the first line of defence of the body; provides protection from mechanical impacts of the environment, limits the influence of variations in the temperature, prevents entrance of chemicals and microorganisms and restricts radiation effect. Skin damage affects all skin functions; therefore, wounds can compromise patient's well-being, self-image, working capacity and independence. Due to all mentioned, a good wound management is necessary not only for the individual but also for the community. Herbal medicines have been used to accelerate wound healing since ancient times. Recently, scientists have been able to employ scientific methods to prove efficacy of many of these herbs and to get a better understanding of mechanisms of their actions. The popularity of herbal medicines may be explained by the perception that herbs cause minimal adverse effects. Preparations from traditional medicinal plants in wound management involve disinfection, debridement and the provision of suitable environment for natural healing process. In this chapter, the field of wound healing is briefly introduced. Further, the crucial information regarding plants, which are effectively used as wound healing agents in traditional medicine are gathered.

Keywords: wound physiology, wound healing, herbs, antimicrobial effect, anti-inflammatory effect, analgesic effect

1. Introduction

The human body consists of several organs, of which the skin is the largest. The human skin plays an important role in the bodies defensive processes, since it represents the first line of defence [1]. Two other important roles of the skin that also contribute to the defensive mechanisms are regulation and sensation. All mentioned provide a crucial set of functions such as enable protection from mechanical impacts and pressure, restrict the influence of temperature changes, lower the potential impact of microorganisms, limit radiation effects and diminish the entrance of different chemicals. Other important skin functions include the regulation of body temperature (e.g. through sweat glands and hair), control over the peripheral circulation and fluid balance, and in the synthesis of vitamin D. Through its extensive nerve cell network, it enables detection and relaying of changes in the environment (e.g. heat/cold, touch and pain). Damage to these networks is called a neuropathy and impairs the sensation of the mentioned functions in the affected areas. The preservation of skin integrity is due to all mentioned functions crucial for maintaining a healthy body [2].

A wound is trauma-induced defect of the human skin, involving a multitude of endogenous biochemical events and cellular reactions of the immune system [3]. Wounds can compromise patient's well-being, self-image, working capacity and independence. Effective wound management is therefore necessary not only for the individual patient, but has an important impact also on the community [4].

2. Mechanism of wound healing

Wound healing is an extremely complex and dynamic process, which includes replacing of devitalized and missing cellular structures and tissue layers. It reflects in a set of biochemical events that integrate into an organized cascade of processes to repair the damaged tissue [5]. Immediately after injury, damaged vessels leak fluid, to which the body responds with haemostasis. Platelets start to aggregate in the wound bed and secrete multiple growth factors that contribute to an effective clot formation to hinder further loss of fluids from the defected area [6]. Simultaneously with the launch of haemostatic mechanisms, the inflammatory phase is induced as well [7]. It is characterized by local vasodilatation, platelet aggregation and phagocytosis, which together with the release of several cytokines, contribute to local inflammation of the wound site. Multiple chemokines, released by platelets, stimulate the immune and other cells (e.g. keratinocytes) to release growth factors and cytokines to regulate various signalling cascades that govern the inflammation and healing in general [8]. Macrophages and other immune cells are stimulated and they migrate towards the wound to dispose cell debris and fight invading bacteria during the wound healing. Angiogenesis occurs at this phase and new blood vessels transport essential nutrients to the wound bed [6]. The next phase in wound healing is the proliferative phase, which is characterized by granulation, wound contraction and epithelialisation. During granulation, fibroblasts form a bed of collagen, followed by the production of new capillaries [7]. During wound contraction, myofibroblasts decrease the size of the wound by gripping the wound edges and pulling them into the wound interior mechanisms that resemble that of smooth muscle cells. After completion of respective processes, unneeded cells undergo apoptosis (controlled cell death) [9]. Epithelialisation is initiated by keratinocytes proliferating and migrating across the wound site [8]. Fibroblasts are activated and differentiated into myofibroblasts that (either indirectly by production of cytokines or directly) regulate other cells to grow and form new epithelial tissue over the wound site. The final wound healing phase is the remodelling

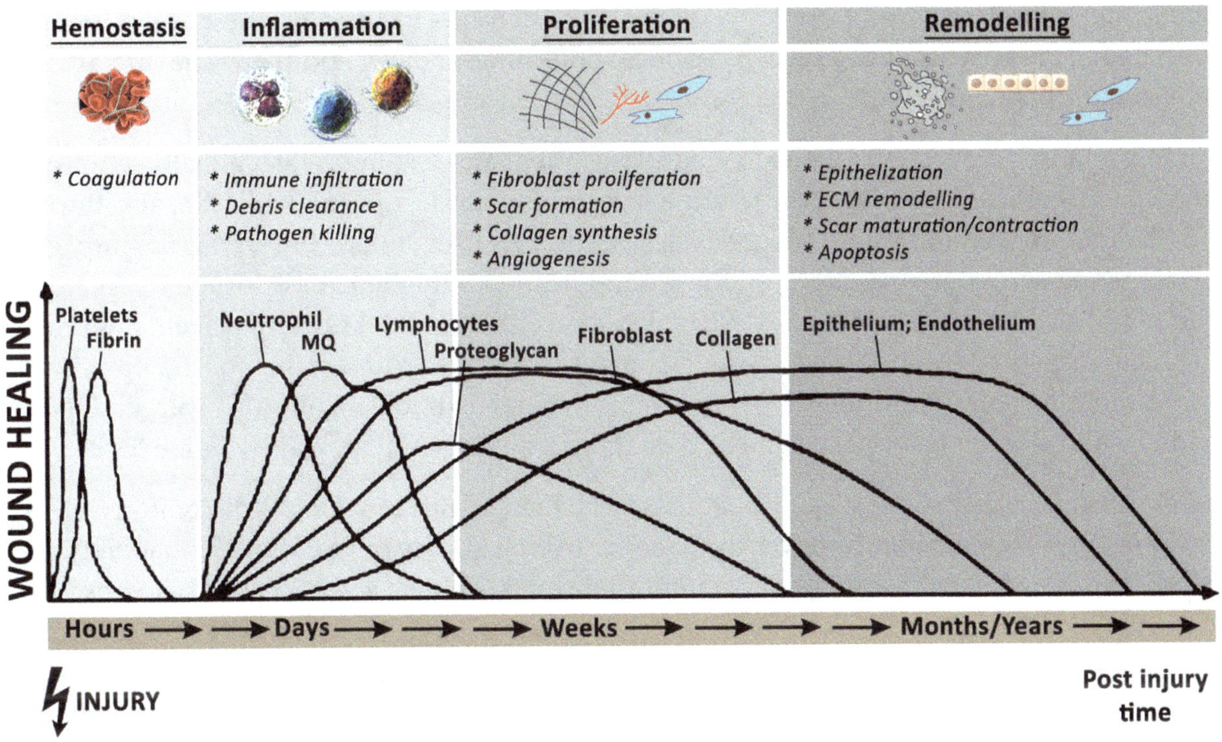

Figure 1. Schematic depiction of distinct phases during wound healing.

phase, which is governed by the rearrangement of the newly formed extracellular matrix (ECM) using increasing amounts of type I collagen. The fibres of collagen rearrange their structures with increasing interfibrillar binding and diameter [10]. The aim of wound treatment can be therefore described as a therapy to either shorten the time required for healing or to minimize the undesired consequences, for example extensive scarring [11]. A general overview of the wound healing is shown in **Figure 1**.

3. Wound healing management

The complex course of the wound healing with the various physiological events that occur simultaneously, as well as consecutively, is vulnerable to possible external interferences (e.g. infections) on one side, as well enables modulation, and hence improvement of the healing performance, through active treatment solutions (e.g. multifunctional wound dressings) [12, 13]. Among the most desired activities are the ones providing anti-inflammatory, antimicrobial, analgesic and antioxidant activities, regardless of the exact underlying mechanism of action [14].

Shortly after the injury, it is during the acute inflammatory response that different cytokines are formed. These are crucial for orchestration of the specific tissue growth, its repair, and hence regeneration [15]. Nevertheless, if this inflammation step persists, it can negatively affect the wound process, namely it leads to vicious cycle of ongoing inflammation, preventing the wound to reach the remodelling phase. If this happens, delays in wound closure occur, which are often accompanied with the increased sensation of pain in the wounded area and its surroundings that can additionally hinder the healing process [16]. Based on these findings about the wound healing physiology, a lot of research has focused on the development of therapeutic approaches that would provide an anti-inflammatory and pain relieving activity to wound dressings [17].

An important complication related to wound treatment and healing is infection. Infections are known to significantly increase the treatment costs of wound care [18], which are also the reason that different strategies are being developed for their prevention [19]. Due to the impact of primary and secondary infections on the wound healing, which increase local inflammation, and hence lead to significant tissue destruction, prevention of their occurrence remains one of the main targets of wound dressing development [20]. An ideal medicine for the prevention of wound infection should therefore have antimicrobial activities, while also stimulating the body's natural immune system without damaging the surrounding healthy tissue [21].

Most wounds induce some level of pain sensation. Pain relates to patient's discomfort, release of stress hormones and often reduces the patients' overall quality of life. Hindered mobility and psychological issues connected with pain-induced stress lead to a less effective wound healing. According to McGuire et al. [22], chronic pain lowers the patients' capability of healing, thereby prolonging the overall recovery process [23]. Suitable and effective pain management can lead to an earlier release from the hospital, stress reduction and a general better reintegration into the community. All mentioned lead to facilitation of wound healing, while at the same time minimizing the risk for development of chronic pain, and finally in lowered treatment costs [24].

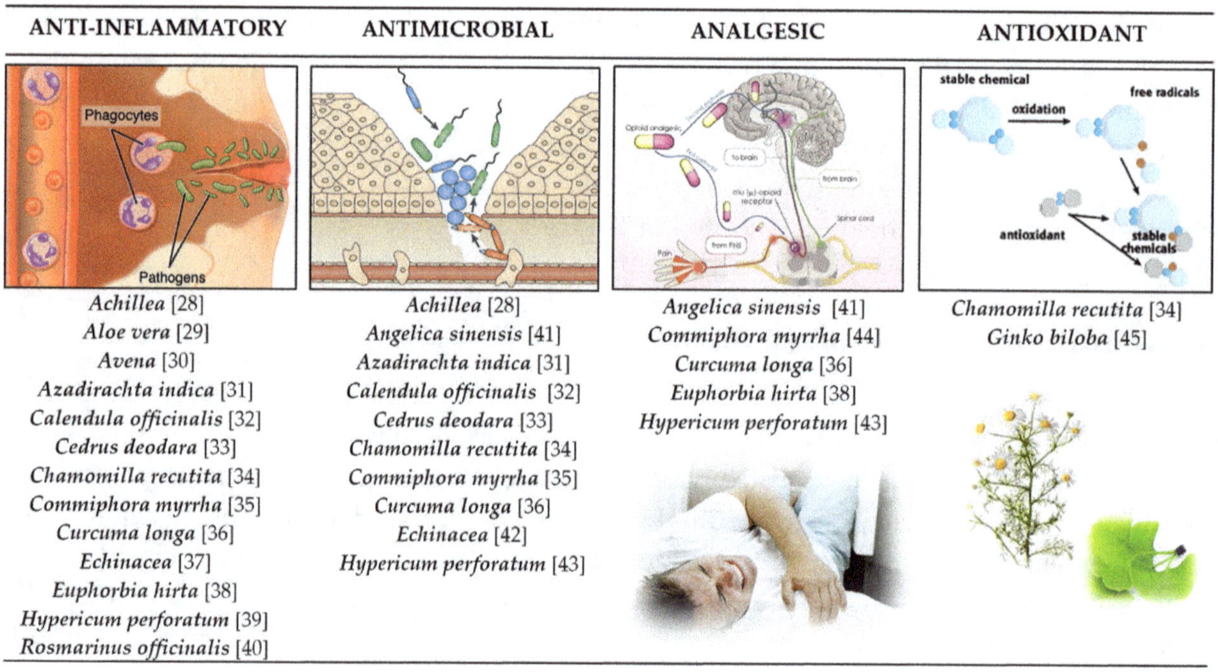

Figure 2. A diagram showing the most important beneficial properties that are desired in wound treatment (and some of the already known plants used in traditional medicine for this purpose). Anti-inflammatory: *Achillea* [28], *Aloe vera* [29], *Avena* [30], *Azadirachta indica* [31], *Calendula officinalis* [32], *Cedrus deodara* [33], *Chamomilla recutita* [34], *Commiphora myrrha* [35], *Curcuma longa* [36], *Echinacea* [37], *Euphorbia hirta* [38], *Hypericum perforatum* [39], *Rosmarinus officinalis* [40]. Antimicrobial: *Achillea* [28], *Angelica sinensis* [41], *Azadirachta indica* [31], *Calendula officinalis* [32], *Cedrus deodara* [33], *Chamomilla recutita* [34], *Commiphora myrrha* [35], *Curcuma longa* [36], *Echinacea* [42], *Hypericum perforatum* [43]. Analgesic: *Angelica sinensis* [41], *Commiphora myrrha* [44], *Curcuma longa* [36], *Euphorbia hirta* [38], *Hypericum perforatum* [43]. Antioxidant: *Chamomilla recutita* [34], *Ginkgo biloba* [45].

Part of the inflammation phase of wound healing causes also a coordinated influx of neutrophils to the wound site. One of the actions of neutrophils is also the activation of the so-called 'respiratory burst', which leads to productions of free radicals [25]. These produce oxidative stress that results in lipid peroxidation, DNA damage, and enzyme inactivation (e.g. free-radical scavenger enzymes and others), even those whose main activity is to limit the effects of reactive oxygen species (ROS). Considering the above mentioned, it is clear that antioxidants may be of therapeutic use in several diseases that are connected with potential pathologic actions of oxidants, including the wound healing [26].

Apart from the above-mentioned wound healing aiding activities, others are also reported in literature, e.g. the astringent activity, stimulated epithelisation and effective hydration of the wound site [27]. The most important properties of plant-derived medicines that are beneficial for the wound healing process are depicted in **Figure 2** together with some examples of plants that were already proven for the mentioned use.

4. Plants with potential use in wound healing

For thousands of years, we looked to nature for various types of medicinal treatments and plant-based systems continue to play an essential role in the primary health care of many less-developed, as well as developing countries [46]. Many plants and various preparations thereof have been used traditionally in relation to wound treatment, especially due to their immense potential to affect the wound healing process [65]. Plant-derived extracts and/or isolates induce healing and tissue regeneration through multiple connected mechanisms, which often have a synergistic effect on the overall healing efficiency [47]. Many plant-derived medicines (commonly called as phytomedicines) are affordable and cause minimal unwanted side effects [48]. Nevertheless, increasing awareness of their potential activities, especially considering the possible combinations of various plant-derived molecules, which could induce toxic effects as well, points out the need for a systematic approach towards their evaluation before efficient introduction to wound care (or other fields of medicine) [49]. In recent years, extensive research has been carried out in the area of wound healing and management through plant-derived medicinal products [38].

The following subchapters review the key details related to the potential use of medicinal plants in wound healing.

4.1. Groups of plant-derived molecules with beneficial effects on wound healing

When we describe the beneficial effects of plant-derived molecules on human health, mostly it is the secondary plant metabolites, producing pharmacological and/or toxicological effects, that we are discussing [48]. Secondary metabolites are produced within the plants and are regarded as by-products of biochemical reactions in the plant cells. As such, these molecules are not part of any crucial daily functioning of the plant, hence are not important for the plants main biosynthetic and metabolic routes that yield products with major significance for the plant growth and/or development [50]. Although this means that these molecules are not key to the plants basic functions, this does not mean that they do not importantly contribute to the success of the plants overall survival in its ecosystem. For example, several of them play important roles in the living plants′ protection, attraction or signalling [51]. It seems that most plant species are capable of producing at least some of these compounds. But before we describe the most important groups of these secondary metabolites, let us first define the related term bioactive compounds. By definition, bioactive compounds in plants are compounds, produced by plants having pharmacological or toxicological effects in man and animals [52].

Bioactive compounds in plants can be classified considering different criteria. A presentation based on clinical function—their pharmacological or toxicological effects—is relevant for the clinician, pharmacist or toxicologist. The botanical approach on the other side considers the plant, from which they originate [53]. Finally, the biochemical approach seems to be the most commonly used. The latter is based on their classification according to the metabolic (biochemical) pathway, by which they are produced [54]. Using this approach, groups are more clearly understandable to most readers with at least basic knowledge in chemistry. The list of possible products is quite long, but since the focus of this chapter is on the ones with a beneficial effect on wound healing, we will focus on the groups, which could benefit the latter also in future clinical applications. The final subchapter summarizes some of the other groups, which might attract more researchers in the future.

4.1.1. Phenolic compounds

Phenolic compounds present secondary metabolites that are known to contribute to several plant functions [55]. Apart from the important functions in relation to the plant host organism, phenolic metabolites (mostly called polyphenols in literature) are among the most important plant-derived molecules with a versatile range of potential beneficial biological properties on the human health [56]. Phenolic compounds were shown to possess beneficial effect on the human health, regardless of the type of intake/application [57]. For example, skin application can alleviate symptoms and inhibit the development of various skin disorders [58]. Because, in nature, there is an abundant source of various polyphenols with proven effect on the skin and due to the already proven low toxicity for many of them, these type of compounds have a great potential in wound healing, including treatment of various skin damage (e.g. wounds and burns) [55]. Polyphenols present an important source for future applications in wound care, ranging from reduction of minor skin problems (e.g., wrinkles, acne) [59] to more severe ones, such as cancer [60].

There are many available studies describing the potential of phenolic compounds to be used in treatment of various skin disorders, including reports about their beneficial influence on wound healing [61]. Phenolic compounds are among the most known plant secondary metabolites mostly due to their broad spectrum of biological properties [62]. The latter were shown to be related to their molecular structure, which consists of the main core, formed by at least one phenol ring, in which hydrogen is usually replaced by a more active moiety (e.g. hydroxyl, methyl or acetyl) [55]. The variability in their biological properties and activities is related to the type and degree of the substitutes on the phenol ring. Since many of the natural phenolic compounds contain more than one phenol ring, such compounds are often called polyphenols [62].

At the moment, we know over 8000 different structures of plant phenolic compounds. Due to this huge number of compounds, it is important to use an effective classification system for their distinction. The most commonly used to distinguish phenolic compounds, groups them initially into flavonoid and non-flavonoid compounds. Both main groups are further divided as presented in **Figure 3**.

4.1.1.1. Flavonoids

Most likely the largest class of polyphenolic compounds found in nature are flavonoids [63]. Over 4000 structurally unique flavonoids were already identified from various plant sources [64]. Primarily, flavonoids were recognized as pigments responsible for many colors that occur in autumn, since they can provide various hues of yellow, orange and red in flowers, vegetables, nuts, seeds, fruits, etc., as well as the color of tea and red wine [65]. Several studies have shown that many plants contain therapeutic amounts of flavonoids [66]. These were (and still are) used in traditional medicine as anti-inflammatory, pain reducing, healing promoting, anti-allergic agents and others [67]. Most of the pharmacological effects found in flavonoids can be related to their (almost common) strong antioxidant activity [68]. They also act as free radical scavengers, can chelate metals, and are able to interact with enzymes, have an action on adenosine receptors and interfere with bio-membranes [69]. Among the main motivations for this review are several studies reporting different flavonoids with beneficial properties for wound-healing [47].

The core molecular structure of flavonoids consists of two aromatic rings connected by a three carbon bridge [70]. In plants, flavonoids often occur in association with sugar moieties

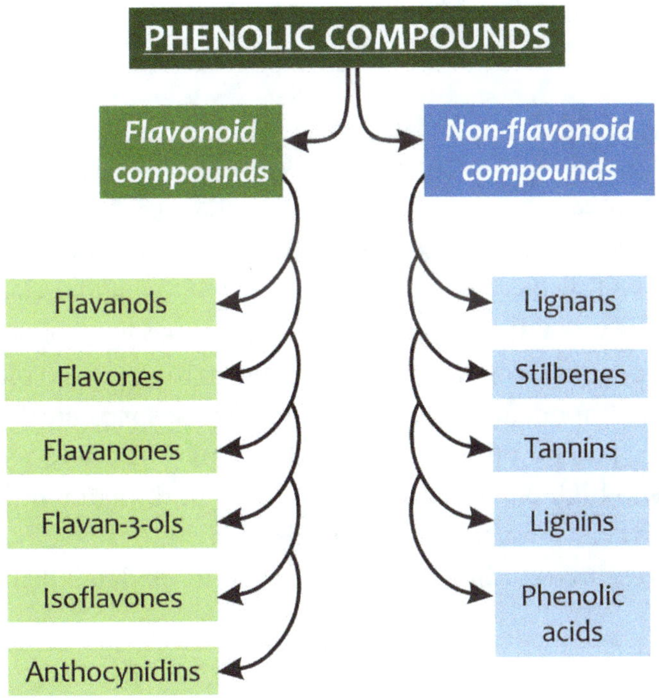

Figure 3. A diagram showing the classification of phenolic compounds.

as glycosides [70]. The main sources of flavonoids in the diet are fruits and vegetables. They occur also in certain grains, seeds, and spices, as well as in wine, tea, coffee, cocoa, and herbal essences [71]. All flavonoid compounds contain phenol-groups, which in general induces an antioxidant activity [72]. Other actions are diverse-several structures reduce inflammation or carcinogenicity [73].

4.1.1.2. Non-flavonoid polyphenols

Non-flavonoid metabolites also comprise several subgroups (**Figure 3**) [74]. Many of these compounds occur mainly as complicated biopolymers. In this, they are different from their flavonoid counterparts by lacking a defined primary carbon base, which results in unique chemical structures for respective polyphenols [75]. An important subgroup of non-flavonoid compounds from plants are phenolic acids, which can be further divided into hydroxycinnamic acids (e.g. caffeic acid, chlorogenic acid, o-, m- and p-coumaric acids, ferulic acids, and sinapic acids), and hydroxybenzoic acids (e.g. gallic acid, p-hydroxybenzoic acid, protocatechuic acid, vanillic and syringic acids) [55]. Both classes often occur in plants in the glycoside form. In plant tissues, phenolic acids can be bound to various compounds, e.g., flavonoids, fatty acids, sterols and cell wall polymers [76]. Another widely distributed group of phenolic compounds in plants are tannins, which may occur as hydrolysable tannins (formed in the pathway of the phenolic acids with sugar polymerization) and condensed tannins (a combination of flavonoids) [77]. Lignans are phenylpropanoid dimers, whereas the most commonly known ones include secoisolariciresinol, lariciresinol, pinoresinol and matairesinol [55]. The most known and researched stilbene is resveratrol, which is present in many edible plant species (e.g. grapes, peanuts, and berries) [78]. Resveratrol plays an important part in the plant defence against mechanical injury, pathogen infection, and UV radiation [78].

4.1.2. Essential oils

By definition, essential oils are concentrated hydrophobic liquids that contain volatile aroma compounds derived from plants [79]. The term essential has not an analogous meaning as in the case of essential amino acids or essential fatty acids. In the latter cases, essential corresponds to a lack of mechanism for their respective synthesis in a specific organism, which also means that these have to be acquired by other means (e.g. diet) [80]. In general, essential oils are extracted by distillation (e.g. by steam). Other processes include expression, solvent extraction, absolute oil extraction, resin tapping and cold pressing [81]. Due to their (often) pleasant fragrance, they are commonly used as components in perfumes, cosmetics, soaps and other products, for flavouring food and drink, and for other similar applications [80]. There are several essential oils derived from plants with high potential to be used in wound treatment [82]. Some of the most important essential oils with proven beneficial effect on wound healing (either in traditional medicine or based on research studies), are described in more detail below.

4.1.2.1. Lavender oil

Lavender (*Lavandula*) oil, derived from lavender flowers, is one of the most commonly used essential oils in various therapies. Due to its antibacterial and antifungal properties, it has been used to treat bites [82]. There are also reports describing its anti-depressant activity, as well as its effect on smooth muscles (acting as a muscle relaxant) [83]. Several researchers have performed many different studies in relation to the potential beneficial effect of lavender oil in various wound care applications [83]. One of these studies, conducted by Kane et al., reports about the significantly reduced pain intensity after aromatherapy using lavender oil during dressing changes in treatment of vascular wounds when compared with control therapies [84]. Another study showing a potential use of lavender oil in wound care is the study by Hartman and Coetzee [85]. They studied the effect of lavender and chamomile essential oils on wound healing in five patients with chronic wounds in a timespan of months. The wounds were graded using the US National Pressure Ulcer Advisory Panel (NPUAP) guidelines based on depth and visual characteristics [85]. The treatment protocol used in this study includes a treatment with a 6 wt.% solution of two drops of lavender oil and one drop of German chamomile, which were applied directly onto the wound, and subsequently covered with a gauze. Their result was that the wounds treated with the oils healed more quickly compared to the control wounds without the additional treatment using the essential oils, which were just covered by the gauze [85].

4.1.2.2. Chamomile oil

The wound healing aiding properties of chamomile (*Matricaria chamomilla* L.) oil, derived from chamomile flowers, were investigated also by Glowania et al. [86]. This double-blind study included 14 patients in which chamomile oil, when added to standard dressings, significantly improved the weeping and drying associated with dermabrasion wounds [86]. Another study that reports evaluation of potential positive effects on wound healing is a review of the bioactivity of chamomile, conducted by McKay et al. [87]. They found a moderate antimicrobial and a significant antiplatelet activity *in vitro*, as well as showed antimutagenic effects in animals [87].

4.1.2.3. Tea tree oil

The tea tree (*Melaleuca alternifolia*) oil is an essential oil derived from the leaves of the tea tree that are used as a complementary therapy in Australia. The latter is mostly related to its known antiseptic, antibacterial, antifungal and anti-inflammatory activities [82]. Several studies report about its potential use in wound healing applications. Halcon and Milkus, for example, tested the tea tree oil as an antimicrobial agent in the case of *Staphylococcus aureus* infections [88]. Although this study was based only on a small clinical trial combined with case studies, the authors nevertheless showed the potential of the tea tree oil treatment of osteomyelitis and in chronic wound healing [88]. Another study was performed by Hammer et al., who investigated the effect of tea tree oil on transient and commensal skin flora *in vitro* [89]. They compared the effectiveness of different concentrations to induce bactericidal action and found the tea tree oil to be effective against *Staphylococcus aureus* and most Gram-negative bacteria (reduction to 0.25%), but was less effective against coagulase-negative staphylococci and micrococci (8%) [89]. Two groups of researchers tested also commercially available products based on tea tree extracts (including the essential oil). Sherry et al. claimed that the antimicrobial preparation from extracts of tea tree oil and eucalyptus showed an activity against methicillin-resistant *Staphylococcus aureus* (MRSA) [90]. Faoagali et al. evaluated the activity of another commercially available tea tree oil-based cream against different bacteria and confirmed its effectiveness against *Staphylococcus aureus* and *Escherichia coli* [91].

4.1.2.4. Thyme oil

Thyme (*Thymus vulgaris*) is an aromatic plant, commonly used in preparation of several dishes, whereas its essential oil has been widely reported to contribute to the healing of burns [82]. Thyme essential oil is derived from the steam distillation of the leaves, stems and flowers of the plant. One of such is the study by Dursun et al., who investigated the impact of thyme oil on the formation of nitric oxide, which is an important inflammatory mediator [92]. They studied the effect of thyme oil on burn wound in rats and showed that it not only decreased the amount of nitric oxide produced in response to the burn, but also facilitated wound healing [92]. Several other studies were conducted in regard of the potential antimicrobial activity of the thyme oil. For example, Bozin et al. showed an effective antibacterial and antifungal activity *in vitro* [93]. Their results are in agreement with another study that was performed by Shin and Kim, who determined a significant inhibitory action of thyme oil against both antibiotic-susceptible and resistant strains of *Streptococci, Staphylococcus aureus* and *Salmonella typhimurium* [94]. With the aim to evaluate the thyme oil's potential antifungal action, Giordani et al. combined it with amphotericin B and showed that it significantly potentiated the effectiveness of the latter [95]. Finally, Komarcevic discussed the available evidence showing that topically applied thyme oil increased collagen deposition, angiogenesis and keratinocyte migration, all together significantly contributing to the efficiency of wound healing [96].

4.1.2.5. Ocimum oil (basil)

Orafidiya et al. performed two studies regarding the potential use of ocimum oil derived from the leaves of *Ocimum basilicum* L. in wound healing applications [97]. First, they studied its potential effect on the healing of full-thickness excisional and incisional wounds in an animal model [97]. They found and improved wound healing performance in wounds treated with the essential oil in comparison with the control [97]. In the second study, Orafidiya et al. demonstrated a significant antiseptic effect of a 2% solution of ocimum oil against strains and isolates from boils, wounds and acne [98]. This group was not the only one testing the potential effect of basil extract. Another similar study was performed by Singh and Majumdar, who studied the potential anti-inflammatory action of ocimum oil. They found a significant inhibition of vascular permeability and leucocyte migration in animal studies [99]. Singh conducted another study, in which he determined that the anti-inflammatory activity of ocimum oil could be related to a blockading of the enzymes cyclooxygenase and lipoxygenase in the arachidonic acid metabolism [100].

4.1.2.6. Other oils

Other less well-known essential oils with a proven beneficial effect on wound healing include the bark oil of *Santiria trimera* (a member of the frankincense family) [101], oils from *Hypericum perforatum* (St. John's Wort) and *Calendula arvensis* [102], oils extracted from *Cinnamomum zeylanicum* (cinnamon) bark [103], and the extract from *Chromolaena odorata* (Siam weed) [104].

An overview of the main chemical components of the above described essential oils is depicted in **Figure 4**.

4.1.3. Other compounds with wound healing properties

Research on plant-derived compounds with potential use in wound healing drugs is a developing area in modern biomedical sciences. Scientists who are trying to develop newer drugs from natural resources are looking towards different regions, where there is a strong evidence of plant in traditional medicine (India, Africa, etc.) [105]. Most of these herbal medicines are not isolated compounds, but rather extracts composed of several constituents, which synergistically aid the wound healing process [106]. Not many have been screened scientifically for the evaluation of their wound healing activity in different pharmacological models and patients, but the potential of most remains unexplored [107]. The most important groups of compounds were described above, whereas we briefly review some of the less commonly used compounds and groups.

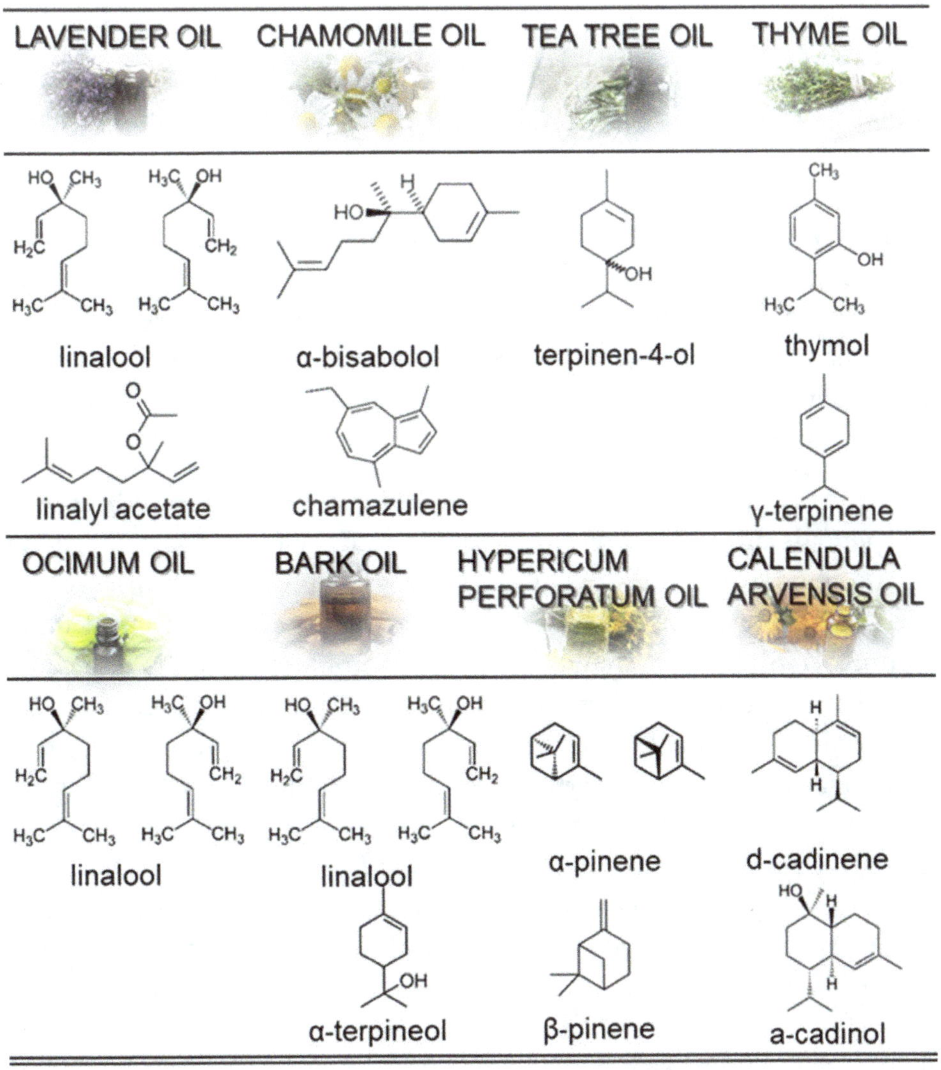

Figure 4. An overview of chemical structures of the above mentioned essential oils.

4.1.3.1. Alkaloids

Alkaloids are heterocyclic compounds that contain a nitrogen atom in at least one of the heterocycles [108]. They usually have various potent biological activities and are of bitter taste [109]. Some synthetic compounds of similar structure are also termed alkaloids. They are not that common in the plant kingdom, are represented by diverse chemical structures, and almost all show interesting properties for therapeutic use [110]. Alkaloids are produced also by other organisms including bacteria, fungi and animals [109]. Although alkaloids are not the first choice of chemicals to be used in relation to wound treatment, there are still some interesting plants that need further analysis due to their already proven potential for this purpose. Among the plants that produce alkaloids with potential beneficial effects on wound healing are the *Papaveraceae* (poppy family) and *Berberidaceae* (barberry family) families [111]. Both produce isoquinoline alkaloids that possess a range of biochemical effects relevant for medical use (e.g. inhibition of pain, growth inhibition of cancer cell growth, and growth of bacterial cells) [111]. Among other indirectly related beneficial properties are also the stimulation of bone marrow leucocytes, which modulate the inflammation phase of wound healing [112].

4.1.3.2. Resins

This group of plant-derived compounds presents a complex mixture of lipid-soluble chemicals [113]. These can be both non-volatile (e.g. diterpenoid and triterpenoid compounds) and volatile (mono- and sesquiterpenoids) [114]. Resins are most commonly found in nature as part of various wood-derived structures, although they are also present in herbaceous plants [115]. Among their common properties are a general stickiness, whereas their fluidity depends on the contents of volatile compounds [115]. When exposed to air they harden. Among their beneficial biological activities for wound healing are the antimicrobial activity, but their actions depend on the composition of the chemical mixture. Resins are generally safe, but contact allergy may occur [116].

The common structural precursor of terpenoids is the five-carbon building block isoprene [117]. Monoterpenoids are formed of two isoprene units, whereas sesquiterpenoids consist of three units. Both mentioned groups are commonly denoted as low-molecular-weight terpenoids, which are one of the most varied groups of plant products that include more than 25,000 compounds [118]. The phenylpropanoid group of terpenoids is less common and is based on a nine-carbon skeleton, whereas their synthesis pathway differs from the other terpenoids [119]. Compounds of all three mentioned groups have often strong odours and flavours, which is related to their properties (e.g. the lipophilicity and volatility) [120]. Since they exhibit various biological activities, they are found in several herbal remedies [121]. Of particular importance in relation to wound healing are their antibacterial and antiviral effects, whereas they possess also other activities like the antineoplastic activity, as well as stimulation gastrointestinal tract [118]. They are not toxic unless they are concentrated as volatile oils [122]. The plant family best known for these compounds is *Lamiaceae* (thyme family).

4.1.3.3. Compounds with antimicrobial activity

Looking at plant extract to find novel antimicrobial compounds is interesting for clinical microbiologists for two reasons, namely, it is very likely that these phytochemicals will be sooner rather than later prescribed as antimicrobial drugs, and the public is becoming increasingly aware of problems with the over prescription and misuse of traditional antibiotics [123]. It is reported that, on average, two or three antibiotics derived from microorganisms are launched each year [124]. Phytochemicals with an antimicrobial activity can be divided into several categories, most of which were already described above. These include phenolics, terpenoids, essential oils and alkaloids [123]. Among the other ones, we will briefly review also the lectins and polypeptides, as well as polyacetylenes.

First antimicrobial peptides were reported back in 1942 [123]. Mostly, these compounds are positively charged and include disulphide bonds in their structure [125]. One of the known possible mechanism of actions involves the formation of ion channels in the microbial membrane [125], while the other is related to a competitive inhibition of adhesion of microbial proteins to host polysaccharide receptors [126]. Some of the most important subgroups of antimicrobial peptides include thionins, which are toxic to yeasts and Gram-negative and Gram-positive bacteria [125].

Polyacetylenes are another group of potential antimicrobial compounds with interesting properties. The compound 8S-heptadeca-2(Z),9(Z)-diene-4,6-diyne-1,8-diol was shown to be effective against *S. aureus* and *B. subtilis* but not to Gram-negative bacteria or yeasts [127]. In Brazil, acetylene compounds and flavonoids derived from single plant extracts traditionally are used for treatment of malaria fever and liver disorders [128].

5. Plants with beneficial effect on wound healing, approved by the Committee on Herbal Medicinal Products (HMPC)

Many plants and their extracts have great potential for the management and treatment of wounds. Natural agents induce healing and regeneration of the lost tissue by multiple mechanisms. The so-called phytomedicines are affordable and they cause minimal adverse effects. However, there is need for scientific standardization, validation and safety evaluation of plants of traditional medicine before these can be recommended for wound healing [49]. Therefore, an extensive research has been carried out in the area of wound healing and management through medicinal plants [38].

The following paragraphs outline some medicinal plants and their properties that exhibit wound healing activity.

Achillea millefolium (Family: *Asteraceae*). Yarrow (a common name of the plant) has been known and used due to its healing effects by many cultures for hundreds of years [129]. Among its proven beneficial effects in wound healing are a good antibacterial activity against *Shigella dysenteriae* [130], moderate activities against *Streptococcus pneumoniae, Clostridium perfringens* and *Candida albicans,* and a weak antibacterial activity against *Mycobacterium smegmatis, Acinetobacter lwoffii* and *Candida krusei* [131]. Yarrow also has a proven anti-inflammatory effect [132].

Aloe vera (Family: *Liliaceae). Aloe vera* has been used for medicinal purposes in several cultures for millennia: Greece, Egypt, India, Mexico, Japan and China [133]. 3500 years ago, Egyptians used this herb in treating burns, infections and parasites [134]. Its gel has the ability to heal different kinds of wounds including ulcers and burns by forming a protective coating on the affected areas and speeding up the healing process. Various constituents of *Aloe vera* stimulate wound healing and have anti-inflammatory activity [29].

Angelica sinensis (Family: *Apiaceae*). Chinese angelica is widely used in Chinese traditional medicine. Its isolate has been found to stimulate wound healing and increase the strength of the healed wounds [135].

Avena sativa (Family: *Poaceae*). The oats has been known for more than 4000 years as a food and the traditional medicinal usage has been documented since the twelfth century. For cutaneous use, mostly fruits of *Avena* are prepared as 'colloidal oatmeal' described in the USP 30 (1990) [136]. *In vitro* investigations are indicative of an anti-inflammatory activity of several oat fruit preparations. Pasta made with oat's flour mixed with beer yeast is used on infected ulcers and wounds, and to facilitate wound healing [137].

Azadirachta indica (Family: *Meliaceae*). Neem has been used in India for over two millennia for many medicinal properties, particularly for skin diseases. Products made from neem trees possess anti-bacterial, anti-fungal, anti-viral and anti-inflammatory activities. Neem oil aids the building of collagen, promotes wound healing and maintains the skin elasticity. It also keeps the wound moist during the healing process. All mentioned mechanisms accelerate wound healing [138].

Calendula officinalis (Family: *Asteraceae*). *In vitro* pharmacological studies confirmed its anti-viral, anti-genotoxic and anti-inflammatory properties [32]. Pot marigold was shown to possess also an antimicrobial activity against *Bacillus subtilis, Escherichia coli, Staphylococcus aureus, Pseudomonas aeruginosa, Candida albicans* [139], *Sarcina lutea, Klebsiella pneumoniae* and *Candida monosa* [140]. Different preparations of pot marigold are known (e.g. suspensions or tinctures) for topical use to reduce inflammation, as well as to control bleeding [141]. It was also shown to inprove the healing of poorly healing wounds [142].

Cedrus deodara (Family: *Pinaceae*). Deodar possesses anti-inflammatory, anti-microbial, astringent and wound healing activities and is therefore particularly useful in treatment of infected wounds [33].

Centella asiatica (Family: *Mackinlayaceae*). Extensive research has been conducted regarding its use in the treatment of leprosy and several other skin conditions, including the treatment of various wounds. For example, centella was used in the treatment of experimentally induced open wounds in rats. In this study, its aqueous extract increased collagen content and the overall thickness of the freshly formed epithelium [143]. Apart from the mentioned, the topical use of its aqueous extract increased proliferation of various cells, improved collagen synthesis at the wound site (all mentioned was proven by increased DNA and protein synthesis in the tested cells), through an increased collagen content in the granulation tissue, and in an improved tensile strength [144]. All mentioned confirms the potential of *Centella asiatica* to promote wound healing and to facilitate repair of the connective tissues [145].

Chamomilla recutita (Family: *Asteraceae*). Chamomile has been used for centuries as an antimicrobial, antioxidant, anti-inflammatory agent, as a mild astringent and a healing medicine [34]. It helps in wound drying and it accelerates epithelization. Chamomile aids wound management also through increased granulation tissue weight, hydroxyproline content, rate of wound contraction and wound-breaking strength [146].

Chromolaena odorata (Family: *Asteraceae*). The aqueous extract and the decoction from the leaves of this plant have been used throughout Vietnam for the treatment of soft tissue and burn wounds. It enhances haemostatic activity, inhibits wound contraction, stimulates granulation tissue and re-epithelization processes and can therefore be of much therapeutic value in the wound healing, minimizing post-burn scar contracture and deformities [147].

Commiphora myrrha (Family: *Burseraceae*). Myrrh is among the oldest known traditional medicines used by humans, with a documented use even in the times of ancient Rome (found in texts written by Hippocrates). In addition, other cultures report its potential medical use. These include the Bible, as well as the Koran [148]. Various pharmacological activities of myrrh are reported (e.g. antibacterial and antifungal effects against several strains, as well as anti-inflammatory, local anaesthetic and analgesic activities). Presently, it is cutaneous used in the form of a tincture in the treatment of minor wounds, abrasions and skin inflammations [35].

Curcuma longa (Family: *Zingiberaceae*). Turmeric possess anti-bacterial, anti-fungal, analgesic and anti-inflammatory activities [149]. Its anti-inflammatory properties, presence of vitamin A, as well as several proteins were shown to have a beneficial effect on the early formation of collagen fibres, which could be related to stimulation of fibroblastic activity [36]. As part of traditional medicines, fresh rhizome juice from turmeric is often used in treatment of fresh wounds, bruises and also leech bites.

Echinacea (Family: *Asteraceae*). *Echinacea* species and various preparations thereof have one of the longest reported histories of use in the American people's medicine [150]. The most used species include *E. purpurea, E. angustifolia, E. palida, E. simulata* and *E. paradoxa* [151]. The documented use of *Echinacea purpurea* dates back to 1787 and includes its use for external application in treatment of wounds, burns and insect bites [152]. Its more specific activities are an antimicrobial activity against *Vesicular Stomatitis virus, Escherichia coli, Pseudomonas aeruginosa, Aspergillus niger, Candida albicans, Staphylococcus aureus, Pseudomonas aeruginosa* [153], *Encephalomyocarditis virus, Vesicular Stomatitis virus* [154], *Saccharomyces cerevisiae, Candida shehata, Candida kefyr, Candida albicans, Candida steatulytica and Candida tropicalis* [42]. Echinacea extracts exhibit also pain reducing effects, which are related to an inhibitory effect on cyclooxygenase-I, cyclooxygenase-II [155] and 5-lipoxygenase [37]. The mentioned activities contribute also to its anti-inflammatory activity. All described properties (e.g. antimicrobial, pain reducing effects, anti-inflammatory activity) present beneficial effects of *Echinacea* for wound healing [37].

Euphorbia hirta (Family: *Euphorbiaceae*). The aqueous extract of the plant shows analgesic, anti-inflammatory activities and an inhibitory action on platelet aggregation. Ethanolic extract of the entire herb was found to possess significant wound healing activity [38].

Ginkgo biloba (Family: *Ginkgoaceae*). Ginkgo leaf extracts have been therapeutically used for hundreds of years [156]. Its pharmacological activities include an increase in blood fluidity, anti-oxidative activity, membrane stabilization, improvement in cognition, and wound healing promotion. Various ginkgo preparations have been shown to improve granulation tissue breaking strength, as well as promote epithelization without influence on wound contraction [45].

Helianthus annuus (Family: *Asteraceae*). In traditional medicine, the sunflower herb is used by Indian tribes for treating inflammation of the eyes, sores, tiger bites, and to treat bone fractures [157]. The alcoholic extract of the whole plant of *Helianthus annuus* applied on the excised wounds of rats led to a significant reduction of the healing period which was indicated by earlier appearance and higher accumulation of mucopolysaccharides [158].

GENUS FAMILY	***Achillea millefolium*** *Asteraceae*	***Angelica sinensis*** *Apiaceae*	***Aloe vera*** *Liliaceae*	***Avena sativa*** *Poaceae*
	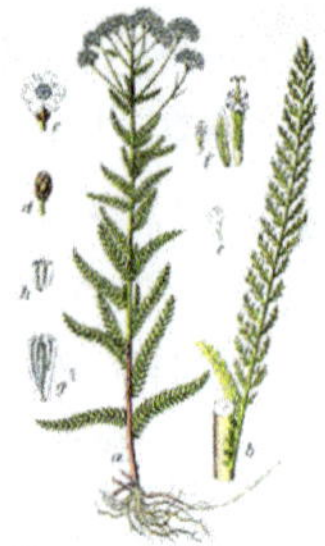	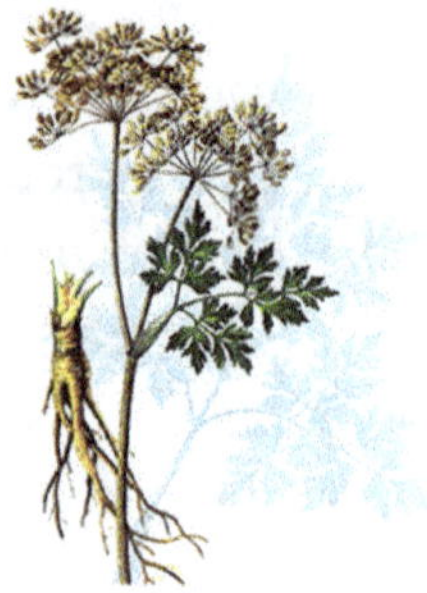	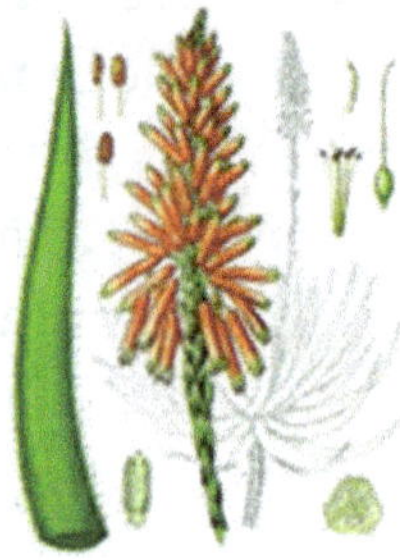	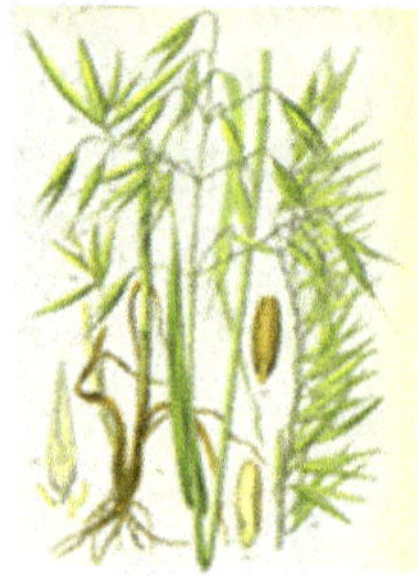
BIOLOGICAL ACTIVITY	Antibacterial activity. Anti-inflammatory activity.	Stimulation of wound healing. Increasing the strength of skin in healed wounds.	Formation of a protective coating on the affected areas. Stimulation and speeding up of a wound healing process. Anti-inflammatory activity.	Anti-inflammatory activity. Facilitation of wound healing.

GENUS FAMILY	***Azardica indica*** *Meliaceae*	***Calendula officinalis*** *Asteraceae*	***Cedrus deodara*** *Pinaceae*	***Centella asiatica*** *Mackinlayaceae*
	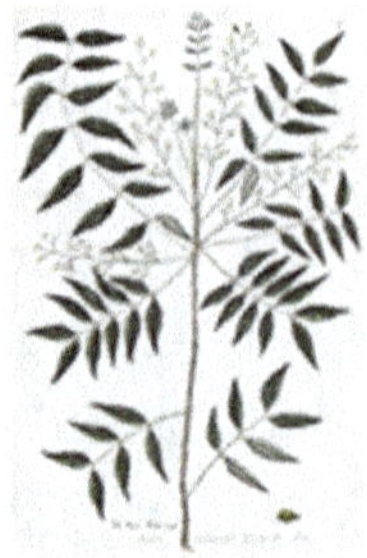	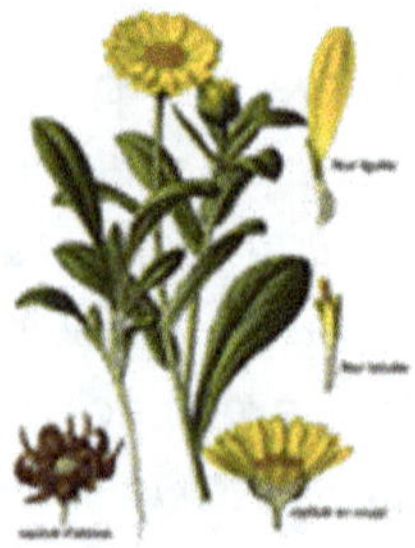	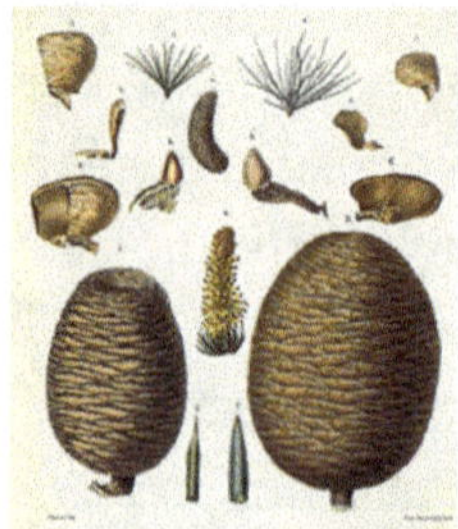	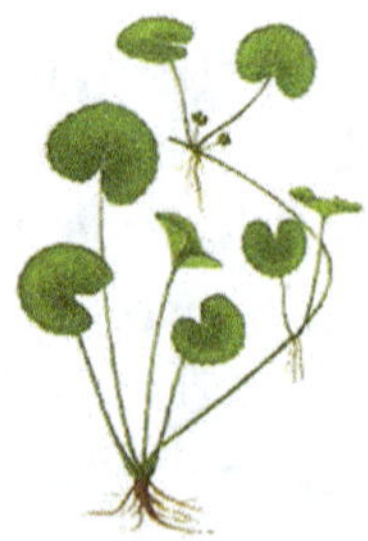
BIOLOGICAL ACTIVITY	Anti-bacterial activity. Anti-fungal activity. Anti-viral activity. Anti-inflammatory activity. Help in collagen forming. Promotion of wound healing.	Anti-viral properties. Anti-inflammatory activity. Antimicrobial activity. Facilitation of healing of poorly healing wound.	Anti-inflammatory activity. Anti-microbial activity. Astringent activity.	Increasing content of collagen and thickness of the epithelium. Increasing cellular proliferation. Promotion of collagen synthesis.

GENUS FAMILY	***Chamomilla recutita*** *Asteraceae*	***Chromolaena odorata*** *Asteraceae*	***Commiphora myrrha*** *Burseraceae*	***Curcuma longa*** *Zingiberaceae*
	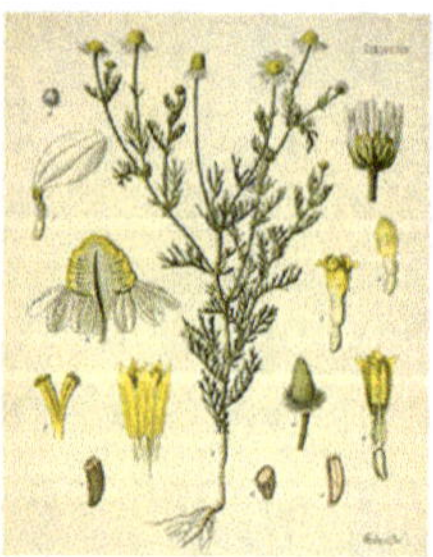	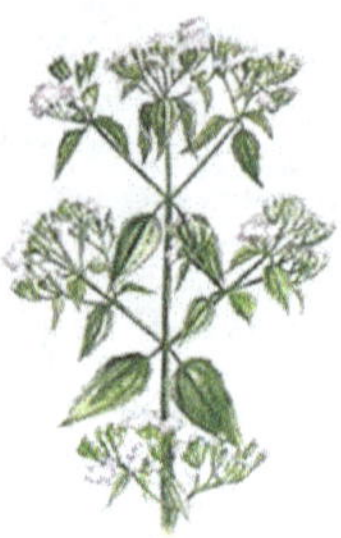	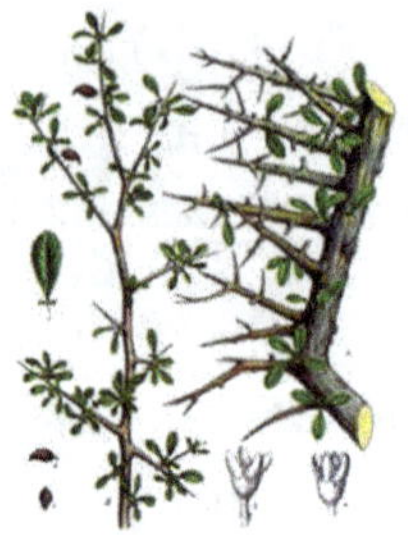	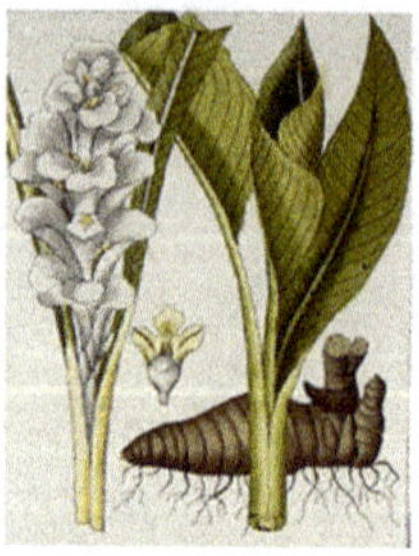
BIOLOGICAL ACTIVITY	Antimicrobial activity. Antioxidant properties. Anti-inflammatory activity. Mild astringent properties. Acceleration of epithelization.	Enhancement of hemostatic activity. Inhibition of wound contraction. Stimulation of granulation tissue synthesis and re-epithelization processes.	Antibacterial and antifungal effects. Anti-inflammatory activity. Local anesthetic and analgesic activity.	Antibacterial and antifungal effects. Anti-inflammatory activity. Analgesic activity. Facilitation of collagen synthesis.

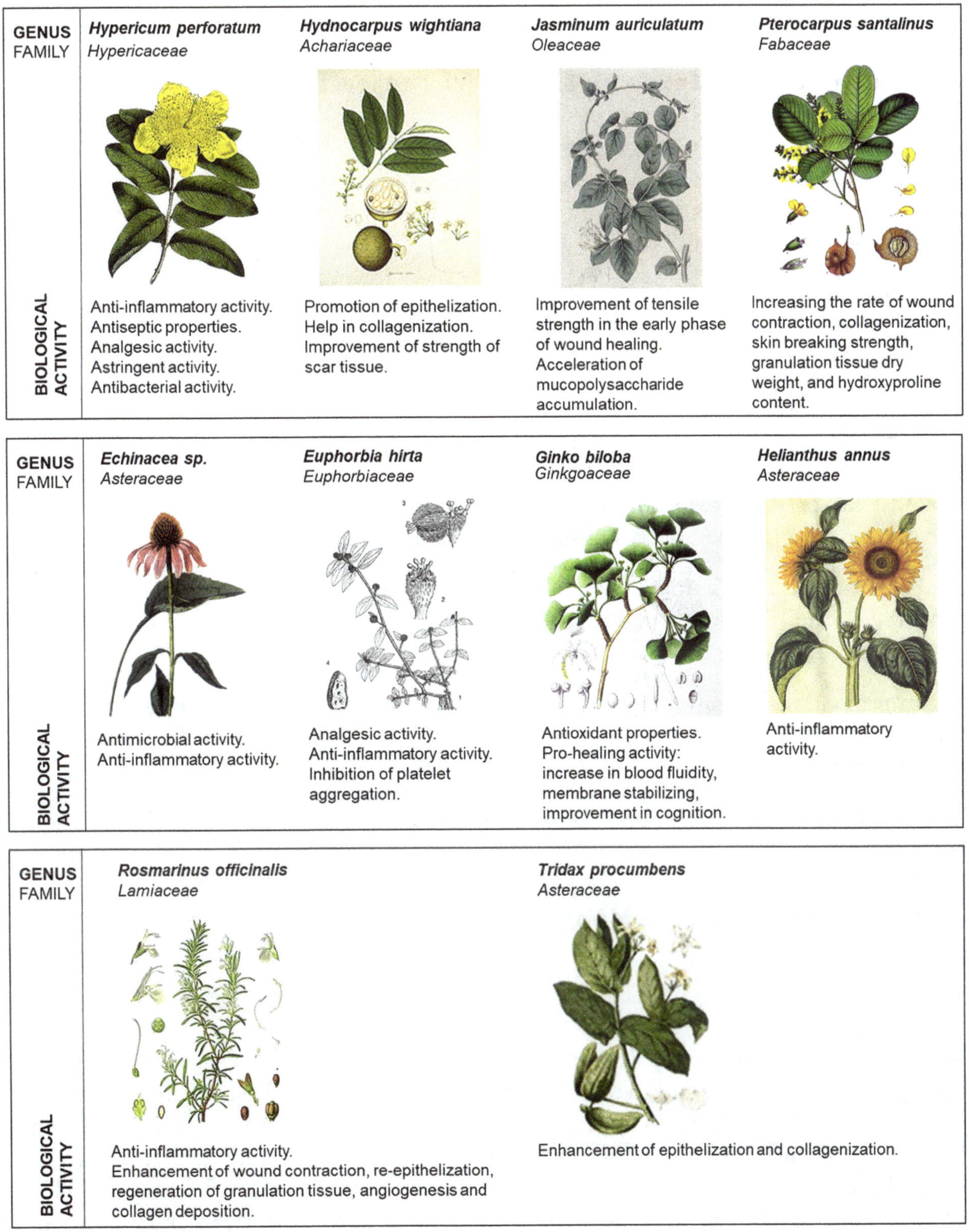

Figure 5. Overview of medical plants traditionally used in wound healing and their pharmacological activities (all plant images were obtained using the Google search engine with the enabled option for 'free use, share and modify').

Hydnocarpus wightiana (Family: *Achariaceae*). The oil from chaulmoogra seeds has been widely used in Indian and Chinese traditional medicine [159]. The wound healing effect is substantiated by improved collagenation and strength of scar tissue, as well as by promoted epithelization [160].

Hypericum perforatum (Family: *Hypericaceae*). Under its traditional names St. John's Wort, this plant has a long history of safe and effective use as part of various folk and herbal remedies. With proven anti-inflammatory [39], antiseptic [161], analgesic, astringent and antibacterial activities [43], it seems an ideal candidate for use in wound treatment. The latter has been confirmed also in different studies, which include its healing promoting action, when used externally on minor wounds [162], as well as through the positive effects of *Hypericum perforatum* tincture on epithelization, an increase in the wound contraction rate and an improved granulation tissue breaking strength [163].

Jasminum auriculatum (Family: *Oleaceae*). The juice of the leaves of *Jasminum auriculatum* was found to promote wound healing through improved tensile strength in the early phase of healing [164] and due to acceleration of mucopolysaccharide accumulation [165].

Pterocarpus santalinus (Family: *Fabaceae*). The wood of the red sanders possesses astringent and tonic properties. Ethanolic extract of the leaf and stem bark of *Pterocarpus santalinus* has demonstrated significant decrease in the period of epithelialisation, an increase: in the rate of wound contraction, the extent of collagenation, in the skin breaking strength, of the granulation tissue dry weight, and of the hydroxyproline content [38].

Rosmarinus officinalis (Family: *Lamiaceae*). Rosemary is used for wound treatment. It reduces inflammation and enhances wound contraction, re-epithelization, and regeneration of granulation tissue, angiogenesis and collagen deposition [40].

Tridax procumbens (Family: *Asteraceae*). The juice of *Tridax procumbens* promotes wound healing by accelerating epithelization and collagenization, resulting in the retardation of scar formation and granulation [166].

Figure 5 presents a summary of plants with proven beneficial effect on wound healing.

6. Outlook and future development

There are many challenges in relation to the potential future use phytochemicals in wound treatment. These are not the same as in the case of use of phytochemicals for other indications, but are still related to the respective compound/extract solubility, biocompatibility with the respective cells of the targeted tissue (in this case the skin with all its components), as well as the lack of preclinical and clinical studies related to its safety and efficiency testing. Poor bioavailability, which is often a limiting factor in the use of phytochemical for other purpose, is mostly not relevant for the case of wound treatment, where were mostly a local activity is enough. Of course, a successful elucidation of molecular targets and mechanisms of phytochemicals is the target for future research. Extensive knowledge about the preclinical performance of extracts, isolated and specific compounds is a prerequisite for successful pre-formulation studies and development of effective materials and prototype products with a high possibility to reach the patient in the near future.

The chemo-preventive properties of many phytochemicals are well known and have been already proven beneficial in treating various disorders, including skin diseases. Different phytochemicals can contribute to the skin protective mechanisms by quenching free radicals and reducing inflammation through the inhibition of cellular and humoral immune responses. In the last decades, several strong research groups performed extensive research with the aim of identifying specific compounds from plant extracts and their molecular targets. This will provide a sound foundation for future clinical trials in the development of phytochemicals as potentially important therapeutic agents.

7. Conclusions

Various plants produce secondary metabolites and other products that have beneficial effects on wound healing, including the enhancement of the skins natural repair mechanisms. Due to the possibility to produce different plant preparations for topical use, these have a huge potential in future therapeutic approach in wound care. Recent developments of novel extraction technologies, newly found knowledge about traditional use of various plants, as well as our steadily improving knowledge about wound healing physiology importantly contribute to the popularization of studies of herbs and herbal materials from the physiological and therapeutic point of view. This in turn contributes also to a steadily increasing number of herbal products for wound treatment. Considering also the increasing number of clinical studies related to the safety and therapeutic efficacy of herbal products, many more herbs have a bright future either in curative or preventative uses in wound healing. Based on our present knowledge, future studies should aim at the isolation and identification of specific active substances from plant extracts, which could also disclose compounds with better therapeutic value. Finally, the combination of traditional and modern knowledge seems to be the best approach to produce novel effective therapeutic interventions for wound healing with a significantly improved treatment efficacy, lowered side effects and costs.

Acknowledgements

The authors acknowledge the financial support from the Slovenian Research Agency for research core funding No. P2-0118 and P3-0036, and for the financial support through the projects No. Z2-8168 and J2-7413.

Author details

Tina Maver[1], Manja Kurečič[1,2], Dragica Maja Smrke[3], Karin Stana Kleinschek[1,2] and Uroš Maver[4,5]*

*Address all correspondence to: uros.maver@um.si

1 Faculty of Mechanical Engineering, Laboratory for Characterisation and Processing of Polymers, University of Maribor, Maribor, Slovenia

2 Institute for Chemistry and Technology of Materials, Graz University of Technology, Graz, Austria

3 University Medical Centre Ljubljana, Ljubljana, Slovenia

4 Faculty of Medicine, Institute of Biomedical Sciences and Institute for Palliative Medicine and Care, University of Maribor, Maribor, Slovenia

5 Faculty of Medicine, Department of Pharmacology, University of Maribor, Maribor, Slovenia

References

[1] Zhang Z, Michniak-Kohn BB. Tissue engineered human skin equivalents. Pharmaceutics. 2012;**4**(1):26-41

[2] QY X, Yang JS, Yang L, Wang YY. Effects of different scraping techniques on body surface blood perfusion volume and local skin temperature of healthy subjects. Journal of traditional Chinese medicine. 2011;**31**(4):316-320

[3] Wang J, Windbergs M. Functional electrospun fibers for the treatment of human skin wounds. European Journal of Pharmaceutics and Biopharmaceutics. 2017;**119**:283-299

[4] Boateng J, Catanzano O. Advanced therapeutic dressings for effective wound healing – A review. Journal of Pharmaceutical Sciences. 2015;**104**(11):3653-3680

[5] Young A, McNaught C-E. The physiology of wound healing. Surgery (Medicine Publishing). 2011;**29**(10):475-479

[6] Cordeiro JV, Jacinto A. The role of transcription-independent damage signals in the initiation of epithelial wound healing. Nature Reviews Molecular Cell Biology. 2013;**14**(4):249

[7] Gantwerker EA, Hom DB. Skin: Histology and physiology of wound healing. Clinics in Plastic Surgery. 2012;**39**(1):85-97

[8] Vukelic S, Stojadinovic O, Pastar I, Rabach M, Krzyzanowska A, Lebrun E, et al. Cortisol synthesis in epidermis is induced by IL-1 and tissue injury. Journal of Biological Chemistry. 2011;**286**(12):10265-10275

[9] Midwood KS, Williams LV, Schwarzbauer JE. Tissue repair and the dynamics of the extracellular matrix. The International Journal of Biochemistry & Cell Biology. 2004; **36**(6):1031-1037

[10] Rieger KA, Birch NP, Schiffman JD. Designing electrospun nanofiber mats to promote wound healing – A review. Journal of Materials Chemistry B. 2013;**1**(36):4531-4541

[11] Myers KA, Marshall RD, Freidin J. Principles of Pathology in Surgery. Boston: Oxford; (Blackwell Scientific: St. Louis, Mo.: Blackwell Mosby Book Distributors). 1980

[12] Maver T, Gradišnik L, Kurečič M, Hribernik S, Smrke DM, Maver U, et al. Layering of different materials to achieve optimal conditions for treatment of painful wounds. International Journal of Pharmaceutics. 2017;**529**(1-2):576-588

[13] Maver T, Maver U, Mostegel F, Grieser T, Spirk S, Smrke D, et al. Cellulose based thin films as a platform for drug release studies to mimick wound dressing materials. Cellulose. 2015;**22**:749-761

[14] Boateng JS, Matthews KH, Stevens HN, Eccleston GM. Wound healing dressings and drug delivery systems: A review. Journal of Pharmaceutical Sciences. 2008;**97**(8):2892-2923

[15] Thomson PD. Immunology, microbiology, and the recalcitrant wound. Ostomy Wound Manage. 2000;**46**(1A Suppl):77S-82S; quiz 3S-4S

[16] Pierce GF. Inflammation in nonhealing diabetic wounds: The space-time continuum does matter. American Journal of Pathology. 2001;**159**(2):399-403

[17] Della Loggia R, Tubaro A, Sosa S, Becker H, Saar S, Isaac O. The role of triterpenoids in the topical anti-inflammatory activity of *Calendula officinalis* flowers. Planta Medica. 1994;**60**(6):516-520

[18] Rijswik L, Harding K, Bacilious N. Issues and clinical implications. Ostomy Wound Management. 2000;**46**:11

[19] de Jonge SW, Boldingh QJJ, Solomkin JS, Allegranzi B, Egger M, Dellinger EP, et al. Systematic review and meta-analysis of randomized controlled trials evaluating prophylactic intra-operative wound irrigation for the prevention of surgical site infections. Surgical Infections. 2017;**18**(4):508-519

[20] Sibbald RG, Orsted H, Schultz GS, Coutts P, Keast D, International Wound Bed Preparation Advisory Board, The Canadian Chronic Wound Advisory Board. Preparing the wound bed 2003: Focus on infection and inflammation. Ostomy/Wound Management. 2003;**49**(11):24-51

[21] Faoagali J. Use of antiseptics in managing difficult wounds. Primary Intention. 1999;**7**:156-160

[22] McGuire L, Heffner K, Glaser R, Needleman B, Malarkey W, Dickinson S, et al. Pain and wound healing in surgical patients. Annals of behavioral medicine. 2006;**31**(2):165-172

[23] Price P, Fogh K, Glynn C, Krasner DL, Osterbrink J, Sibbald RG. Why combine a foam dressing with ibuprofen for wound pain and moist wound healing? International Wound Journal. 2007;**4**(Suppl 1):1-3

[24] Pediani R. What has pain relief to do with acute surgical wound healing. World Wide Wounds. 2001;**50**(2):76

[25] Babior BM. Oxygen-dependent microbial killing by phagocytes (second of two parts). The New England Journal of Medicine. 1978;**298**(13):721-725

[26] Yeoh S. The influence of iron and free radicals on chronic leg ulceration. Primary Intention. 2000;**8**:47-55

[27] Sibbald RG, Williamson D, Orsted HL, Campbell K, Keast D, Krasner D, et al. Preparing the wound bed – Debridement, bacterial balance, and moisture balance. Ostomy/Wound Management 2000;**46**(11):14-22. 4-8, 30-5; quiz 6-7

[28] Benedek B, Kopp B, Melzig MF. *Achillea millefolium* L. s.l. – is the anti-inflammatory activity mediated by protease inhibition? Journal of Ethnopharmacology. 2007;**113**(2):312-317

[29] Schmidt JM, Greenspoon JS. Aloe Vera dermal wound gel is associated with a delay in wound-healing. Obstetrics and Gynecology. 1991;**78**(1):115-117

[30] Laekeman G, Vlietinck A. Assesment Report on *Avena sativa* L., Herba and *Avena sativa* L., Fructus. London, UK: European Medicines Agency; 2008. Contract No.: EMEA/HMPC/202967/2007

[31] Ilango K, Maharajan G, Narasimhan S. Anti-nociceptive and anti-inflammatory activities of *Azadirachta indica* fruit skin extract and its isolated constituent azadiradione. Natural Product Research. 2013;**27**(16):1463-1467

[32] Jimenez-Medina E, Garcia-Lora A, Paco L, Algarra I, Collado A, Garrido FA. New extract of the plant *Calendula officinalis* produces a dual in vitro effect: Cytotoxic anti-tumor activity and lymphocyte activation. BMC Cancer. 2006;**6**:119

[33] Coppen JJW, Food, Agriculture Organization of the United Nations. Flavours and Fragrances of Plant Origin. Rome: Food and Agriculture Organization of the United Nations; 1995

[34] Petronilho S, Maraschin M, Coimbra MA, Rocha SM. In vitro and in vivo studies of natural products: A challenge for their valuation. The case study of chamomile (*Matricaria recutita* L.). Industrial Crops and Products. 2012;**40**:1-12

[35] Barnes J, Anderson LA, Phillipson JD. Herbal Medicines. London; Grayslake, IL: Pharmaceutical Press; 2007

[36] Kumar A, Sharma VK, Singh HP, Prakash P, Singh SP. Efficacy of some indigenous drugs in tissue-repair in buffalos. Indian Veterinary Journal. 1993;**70**(1):42

[37] Merali S, Binns S, Paulin-Levasseur M, Ficker C, Smith M, Baum B, et al. Antifungal and anti-inflammatory activity of the genus Echinacea. Pharmaceutical Biology. 2003;**41**(6):412-420

[38] Nagori BP, Solanki R. Role of medical plants in wound healing. Research Journal of Medicinal Plant. 2011;**5**(4):392-405

[39] Sosa S, Pace R, Bornancin A, Morazzoni P, Riva A, Tubaro A, et al. Topical anti-inflammatory activity of extracts and compounds from *Hypericum perforatum* L. Journal of Pharmacy and Pharmacology. 2007;**59**(5):703-709

[40] Abu-Al-Basal MA. Healing potential of *Rosmarinus officinalis* L. on full-thickness excision cutaneous wounds in alloxan-induced-diabetic BALB/c mice. Journal of Ethnopharmacology. 2010;**131**(2):443-450

[41] Hook IL. Danggui to *Angelica sinensis* root: Are potential benefits to European women lost in translation? A review. Journal of Ethnopharmacology. 2014;**152**(1):1-13

[42] Binns SE, Purgina B, Bergeron C, Smith ML, Ball L, Baum BR, et al. Light-mediated antifungal activity of Echinacea extracts. Planta Medica. 2000;**66**(3):241-244

[43] Gibbons S, Ohlendorf B, Johnsen I. The genus Hypericum – A valuable resource of anti-staphylococcal leads. Fitoterapia. 2002;**73**(4):300-304

[44] European Scientific Cooperative on Phytotherapy. E/S/C/O/P Monographs: The Scientific Foundation for Herbal Medicinal Products. Exeter, UK; Stuttgart, Germany; New York: European Scientific Cooperative on Phytotherapy; Thieme; 2003

[45] Bairy K, Rao C. Wound healing profiles of *Ginkgo biloba*. Journal of Natural Remedies. 2001;**1**(1):25-27

[46] De Smet PA. The role of plant-derived drugs and herbal medicines in healthcare. Drugs. 1997;**54**(6):801-840

[47] Maver T, Maver U, Stana Kleinschek K, Smrke DM, Kreft SA. Review of herbal medicines in wound healing. International Journal of Dermatology. 2015;**54**(7):740-751

[48] Ekor M. The growing use of herbal medicines: Issues relating to adverse reactions and challenges in monitoring safety. Frontiers in Pharmacology. 2013;**4**:177

[49] Gupta N, Jain UK. Prominent wound healing properties of indigenous medicines. Journal of Natural Pharmaceuticals. 2010;**1**(1):2-13

[50] Smetanska I. Production of secondary metabolites using plant cell cultures. Advances in Biochemical Engineering/Biotechnology. 2008;**111**:187-228

[51] Bartwal A, Mall R, Lohani P, Guru S, Arora S. Role of secondary metabolites and brassinosteroids in plant defense against environmental stresses. Journal of Plant Growth Regulation. 2013;**32**(1):216-232

[52] Rao SR, Ravishankar GA. Plant cell cultures: Chemical factories of secondary metabolites. Biotechnology Advances. 2002;**20**(2):101-153

[53] Wink M. Evolution of secondary metabolites from an ecological and molecular phylogenetic perspective. Phytochemistry. 2003;**64**(1):3-19

[54] Wink M. Introduction: Biochemistry, physiology and ecological functions of secondary metabolites. In: Annual Plant Reviews. Vol. 40. Biochemistry of Plant Secondary Metabolism. 2nd ed. Wiley-Blackwell. 2010. pp. 1-19

[55] Działo M, Mierziak J, Korzun U, Preisner M, Szopa J, Kulma A. The potential of plant phenolics in prevention and therapy of skin disorders. International Journal of Molecular Sciences. 2016;**17**(2):160

[56] Ganesan K, Xu B. A critical review on polyphenols and health benefits of black soybeans. Nutrients. 2017;**9**(5):455-472

[57] Rimbach G, Melchin M, Moehring J, Wagner AE. Polyphenols from cocoa and vascular health – A critical review. International Journal of Molecular Sciences. 2009;**10**(10):4290-4309

[58] Shaw JC. Green tea polyphenols may be useful in the treatment of androgen-mediated skin disorders. Archives of Dermatology. 2001;**137**(5):664

[59] Saric S, Notay M, Sivamani RK. Green tea and other tea polyphenols: Effects on sebum production and acne vulgaris. Antioxidants (Basel). 2016;**6**(1):2-18

[60] Vittorio O, Curcio M, Cojoc M, Goya GF, Hampel S, Iemma F, et al. Polyphenols delivery by polymeric materials: Challenges in cancer treatment. Drug Delivery. 2017;**24**(1):162-180

[61] Kostyuk VA, Potapovich AI, Lulli D, Stancato A, De Luca C, Pastore S, et al. Modulation of human keratinocyte responses to solar UV by plant polyphenols as a basis for chemoprevention of non-melanoma skin cancers. Current Medicinal Chemistry. 2013;**20**(7):869-879

[62] Dai J, Mumper RJ. Plant phenolics: Extraction, analysis and their antioxidant and anticancer properties. Molecules. 2010;**15**(10):7313

[63] Terahara N. Flavonoids in foods: A review. Natural Product Communications. 2015;**10**(3):521-528

[64] Srivastava JK, Gupta S. Extraction, characterization, stability and biological activity of flavonoids isolated from chamomile flowers. Molecular and Cellular Pharmacology. 2009;**1**(3):138

[65] Santos-Buelga C, Mateus N, De Freitas V. Anthocyanins. Plant Pigments and Beyond. Journal of Agricultural and Food Chemistry. 2014;**62**(29):6879-6884

[66] Hughes SD, Ketheesan N, Haleagrahara N. The therapeutic potential of plant flavonoids on rheumatoid arthritis. Critical Reviews in Food Science and Nutrition. 2017;**57**(17):3601-3613

[67] Salaritabar A, Darvishi B, Hadjiakhoondi F, Manayi A, Sureda A, Nabavi SF, et al. Therapeutic potential of flavonoids in inflammatory bowel disease: A comprehensive review. World Journal of Gastroenterology. 2017;**23**(28):5097-5114

[68] Nijveldt RJ, van Nood E, van Hoorn DE, Boelens PG, van Norren K, van Leeuwen PA. Flavonoids: A review of probable mechanisms of action and potential applications. The American Journal of Clinical Nutrition. 2001;**74**(4):418-425

[69] Peluso I, Miglio C, Morabito G, Ioannone F, Serafini M. Flavonoids and immune function in human: A systematic review. Critical Reviews in Food Science and Nutrition. 2015;**55**(3):383-395

[70] Kumar S, Pandey AK. Chemistry and biological activities of flavonoids: An overview. The Scientific World Journal. 2013;**2013**:1-16

[71] Pallauf K, Duckstein N, Rimbach G. A literature review of flavonoids and lifespan in model organisms. The Proceedings of the Nutrition Society. 2017;**76**(2):145-162

[72] Chen X, Mukwaya E, Wong MS, Zhang Y. A systematic review on biological activities of prenylated flavonoids. Pharmaceutical Biology. 2014;**52**(5):655-660

[73] Sak K. Epidemiological evidences on dietary flavonoids and breast cancer risk: A narrative review. Asian Pacific Journal of Cancer Prevention. 2017;**18**(9):2309-2328

[74] Manach C, Scalbert A, Morand C, Remesy C, Jimenez L. Polyphenols: Food sources and bioavailability. The American Journal of Clinical Nutrition. 2004;**79**(5):727-747

[75] Le Floch A, Jourdes M, Teissedre P-L. Polysaccharides and lignin from oak wood used in cooperage: Composition, interest, assays: A review. Carbohydrate Research. 2015; **417**(Supplement C):94-102

[76] Heleno SA, Martins A, Queiroz MJ, Ferreira IC. Bioactivity of phenolic acids: Metabolites versus parent compounds: A review. Food Chemistry. 2015;**173**:501-513

[77] Okuda T, Ito H. Tannins of constant structure in medicinal and food plants – Hydrolyzable tannins and polyphenols related to tannins. Molecules. 2011;**16**(3):2191

[78] Stervbo U, Vang O, Bonnesen C. A review of the content of the putative chemopreventive phytoalexin resveratrol in red wine. Food Chemistry. 2007;**101**(2):449-457

[79] Pisseri F, Bertoli A, Pistelli L. Essential oils in medicine: Principles of therapy. Parassitologia. 2008;**50**(1-2):89-91

[80] Ali B, Al-Wabel NA, Shams S, Ahamad A, Khan SA, Anwar F. Essential oils used in aromatherapy: A systemic review. Asian Pacific Journal of Tropical Biomedicine. 2015; **5**(8):601-611

[81] Tongnuanchan P, Benjakul S. Essential oils: Extraction, bioactivities, and their uses for food preservation. Journal of Food Science. 2014;**79**(7):R1231-R1R49

[82] Woollard AC, Tatham KC, Barker S. The influence of essential oils on the process of wound healing: A review of the current evidence. Journal of Wound Care. 2007;**16**(6):255-257

[83] Cavanagh HM, Wilkinson JM. Biological activities of lavender essential oil. Phytotherapy Research. 2002;**16**(4):301-308

[84] Kane FM, Brodie EE, Coull A, Coyne L, Howd A, Milne A, et al. The analgesic effect of odour and music upon dressing change. British Journal of Nursing. 2004;**13**(Suppl 4):S4-S12

[85] Hartman D, Coetzee JC. Two US practitioners' experience of using essential oils for wound care. Journal of Wound Care. 2002;**11**(8):317-320

[86] Glowania HJ, Raulin C, Swoboda M. Effect of chamomile on wound healing-a clinical double-blind study. Zeitschrift für Hautkrankheiten. 1987;**62**(17):1262 7-71

[87] McKay DL, Blumberg JBA. Review of the bioactivity and potential health benefits of chamomile tea (*Matricaria recutita* L.). Phytotherapy Research. 2006;**20**(7):519-530

[88] Halcón L, Milkus K. *Staphylococcus aureus* and wounds: A review of tea tree oil as a promising antimicrobial. American Journal of Infection Control. 2004;**32**(7):402-408

[89] Hammer KA, Carson CF, Riley TV. Susceptibility of transient and commensal skin flora to the essential oil of *Melaleuca alternifolia* (tea tree oil). American Journal of Infection Control. 1996;**24**(3):186-189

[90] Sherry E, Boeck H, Warnke PH. Percutaneous treatment of chronic MRSA osteomyelitis with a novel plant-derived antiseptic. BMC Surgery. 2001;**1**:1

[91] Faoagali J, George N, Leditschke JF. Does tea tree oil have a place in the topical treatment of burns? Burns. 1997;**23**(4):349-351

[92] Farnan TB, McCallum J, Awa A, Khan AD, Hall SJ. Tea tree oil: In vitro efficacy in otitis externa. The Journal of Laryngology & Otology. 2005;**119**(3):198-201

[93] Bozin B, Mimica-Dukic N, Simin N, Anackov G. Characterization of the volatile composition of essential oils of some Lamiaceae spices and the antimicrobial and antioxidant activities of the entire oils. Journal of Agricultural and Food Chemistry. 2006;**54**(5):1822-1828

[94] Shin S, Kim JH. Vitro inhibitory activities of essential oils from two Korean Thymus species against antibiotic-resistant pathogens. Archives of Pharmacal Research. 2005; **28**(8):897

[95] Giordani R, Regli P, Kaloustian J, Mikaïl C, Abou L, Portugal H. Antifungal effect of various essential oils against Candidaalbicans. Potentiation of antifungal action of amphotericin B by essential oil from Thymus Vulgaris. Phytotherapy Research. 2004;**18**(12):990-995

[96] Komarčević A. Modern approach to wound management. Medicinski Pregled. 2000;**53**(7-8): 363-368

[97] Orafidiya L, Agbani E, Abereoje O, Awe T, Abudu A, Fakoya F. An investigation into the wound-healing properties of essential oil of *Ocimum gratissimum* Linn. Journal of Wound Care. 2003;**12**(9):331-334

[98] Orafidiya LO, Oyedele AO, Shittu AO, Elujoba AA. The formulation of an effective topical antibacterial product containing *Ocimum gratissimum* leaf essential oil. International Journal of Pharmaceutics. 2001;**224**(1):177-183

[99] Singh S, Majumdar DK. Effect of *Ocimum sanctum* fixed oil on vascular permeability and leucocytes migration. Indian Journal of Experimental Biology. 1999;**37**(11):1136-1138

[100] Singh S. Mechanism of action of antiinflammatory effect of fixed oil of *Ocimum basilicum* Linn. Indian Journal of Experimental Biology. 1999;**37**(3):248-252

[101] Martins A, Salgueiro L, Goncalves M, da Cunha AP, Vila R, Canigueral S. Essential oil composition and antimicrobial activity of Santiria trimera bark. Planta Medica. 2003;**69**(01):77-79

[102] Lavagna SM, Secci D, Chimenti P, Bonsignore L, Ottaviani A, Bizzarri B. Efficacy of Hypericum and calendula oils in the epithelial reconstruction of surgical wounds in childbirth with caesarean section. Il Farmaco. 2001;**56**(5):451-453

[103] Kamath JV, Rana A, Roy Chowdhury A. Pro-healing effect of *Cinnamomum zeylanicum* bark. Phytotherapy Research. 2003;**17**(8):970-972

[104] Phan TT, Hughes MA, Cherry GW. Enhanced proliferation of fibroblasts and endothelial cells treated with an extract of the leaves of *Chromolaena odorata* (Eupolin), an herbal remedy for treating wounds. Plastic and Reconstructive Surgery. 1998;**101**(3):756-765

[105] Xu X, Li X, Zhang L, Liu Z, Pan Y, Chen D, et al. Enhancement of wound healing by the traditional Chinese medicine herbal mixture Sophora Flavescens in a rat model of perianal ulceration. In Vivo. 2017;**31**(4):543-549

[106] Jahandideh M, Hajimehdipoor H, Mortazavi SA, Dehpour A, Hassanzadeh GA. Wound healing formulation based on Iranian traditional medicine and its HPTLC fingerprint. Iranian Journal of Pharmaceutical Research. 2016;**15**(Suppl):149-157

[107] Biswas TK, Mukherjee B. Plant medicines of Indian origin for wound healing activity: A review. The International Journal of Lower Extremity Wounds. 2003;**2**(1):25-39

[108] Hoffmann D. Medical Herbalism: The Science and Practice of Herbal Medicine. Rochester, Vt.: Healing Arts Press; 2003. 666 p

[109] Numata A, Ibuka T. Chapter 6: Alkaloids from ants and other insects. In: Brossi A, editor. The Alkaloids: Chemistry and Pharmacology. Vol. 31. Academic Press, Elsevier, NL; 1987. pp. 193-315

[110] Cushnie TPT, Cushnie B, Lamb AJ. Alkaloids: An overview of their antibacterial, antibiotic-enhancing and antivirulence activities. International Journal of Antimicrobial Agents. 2014;**44**(5):377-386

[111] Qing Z-X, Huang J-L, Yang X-Y, Liu J-H, Cao H-L, Xiang F, Cheng P, Zeng J-G. Anticancer and reversing multidrug resistance activities of natural isoquinoline alkaloids and their structure-activity relationship. Current Medicinal Chemistry. 2017. DOI: 10.2174/0929867324666170920125135

[112] Sobarzo-Sanchez E, Soto PG, Valdes Rivera C, Sanchez G, Hidalgo ME. Applied biological and physicochemical activity of isoquinoline alkaloids: Oxoisoaporphine and boldine. Molecules. 2012;**17**(9):10958-10970

[113] Dunning T. Aromatherapy: Overview, safety and quality issues. OA alternative. Medicine. 2013;**1**(1):6

[114] Paiva LAF, de Alencar Cunha KM, Santos FA, Gramosa NV, Silveira ER, Rao VSN. Investigation on the wound healing activity of oleo-resin from *Copaifera langsdorffi* in rats. Phytotherapy Research. 2002;**16**(8):737-739

[115] Langenheim JH. Plant Resins: Oregon, etc. USA: Timber Press Inc.; 2003

[116] Wilson MB, Spivak M, Hegeman AD, Rendahl A, Cohen JD. Metabolomics reveals the origins of antimicrobial plant resins collected by honey bees. PLoS One. 2013;**8**(10):e77512

[117] Skalicka-Wozniak K, Garrard I. Counter-current chromatography for the separation of terpenoids: A comprehensive review with respect to the solvent systems employed. Phytochemistry Reviews. 2014;**13**:547-572

[118] Morikawa T, Matsuda H, Yoshikawa M. A review of anti-inflammatory Terpenoids from the incense gum resins frankincense and myrrh. Journal of Oleo Science. 2017; **66**(8):805-814

[119] Seo KH, Nam YH, Lee DY, Ahn EM, Kang TH, Baek NI. Recovery effect of phenylpropanoid glycosides from *Magnolia obovata* fruit on alloxan-induced pancreatic islet damage in zebrafish (Danio rerio). Carbohydrate Research. 2015;**416**:70-74

[120] Joshi S, Chanotiya CS, Agarwal G, Prakash O, Pant AK, Mathela CS. Terpenoid compositions, and antioxidant and antimicrobial properties of the rhizome essential oils of different Hedychium species. Chemistry & Biodiversity. 2008;**5**(2):299-309

[121] JJ L, Dang YY, Huang M, WS X, Chen XP, Wang YT. Anti-cancer properties of terpenoids isolated from Rhizoma Curcumae – A review. Journal of Ethnopharmacology. 2012;**143**(2):406-411

[122] Castilhos R, Grützmacher A, Coats J. Acute Toxicity and Sublethal Effects of Terpenoids and Essential Oils on the Predator *Chrysoperla externa* (Neuroptera: Chrysopidae). Neotropical Entomology. 2017. DOI: 10.1007/s13744-017-0547-6

[123] Cowan MM. Plant products as antimicrobial agents. Clinical Microbiology Reviews. 1999;**12**(4):564-582

[124] Clark AM. Natural products as a resource for new drugs. Pharmaceutical Research. 1996;**13**(8):1133-1141

[125] Zhang Y, Lewis K. Fabatins: New antimicrobial plant peptides. FEMS Microbiology Letters. 1997;**149**(1):59-64

[126] Sharon N. Lectins: Carbohydrate-specific reagents and biological recognition molecules. Journal of Biological Chemistry. 2007;**282**(5):2753-2764

[127] Estevez-Braun A, Estevez-Reyes R, Moujir L, Ravelo A, Gonzalez A. Antibiotic activity and absolute configuration of 8S-heptadeca-2 (Z), 9 (Z)-diene-4, 6-diyne-1, 8-diol from *Bupleurum salicifolium*. Journal of Natural Products. 1994;**57**(8):1178-1182

[128] Brandao MG, Krettli AU, Soares LS, Nery CG, Marinuzzi HC. Antimalarial activity of extracts and fractions from *Bidens pilosa* and other Bidens species (Asteraceae) correlated with the presence of acetylene and flavonoid compounds. Journal of Ethnopharmacology. 1997;**57**(2):131-138

[129] Budavari S. The Merck Index. Whitehouse Station, NJ; London: Merck; Stationery Office; 2000

[130] Caceres A, Cano O, Samayoa B, Aguilar L. Plants used in Guatemala for the treatment of gastrointestinal disorders. 1. Screening of 84 plants against enterobacteria. Journal of Ethnopharmacology. 1990;**30**(1):55-73

[131] Candan F, Unlu M, Tepe B, Daferera D, Polissiou M, Sokmen A, et al. Antioxidant and antimicrobial activity of the essential oil and methanol extracts of *Achillea millefolium* subsp. millefolium Afan. (Asteraceae). Journal of Ethnopharmacology. 2003;**87**(2-3): 215-220

[132] Goldberg AS, Mueller EC, Eigen E, Desalva SJ. Isolation of the anti-inflammatory principles from *Achillea millefolium* (Compositae). Journal of Pharmaceutical Sciences. 1969;**58**(8):938-941

[133] Bruster S, Jarman B, Bosanquet N, Weston D, Erens R, Delbanco TL. National survey of hospital patients. British Medical Journal. 1994;**309**(6968):1542-1546

[134] Davis RH, Leitner MG, Russo JM, Maro NP. Biological-activity of Aloe-Vera. Medical Science Research-Biochemistry. 1987;**15**(5-6):235

[135] Zhao H, Deneau J, Che GO, Li S, Vagnini F, Azadi P, et al. *Angelica sinensis* isolate SBD.4: Composition, gene expression profiling, mechanism of action and effect on wounds, in rats and humans. European Journal of Dermatology. 2012;**22**(1):58-67

[136] Laekeman G, Vlietinck A. Assessment Report on *Avena Sativa* L. Herba and Avena Sativa L, Fructus London: European Medicines Agency. 2008. pp. 11-12

[137] Fabre B. *Avena sativa,* demande d'inscription en usage topique. Pierre Fabre Innovation Developpement. Concept paper; 2004

[138] Raina R, Parwez S, Verma P, Pankaj N. Medicinal plants and their role in wound healing. Online Veterinary J. 2008;**3**:21

[139] Janssen A, Chin N, Scheffer J, Svendsen A. Screening for antimicrobial activity of some essential oils by the agar overlay technique. Pharmacy World & Science. 1986;**8**(6): 289-292

[140] Tarle D, Dvorzak I. Antimicrobial substances in Flos Calendulae. Farmacevtski Vestnik. 1989;**40**:117-120

[141] Duran V, Matic M, Jovanovc M, Mimica N, Gajinov Z, Poljacki M, et al. Results of the clinical examination of an ointment with marigold (*Calendula officinalis*) extract in the treatment of venous leg ulcers. International Journal of Tissue Reactions. 2005;**27**(3):101-106

[142] Blumenthal M, Busse WR, Bundesinstitut für Arzneimittel und Medizinprodukte. The complete German Commission E monographs, therapeutic guide to herbal medicines. Austin, Tex.; Boston: American Botanical Council; Integrative Medicine Communications; 1998

[143] Vishnu RG, Shivakumar H, Parthasarathi G. Influence of aqueous extract of *Centella asiatica* (Brahmi) on experimental wounds in albino rats. Indian Journal of Pharmacology. 1996;**28**(4):249

[144] Suguna L, Sivakumar P, Chandrakasan G. Effects of *Centella asiatica* extract on dermal wound healing in rats. Indian Journal of Experimental Biology. 1996;**34**(12):1208-1211

[145] Shukla A, Rasik AM, Jain GK, Shankar R, Kulshrestha DK, Dhawan BN. In vitro and in vivo wound healing activity of asiaticoside isolated from *Centella asiatica.* Journal of Ethnopharmacology. 1999;**65**(1):1-11

[146] Srivastava JK, Shankar E, Gupta S. Chamomile: A herbal medicine of the past with bright future. Molecular Medicine Reports. 2010;**3**(6):895-901

[147] Phan TT, Allen J, Hughes MA, Cherry G, Wojnarowska F. Upregulation of adhesion complex proteins and fibronectin by human keratinocytes treated with an aqueous extract from the leaves of *Chromolaena odorata* (Eupolin). European Journal of Dermatology. 2000;**10**(7):522

[148] Anderberg K. Folk uses and history of medicinal uses of nettles. 2012 August 19. Available from: http://users.resist.ca/~kirstena/pagenettles.html

[149] Srimal RC, Khanna NM, Dhawan SA. Preliminary report on anti-inflammatory activity of curcumin. Indian Journal of Pharmacology. 1971;**3**:10

[150] Wishart DJ. Encyclopedia of the Great Plains Indians. Vol. viii. Lincoln: University of Nebraska Press; 2007. 252 p

[151] Bauer R, Foster S. Analysis of alkamides and caffeic acid derivatives from *Echinacea simulata* and *E. paradoxa* roots. Planta Medica. 1991;**57**(5):447-449

[152] Hostettmann K. Geschichte einer Pflanze am Beispiel von Echinacea. Forschende Komplementärmedizin und klassische Naturheilkunde = Research in Complementary and Natural Classical Medicine. 2003;**10**:9-12

[153] Reisch J, Spitzner W, Schulte KE. On the problem of the microbiological activity of simple acetylene compounds. Arzneimittel-Forschung. 1967;**17**(7):816-825

[154] Skwarek T, Tynecka Z, LGlowniak K, Lutostanska E. Echinacea – inducer of interferons. Herba Polonica. 1996;**42**:110-117

[155] Clifford LJ, Nair MG, Rana J, Dewitt DL. Bioactivity of alkamides isolated from *Echinacea purpurea* (L.) Moench. Phytomedicine. 2002;**9**(3):249-253

[156] Newall CA, Anderson LA, Phillipson JD. Herbal Medicines : A Guide for Health-Care Professionals. London: Pharmaceutical Press; 1996

[157] Jain SK, Tarafdar CR. Medicine plant love of Sautals (A review of P.O. Bodding's work). Economic Botany. 1970;**24**:241

[158] Deshpande PJ, Pathak SN, Shankaran PS. Healing of experimental wounds with *Helianthus annus*. The Indian Journal of Medical Research. 1965;**53**:539-544

[159] Norton SA. Useful plants of dermatology. I. Hydnocarpus and chaulmoogra. Journal of the American Academy of Dermatology. 1994;**31**(4):683-686

[160] Oommen ST. The effect of oil of hydnocarpus on excision wounds. International Journal of Leprosy and Other Mycobacterial Diseases. 2000;**68**(1):69-70

[161] Saddiqe Z, Naeem I, Maimoona A. A review of the antibacterial activity of *Hypericum perforatum* L. Journal of Ethnopharmacology. 2010;**131**(3):511-521

[162] Panossian AG, Gabrielian E, Manvelian V, Jurcic K, Wagner H. Immunosuppressive effects of hypericin on stimulated human leukocytes: Inhibition of the arachidonic acid release, leukotriene B4 and interleukin-Iα production, and activation of nitric oxide formation. Phytomedicine. 1996;**3**(1):19-28

[163] Aye R-D, Hamacher H. Selbstmedikation: Arzneimittelinformation und Beratung in der Apotheke. 2, [Grundwerk]. Stuttgart: Dt. Apotheker-Verl.; 2011

[164] Desphande PJ, Pathak SN. Effect of ghee medicated with *Jasminum auriculatum* on experimental wound. Indian Journal of Medical Research. 1966;**1**:81

[165] Desphande PJ, Pathak SN. Influence of juice of leaves of *Jasminum auriculatum* on experimental wounds in albino rats. Medical Surgery. 1966;**6**:21

[166] Diwan PV, Tilloo LD, Kulkarni DR. Steroid depressed wound healing and *Tridax procumbens*. Indian Journal of Physiology and Pharmacology. 1983;**27**(1):32-36

9

Plants Secondary Metabolites: The Key Drivers of the Pharmacological Actions of Medicinal Plants

Rehab A. Hussein and Amira A. El-Anssary

Abstract

The vast and versatile pharmacological effects of medicinal plants are basically dependent on their phytochemical constituents. Generally, the phytochemical constituents of plants fall into two categories based on their role in basic metabolic processes, namely primary and secondary metabolites. Primary plant metabolites are involved in basic life functions; therefore, they are more or less similar in all living cells. On the other hand, secondary plant metabolites are products of subsidiary pathways as the shikimic acid pathway. In the course of studying, the medicinal effect of herbals is oriented towards the secondary plant metabolites. Secondary plant metabolites played an important role in alleviating several aliments in the traditional medicine and folk uses. In modern medicine, they provided lead compounds for the production of medications for treating various diseases from migraine up to cancer. Secondary plant metabolites are classified according to their chemical structures into various classes. In this chapter, we will be presenting various classes of secondary plant metabolites, their distribution in different plant families and their important medicinal uses.

Keywords: secondary plant metabolites, phenolics, alkaloids, saponins, terpenes

1. Introduction

Plant chemistry is the basis of the therapeutic uses of herbs. A good knowledge of the chemical composition of plants leads to a better understanding of its possible medicinal value. Modern chemistry has described the role of primary plant metabolites in basic life functions such as cell division and growth, respiration, storage and reproduction. They include the components of processes such as glycolysis, the Krebs or citric acid cycle, photosynthesis and associated pathways. Primary metabolites include small molecules such as sugars, amino acids, tricarboxylic acids, or Krebs cycle intermediates, proteins, nucleic acids and polysaccharides. Eventually, the primary metabolites are similar in all living cells [1].

Secondary plant metabolites are numerous chemical compounds produced by the plant cell through metabolic pathways derived from the primary metabolic pathways. The concept of secondary metabolite was first defined by Albrecht Kossel, Nobel Prize winner for physiology or medicine in 1910 [2]. Thirty years later, Czapek described them as end-products [3]. According to him, these products are derived from nitrogen metabolism by what he called 'secondary modifications' such as deamination. In the middle of the twentieth century, advances of analytical techniques such as chromatography allowed the recovery of more and more of these molecules, and this was the basis for the establishment of the discipline of phytochemistry.

Secondary metabolites have shown to possess various biological effects, which provide the scientific base for the use of herbs in the traditional medicine in many ancient communities. They have been described as antibiotic, antifungal and antiviral and therefore are able to protect plants from pathogens. Besides, they constitute important UV absorbing compounds, thus preventing serious leaf damage from the light. It was noticed that some herbs as forage grasses such as clover or alfalfa can express estrogenic properties and interact with fertility of animals [4].

Secondary plant metabolites are classified according to their chemical structures into several classes. In this chapter, the nature of secondary plant metabolites will be discussed as a foundation for a review of the main categories of constituents considered to be of therapeutic importance. Each section includes an overview of a class of the secondary plant metabolites regarding structure, botanical distribution and generalizations about pharmacology, followed by examples of representative molecules. The classes of secondary plant metabolites include:

- Phenolics
- Alkaloids
- Saponins
- Terpenes
- Lipids
- Carbohydrates

2. Phenolics

Phenolics probably constitute the largest group of plant secondary metabolites. They share the presence of one or more phenol groups (**Figure 1**) as a common characteristic and range from simple structures with one aromatic ring to highly complex polymeric substances. They are widespread in plants where they contribute significantly to the color, taste and flavor of many herbs, foods and drinks. Some phenolics are valued pharmacologically for their

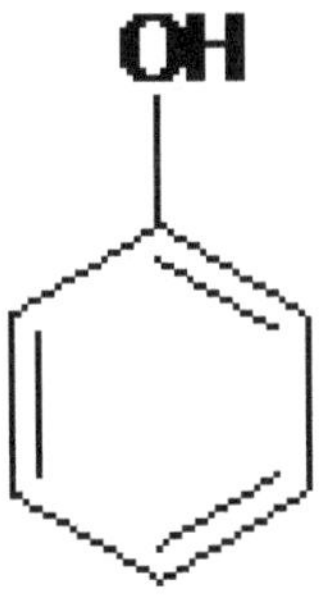

Figure 1. Phenol.

anti-inflammatory activities such as quercetin or antihepatotoxic properties such as silybin. Others exert phytoestrogenic activity as genistein and daidzein, while others are insecticidal as naringenin [5]. Many of the phenolic molecules are also effective antioxidants and free radical scavengers, especially flavonoids. Phenolics can be classified according to their structure or biosynthetic origin. According to their structures, phenolics can be classified into:

- Simple phenolics
- Tannins
- Coumarins
- Flavonoids
- Chromones and xanthones
- Stilbenes
- Lignans

2.1. Simple phenolics

Phenolic acids are ubiquitous among plants; although free phenols are rare, gallic acid is relatively widespread and is the parent compound of the gallotannins (**Figure 2**). Gallic acid is well known for its astringent properties but has demonstrated many other activities in vitro, including antibacterial, antiviral, antifungal, anti-inflammatory, antitumor, antianaphylactic, antimutagenic, choleretic and bronchodilatory actions. It also inhibits insulin degradation and promotes smooth muscle relaxation [6]. The phenolic compounds in this group vary according to their functional group, which may be hydroxyl, aldehydic, or carboxylic group; these include eugenol (a phenolic phenylpropane), vanillin (a phenolic aldehyde) and salicylic, ferulic and caffeic acids (phenolic acids). Hydroquinone is also among the most widely distributed of the simple phenols, occurring in a number of plants as the glycoside arbutin. Glycoside formation is common, and the widely distributed glycoside coniferin and other derivatives of phenolic cinnamic alcohols are precursors of lignin [7, 8].

The pharmacological properties of these widely found constituents are probably best demonstrated by the urinary tract antimicrobial arbutin [9] and the anti-inflammatory salicylates [10]. A property shared by all phenols is antimicrobial activity. In fact, phenol itself was the first antiseptic used in surgery [11].

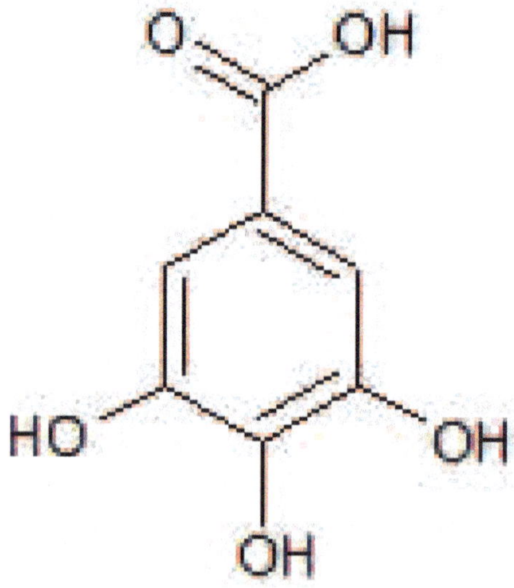

Figure 2. Gallic acid.

The pharmacological activities of many plants are attributed to simple phenolics among which the antimicrobial and diuretic activities of *Arctostaphylos uva-ursi* were attributed to its phenolic content [12]. *Capsicum* spp. showed circulatory stimulant, rubefacient and analgesic activities due to the presence of capsaicinoids, which are simple phenolic compounds [13]. Moreover, the cholagogue activity of *Cynara scolymus*, the anthelmintic activity of *Dryopteris filix-mas*, the anti-inflammatory analgesic activity of *Filipendula ulmaria* as well as the anticatarrhal and diuretic activities of *Solidago virgaurea* are all attributed to the action of simple phenolics [8]. **Figure 3** illustrates some examples of simple phenolics.

2.2. Tannins

Tannins are polyphenols which have the ability to precipitate protein. These compounds have been used for decades to convert raw animal hides into leather. In this process, tannin molecules crosslink the protein and make it more resistant to bacterial and fungal attack. Today, however, many substances considered to be tannins by virtue of their structure and biosynthetic origin have limited, if any, ability to make leather [14]. There are two major types of tannins: hydrolyzable tannins and condensed tannins. Hydrolyzable tannins are formed from several molecules of phenolic acids such as gallic and hexahydroxydiphenic acids, which are united by ester linkages to a central glucose molecule. Two principal types of hydrolysable tannins are gallotannins and ellagitannins, which are, respectively, composed of gallic acid and ellagic acid units. Ellagitannins found in plants of medicinal interest and for which structures have been elucidated include geraniin (isolated from *Geranium robertianum* (Herb Robert) and *Geranium maculatum* (American cranesbill) [15]) and tellimagrandins 1 and 2 [16] (isolated from *Quercus alba* (Oak bark), *Punica granatum* (pomegranate) and *Filipendula ulmaria* (Meadowsweet)) [7].

Condensed tannins, or proanthocyanidins, are compounds whose structures are based on oligomeric flavonoid precursors and vary in the type of linkages between flavonoid units; hydroxylation patterns; stereochemistry of carbons 2, 3 and 4 of the pyran ring and the

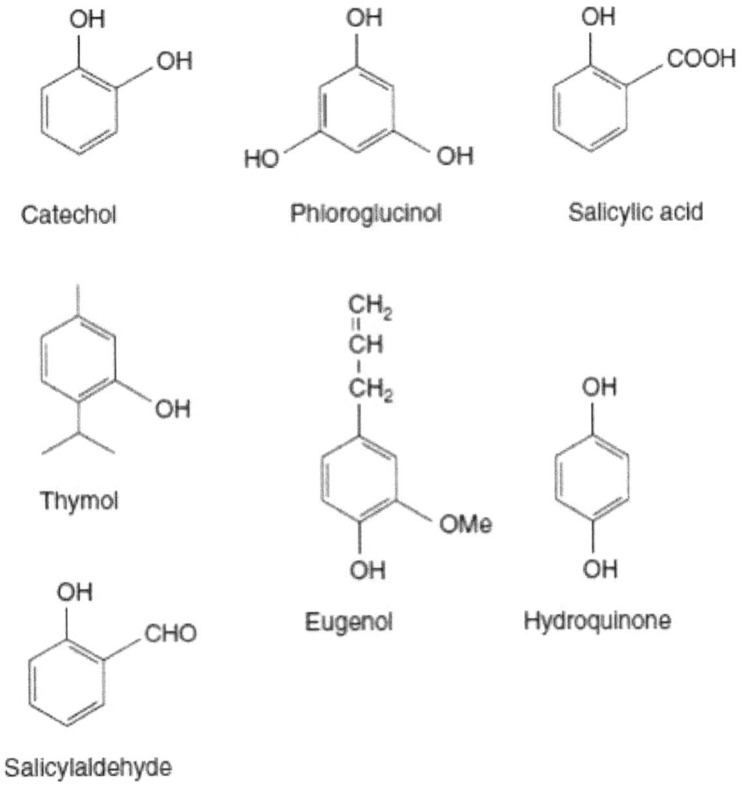

Figure 3. Examples of simple phenolics.

presence of additional substituents. Some drugs (e.g., *Camellia sinensis* (tea), *Hamamelis virginiana* leaves and bark) contain both hydrolyzable and condensed tannins [17].

Tannin-containing drugs act as antidiarrhoeals and have been employed as antidotes in poisoning by heavy metals and alkaloids. Epigallocatechin-3-gallate, the active principal in tea, has been shown to be antiangiogenic in mice. *Vaccinium oxycoccos* (cranberry) juice has long been used as urinary antiseptic [18], which was scientifically proven in a randomized, double-blind, placebo-controlled trial that has been carried out on 153 elderly women [19]. **Figure 4** illustrates some examples of hydrolysable tannins.

2.3. Coumarins

Coumarins are derivatives of benzo-α-pyrone, the lactone of *O*-hydroxycinnamic acid, coumarin. Some 1000 natural coumarins have been isolated. Coumarin itself has been found in about 150 species belonging to over 30 different families. The richest sources of coumarin are sweet clover or melilot (*Melilotus* spp.), *Dipteryx odorata* (tonka bean) and *Galium odoratum* (sweet woodruff) [8]. Aesculetin, umbelliferone and scopoletin are common coumarins present in plants both in the free state and as glycosides. Plants rich in coumarins include *Atropa belladonna, Datura stramonium* (Solanaceae), *Daphne mezereum* (Thymeliaceae), *Ruta graveolens* (Umbelliferae) and certain *Aesculus hippocastanum* (Horse-chestnut) (Hippocastanaceae) and certain Rosaceae [7]. Anti-inflammatory, anticoagulant, anticancer and anti-Alzheimer's activities are the most important biological activities reported for coumarins [20]. Examples of coumarins are shown in **Figure 5**.

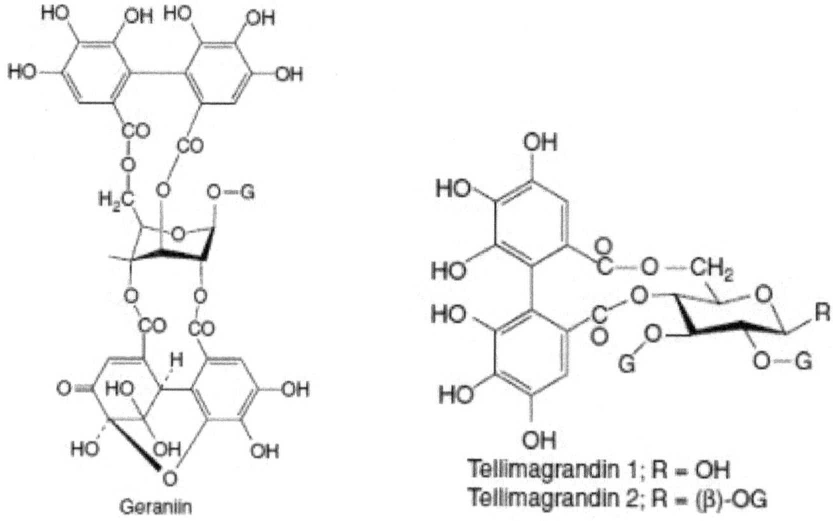

Figure 4. Examples of hydrolysable tannins.

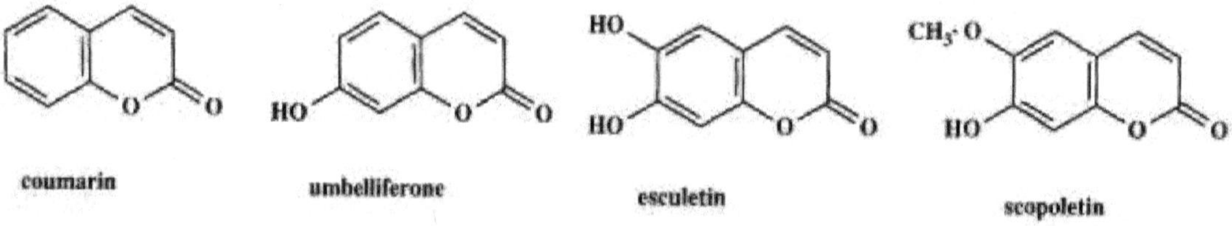

Figure 5. Examples of coumarins.

2.4. Flavonoids

Flavonoids are the largest group of naturally occurring phenols. More than 2000 of these compounds are now known, with nearly 500 occurring in the free state [7]. The structural skeleton of flavonoids includes a chroman ring bearing an aromatic ring in position 2, 3 or 4. Flavonoids may be divided into various classes according to the oxidation level of the central ring (ring C). The most common of these are anthocyanins, flavones and flavonols. The flavones and their close relations are often yellow (Latin *flavus*, yellow). They are widely distributed in nature but are more common in the higher plants and in young tissues, where they occur in the cell sap. They are abundant in the Polygonaceae, Rutaceae, Leguminosae, Umbelliferae and Compositae. Recent researches have demonstrated the medicinal action of drugs containing flavonoids such as *Glycyrrhiza glabra* (liquorice root), *Chamaemelum nobile* (Roman chamomile) and *Ginkgo biloba* (gingko). A number of flavonoid-containing herbs have now been included in the *British Pharmacopeia*, examples are *Betula pendula* (Birch Leaf), *Calendula officinalis* Flower, *Sambucus nigra* (ElderFlower), *Equisetum ramosissimum* (Horsetail), *Tilia cordata* (Lime Flower), *Leonurus cardiaca* (Motherwort) and *Passiflora edulis* (passion flower). The group is known for its anti-inflammatory and anti-allergic effects, for antithrombotic and vasoprotective properties, for inhibition of tumor promotion and as a protective for the gastric mucosa [21, 22]. Examples of flavonoids are shown in **Figure 6**.

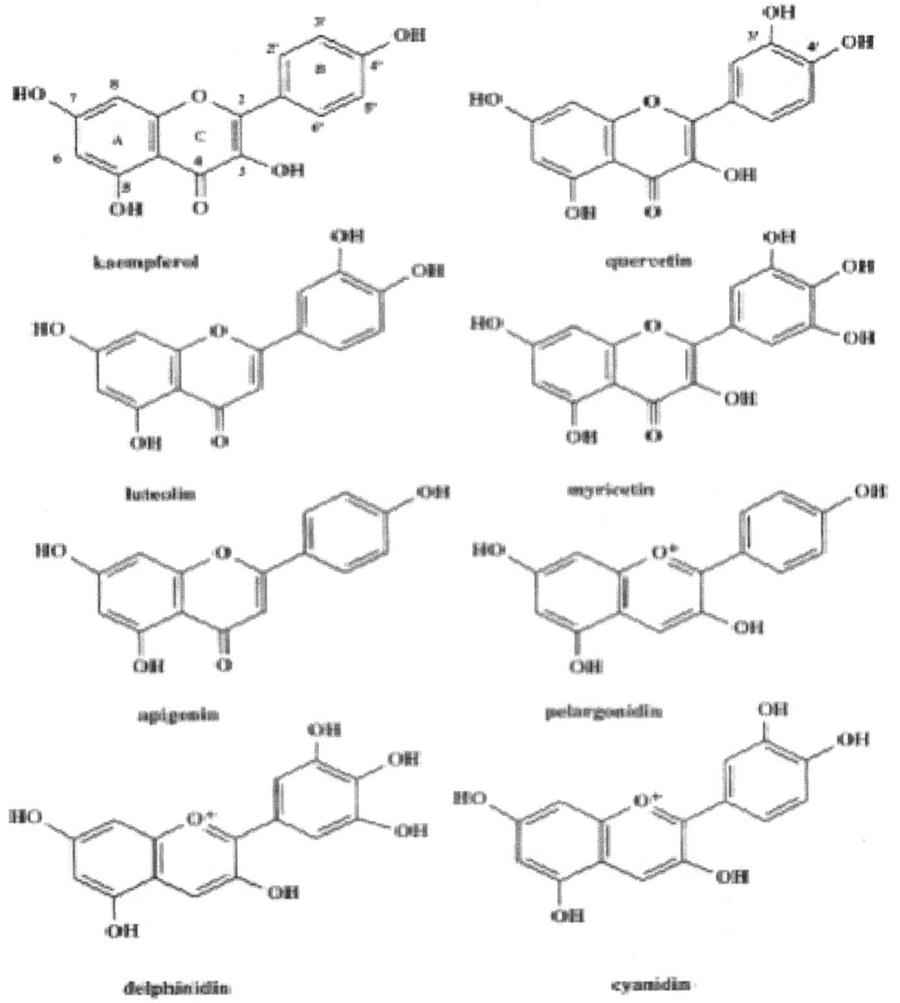

Figure 6. Examples of flavonoids.

2.5. Chromones and xanthones

These compounds are structural derivatives of benzo-γ-pyrone, and although not of great pharmaceutical importance, a few compounds are worthy of mention; eugenin is found in the clove plant and khellin from mustard seeds [7]. More complex are the furanochromones, the active constituents of the fruits of *Ammi visnaga*. Xanthones are found mainly in the Gentianaceae and Guttiferae, otherwise scattered sporadically throughout the plant kingdom as in the Moraceae and Polygalaceae. *Polygala nyikensis* is used by the highlanders of Malawi and bordering countries to treat various skin problems of fungal origin. The root of the plant was recently shown to exert its antifungal activity owing to the presence of xanthones [23].

2.6. Stilbenes

Stilbenes are a relatively small, but widely distributed, group of plant secondary metabolites found mostly as heartwood constituents in a heterogeneous assembly of plant species. They are especially important in the heartwood of trees of the genera *Pinus* (Pinaceae), *Eucalyptus*

(Myrtaceae) and *Madura* (Moraceae) [1]. The *para-hydroxylated* compound, resveratrol, is the most widespread stilbene in nature. Resveratrol possesses estrogen-like activity and occurs in *Picea*, *Pinus*, the Fabaceae, Myrtaceae and the Vitaceae [24].

2.7. Lignans

Lignans are dimeric compounds formed essentially by the union of two molecules of a phenylpropene derivative reported from the members of Asteraceae (e.g., *Achillea lingulata* [25]), Pinaceae (e.g., *Cedrus deodara* [26]) and Rutaceae (e.g., *Fagara heitzii*) [27]. Four major subtypes occur: dibenzylbutane derivatives, dibenzylbutryolactones (lignanolides or derivatives of butanolide), monoepoxy lignans or derivatives of tetrahydrofuran and bisepoxylignans or derivatives of 3,7-dioxabicyclo(3.3.0)-octane. Many of these compounds showed antimicrobial and antifungal activities [1], while others showed cytotoxic activities such as wikstromal, matairesinol and dibenzyl butyrolactol from *Cedrus deodara* [26].

3. Alkaloids

Alkaloids are organic compounds with at least one nitrogen atom in a heterocyclic ring. Their definition is problematic, as they do not represent a homogeneous group of compounds from any standpoint, whether chemical, biochemical, or physiological. Except for the fact that they are all nitrogen-containing compounds, no general definition fits all alkaloids. Alkaloids can be divided according to their basic chemical structure into different types. The following are basic types of alkaloids: acridones, aromatics, carbolines, ephedras, ergots, imidazoles, indoles, bisindoles, indolizidines, manzamines, oxindoles, quinolines, quinozolines, phenylisoquinolines, phenylethylamines, piperidines, purines, pyrrolidines, pyrrolizidines, pyrroloindoles, pyridines and simple tetrahydroisoquinolines [28].

Although plants containing alkaloids have been used by man for at least 3000 years as medicines, teas and potions, the compounds responsible for activity were not isolated and characterized until the nineteenth century [1]. Alkaloids are not common in lower plants. Lysergic acid derivatives and sulfur-containing alkaloids, e.g., the gliotoxins, are detected in fungi. Concerning the pteridophytes and gymnosperms alkaloids reported for their medicinal uses include the lycopodium, ephedra and *Taxus* alkaloids. Alkaloids are unevenly distributed among the angiosperms. The following are the orders reported to be rich in alkaloids: Centrospermae (Chenopodiaceae), Magnoliales (Lauraceae, Magnoliaceae), Ranunculales (Berberidaceae, Menispermaceae, Ranunculaceae), Papaverales (Papaveraceae, Fumariaceae), Rosales (Leguminosae, subfamily Papilionaceae), Rutales (Rutaceae), Gentiales (Apocynaceae, Loganiaceae, Rubiaceae), Tubiflorae (Boraginaceae, Convolvulaceae, Solanaceae) and Campanulales (Campanulaceae, sub-family Lobelioideae; Compositae, subfamily Senecioneae). However, there is no report for the presence of alkaloids in Salicales, Fagales, Cucurbitales and Oleales dicot orders till the present time [7].

Alkaloids demonstrate a diverse array of pharmacological actions including analgesia, local anesthesia, cardiac stimulation, respiratory stimulation and relaxation, vasoconstriction, muscle relaxation and toxicity, as well as antineoplastic, hypertensive and hypotensive properties. The activity of alkaloids against herbivores, toxicity in vertebrates, cytotoxic activity, the molecular targets of alkaloids, mutagenic or carcinogenic activity, antibacterial, antifungal, antiviral and allelopathic properties have been reported in literature. Many alkaloids are sufficiently toxic to animals to cause death if eaten. Several (e.g., nicotine and anabasine) are used as insecticides [1, 8].

Examples of some alkaloids:

3.1. Nicotine

Nicotine is found in the tobacco plant (*Nicotiana tabacum*) and other *Nicotiana* species; it has tranquilizing properties and is the addictive component of tobacco. It is also extremely toxic, causing respiratory paralysis at high doses (**Figure** 7). Nicotine is a ganglion cholinergic-receptor agonist with complex pharmacological actions, including effects mediated by binding to receptors in the autonomic ganglia, the adrenal medulla, the neuromuscular junction and the brain [29].

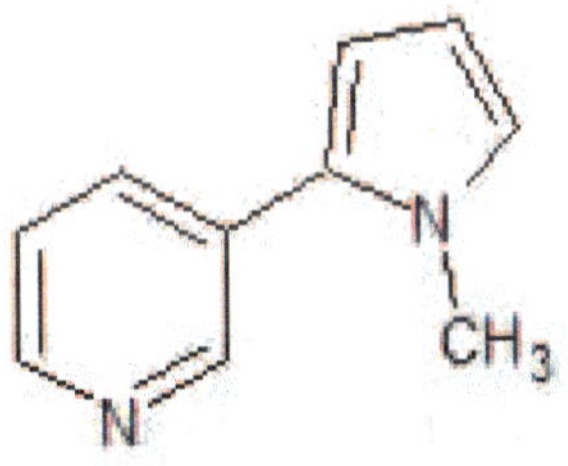

Nicotine

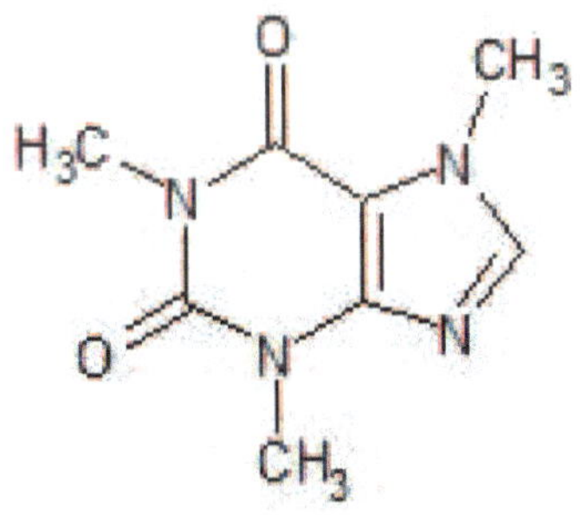

Caffeine

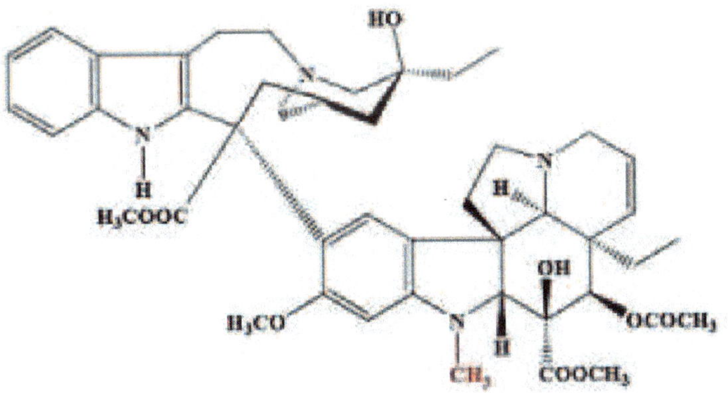

Vinblastine

Figure 7. Examples of alkaloids.

3.2. Caffeine

Caffeine occurs in a number of botanically unrelated species, including coffee (*Coffea* spp.), tea (*Camellia sinensis*), mate (*Ilex paraguariensis*), guarana (*Paullinia cupana*) and kola (*Cola acuminata*) (**Figure 7**). Caffeine is bound to chlorogenic acid in raw coffee beans. The roasting process liberates the caffeine and other compounds that contribute to the aroma of coffee. Caffeine is a diuretic and has stimulant effects on the respiratory, cardiovascular and central nervous systems [30].

3.3. Vinblastine

Vinblastine is isolated from *Catharanthus roseus* G. (**Figure 7**) and has been used to treat diabetes and high blood pressure and as disinfectant. Nevertheless, Vinblastine is so important for being cancer fighters. It is used along with the other vinca alkaloids vinorelbine, vincristine and vindesine, which are in clinical use in the United States and Europe [31].

4. Saponins

Saponins are compounds that possess a polycyclic aglycone moiety with either a steroid (steroidal saponins) or triterpenoid (triterpenoidal saponins) attached to a carbohydrate unit (a monosaccharide or oligosaccharide chain) (examples illustrated in **Figures 8** and **9**). These sugar units are composed variously of pentoses, hexoses, or uronic acids. This hydrophobic-hydrophilic asymmetry means that these compounds have the ability to lower surface tension and are soap-like. They form foam in aqueous solutions and cause hemolysis of blood erythrocytes in vitro. The aglycone portion of the saponin molecule is called the *genin* or *sapogenin*. Saponins are widespread among plants, having been reported from more than 500 plants from at least 90 different families; these substances have been isolated from all parts of

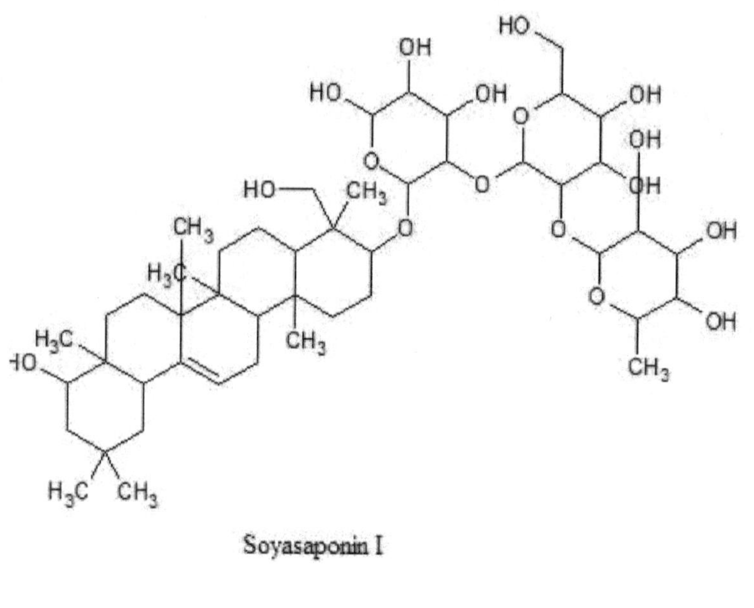

Figure 8. Example of triterpenoidal saponin.

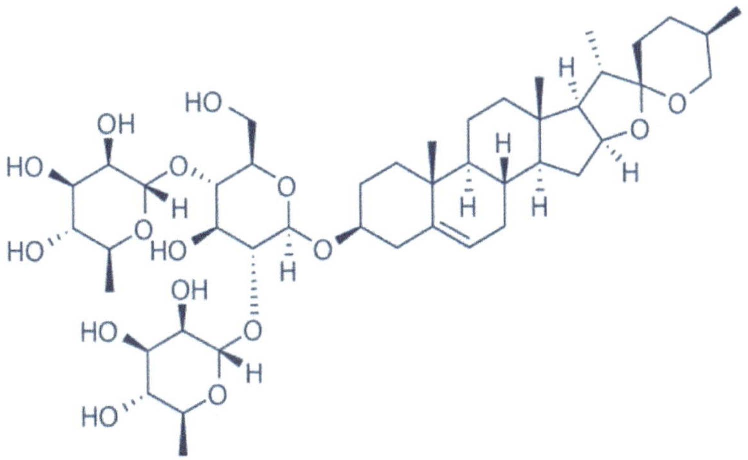

Dioscin

Figure 9. Example of steroidal saponin.

plants: leaves, stems, roots bulbs, flowers and fruits, although they tend to be concentrated in the roots of many species such as *Digitalis purpurea* (*foxglove*), *Dioscorea villosa* (*wild yam*), *Eleutherococcus senticosus* (*Siberian ginseng*), *Gentiana lutea* (*gentian*), *Glycyrrhiza* spp. (*licorice*) and *Panax ginseng* (*Korean ginseng*) [32].

Saponins have demonstrated numerous pharmacological properties. Some saponins have antitumor, piscicidal, molluscicidal, spermicidal, sedative, expectorant and analgesic properties. Glycyrrhizin from *glycyrrhizae radix* (from *Glycyrrhiza glabra*, Fabaceae) is useful as expectorant and antitussive agent. It is also used to treat chronic hepatitis and cirrhosis. Some saponins have anti-inflammatory properties as the saponins from *Bupleurum falcatum* (Apiaceae). *Phytolacca americana* roots are reputed to possess anti-inflammatory properties in Korean medicine. Similar properties have been demonstrated for a number of other saponins, for example aescin, from horse chestnut (*Aesculus hippocastanum*), has been shown to be 600 times more effective than rutin in reducing rat paw edema [33].

5. Terpenes

Terpenes are the largest and most diverse group of plant secondary compounds. The name "terpene" is derived from the word "turpentine," which in turn comes from the old French *ter(e)bintb*, meaning "resin." They are all derived chemically from 5-carbon isoprene units assembled in different ways [8]. Terpenes are classified according to the number of isoprene units in the molecule; a prefix in the name indicates the number of terpene units as follows.

5.1. Hemiterpenes

They consist of *a single isoprene* unit. Isoprene itself is considered the only hemiterpene, but oxygen-containing derivatives such as angelic acid isolated from *Angelica archangelica* and isovaleric acid from *Vaccinium myrtillus* are hemiterpenoids [1].

5.2. Monoterpenes

They consist of *two isoprene* units and have the molecular formula $C_{10}H_{16}$ (see **Figure 10**). They are important components of plant essential oils or volatile oils. Monoterpenes tend to occur in members of certain plant families, such as Lamiaceae, Pinaceae, Rutaceae and Apiaceae, from which many essential oils are commercially produced. Some of these compounds, such as geraniol, are almost ubiquitous and can be found in small amounts in the volatile secretions of most plants. Monoterpenes are further classified into unsaturated hydrocarbons (e.g., limonene), alcohols (e.g., linalool), alcohol esters (e.g., linalyl acetate), aldehydes (e.g., citronellal) and ketones (e.g., Carvone). Monoterpenes and other volatile terpenes have a number of widespread medicinal uses. Compounds such as camphor and menthol are used as counterirritants analgesics and anti-itching agents. Many monoterpenes have been used as anthelmintics. A series of monoterpene glycosides appear to have vasodilation effect on coronary vessels and the femoral vascular bed [16].

5.3. Sesquiterpenes

They consist of *three isoprene* units and have the molecular formula $C_{15}H_{24}$ (see **Figure 11**). Based on biogenetic origin, there are more than 200 different structural types of sesquiterpenes, and several thousand such compounds are known. These compounds can be conveniently classified into three main groups according to structure: acyclic (e.g., farnesol), monocyclic (e.g., bisabolol) and bicyclic (e.g., caryophyllene). A number of sesquiterpene lactones show antibacterial, antifungal and antiprotozoan activities. Sesquiterpenes from *Vernonia colorata* inhibit *Entamoeba histolytica* at concentrations comparable to metronidazole, an antiamoebic drug. Helenalin and a series of related compounds are responsible for the cardiotonic properties of *Arnica montana* flowers. *Atractylodis rhizoma*, from *Atractylodis macrocephala* (Asteraceae), is clinically used as diuretic, analgesic and anti-inflammatory. The activity is related to the presence of active compounds including eudesma-4(14)-7(1 l)-dien-8-one and atractylenolide I. Several related medicinal plants are also used for the same purposes due to the presence of sesquiterpenes [1, 34].

5.4. Diterpenes

They are composed of *four isoprene* units and have the molecular formula $C_{20}H_{32}$ (see **Figure 12**). Diterpenes are classified into acyclic and macrocyclic compounds. Moreover, macrocyclic

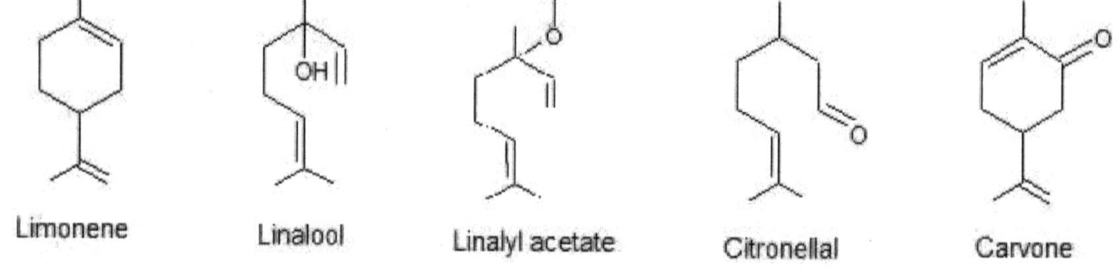

Figure 10. Examples of monoterpenes.

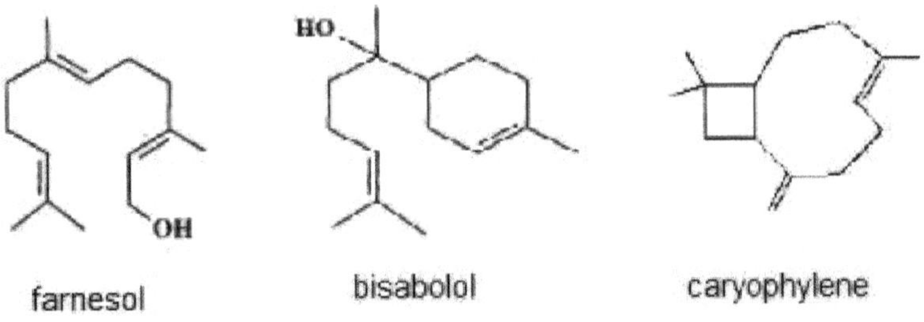

Figure 11. Examples of sesquiterpenes.

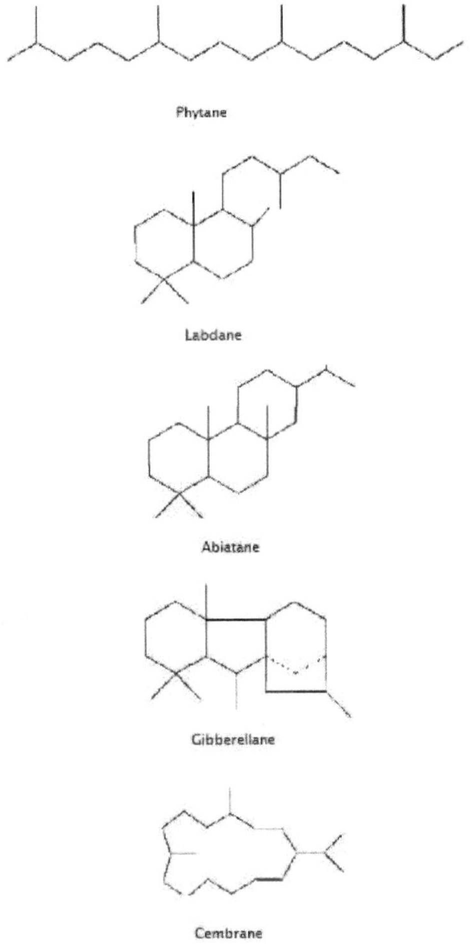

Figure 12. Examples of diterpenes.

diterpenes are classified according to the number of ring systems present. Diterpenes may be 6-membered ringed structures or they may have fused 5- and 7-membered ringed structures. In addition, many diterpenes have additional ring systems. These occur as side substitutions as esters or epoxides [8]. Diterpenoids constitute the active constituents of a number of medicinal plants. Vitamin K1, an antihemorrhagic compound, first discovered in plants in 1929, is a diterpene. Vitamin A, a diterpenoid, is referred to, together with the related compounds, as "carotenes." The bitter principles of *Jateorhiza palmata* (calumba root) belong to furanoditerpenes. *Teucrium chamaedrys* (wall germander) and *T. scorodonia* (wood sage) family

Labiatae, both produce diterpenes of the neoclerodane type. They are used in herbal medicine as diaphoretics and antirheumatics [35]. Like all groups of terpenes, diterpenes have demonstrated a range of pharmacological properties including: analgesic, antibacterial, antifungal, anti-inflammatory, antineoplastic and antiprotozoal activities [8]. Some diterpenes from *Kalmia latifolia* (Ericaceae) have antifeedant properties with respect to the gypsy moth. The gibberellins, first obtained from fungi of the genus *Gibberella* but also found in higher plants, are diterpenoid acids, which have a marked effect on growth of seedlings [7].

5.5. Sesterterpenes

Terpenes having 25 carbons and *five isoprene* units are rare relative to the other sizes (the *sester-* prefix means half to three, i.e. two and a half). An example of a sesterterpenoid is geranyl farnesol isolated from seed oils of *Camellia sasanqua* (sasanqua) and *Camellia japonica* (camellia), family Theaceae [36]. Geranyl farnesol showed cytotoxic activity in mouse leukemic M1 cells [37].

5.6. Triterpenes

They consist of *six isoprene* units and have the molecular formula $C_{30}H_{48}$ (see **Figure 13**). The linear triterpene squalene, the major constituent of shark liver oil, is derived from the reductive coupling of two molecules of farnesyl pyrophosphate. Triterpenes constitute a significant portion of the lipid substances of all plants; more than 4000 triterpenoids have been isolated. These compounds are precursors to steroids in both plants and animals. Both triterpenes and steroids occur free, as glycosides or in other combined forms. The structures of triterpenes and steroids may be subdivided into about 40 major types [1]. β-Boswellic acids (ursane-type triterpene) and α-boswellic acids (oleanane-type triterpene) that are isolated from the oleo-gum-resin of *Boswellia carterii* are known for their anti-inflammatory and anti-rheumatic activities [38].

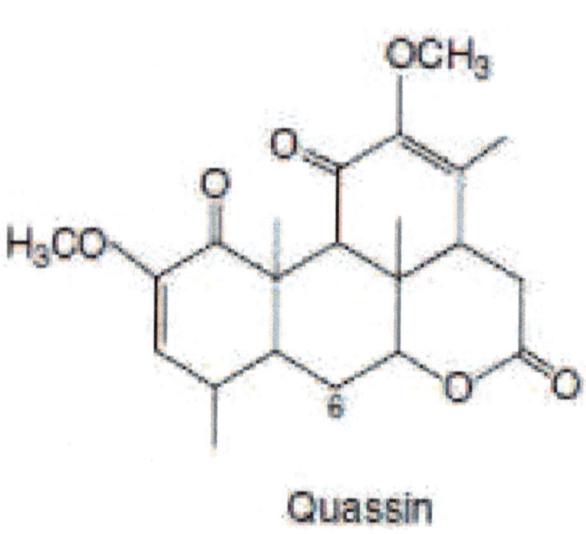

Figure 13. Example of triterpene.

One group of compounds showing a range of interesting biological activity is the quassinoids isolated from *Quassia amara*. These are degradation and rearrangement products of triterpenes. Quassia is used as a bitter tonic, as an insecticide and as an enema for the expulsion of thread worms.

Terpenes also include sesquarterpenes (*seven isoprene* units, $C_{35}H_{56}$), tetraterpenes (*eight isoprene* units, $C_{40}H_{64}$) as well as polyterpenes and norisoprenoids (long chains of *many isoprene* units.

6. Lipids

Lipids comprise a group of naturally occurring molecules that include fixed oils, waxes, essential oils, sterols, fat-soluble vitamins (such as vitamins A, D, E and K), phospholipids and others. Lipids serve various biological actions as major structural components of all biological membranes and as energy reservoirs and fuel for cellular activities in addition to being vitamins and hormones [39, 40]. Although lipids are considered primary plant metabolites, recent studies revealed pharmacological activities to members of this class of phytochemicals.

6.1. Fixed oils

Fixed oils constitute of high molecular aliphatic long-chain fatty acids, such as palmitic, stearic and oleic acids, esterified with glycerol. Fixed oils contain a relatively higher percentage of liquid glycerides (polyunsaturated) such as glycerin oleate, while fats are rich in solid glycerides such as glycerin stearate. [39]. Flax and linseed and its oil are obtained from *Linum usitatissimum*, family Linaceae. Polyunsaturated fatty acids in some fixed oils cause reduced excretion of lipid peroxidation products and hence are potent antioxidants and anti-inflammatory. They are used as prophylactic to decrease the risk of atherosclerosis and cardiovascular disease [41].

6.2. Waxes

Waxes are lipoidal matter constituting mainly from long aliphatic chains that may contain one or more functional groups. They may contain hydroxyl groups as in the case of primary and secondary long-chain alcohols that are frequently present in the form of esters. Others contain unsaturated bonds, aromatic systems, amide, ketonic, aldehydic or carboxylic functional groups. On the other hand, synthetic waxes constitute of long-chain hydrocarbons (alkanes or paraffins) that lack functional groups. They are similar to the fixed oils and fats since they are esters of fatty acids, but with the difference that the alcohol is not glycerin. The seeds of *Simmondsia chinensis* yield the liquid wax, jojoba wax, which consists of straight chain esters of fatty acids and alcohols [42]. Jojoba wax has anti-inflammatory, anti-aging and wound healing activities, and hence it can be utilized in several skin conditions. Jojoba wax has also been used in topical medications to enhance drug absorption. In addition, it is used in skin care products and in cosmetics such as sunscreens and moisturizers [43].

6.3. Essential oils

Essential oils are volatile aromatic complex mixtures of relatively low molecular weight compounds. Although they may contain up to 60 components, yet they are characterized by the presence of two or three major components at fairly high concentrations (20–70%) compared to other components present in trace amounts. For example, *Origanum compactum* essential oil contains carvacrol (30%) and thymol (27%) as major components. Linalol is the major component of *Coriandrum sativum* essential oil reaching up to 68%. Other examples are *Artemisia herba-alba* essential oil which contains α- and β-thuyone (57%) and camphor (24%) as major constituent, *Cinnamomum camphora* essential oil with 1,8-cineole (50%) as major constituent and finally *Mentha piperita* essential oil with menthol (59%) and menthone (19%) being the major constituent. Generally, these major components determine the biological properties of the essential oils [44]. They have many and important medical uses such as antiseptic, antimicrobial, analgesic, sedative, anti-inflammatory, spasmolytic and locally anesthesic remedies. They are also used as fragrances in embalmment and in food preservation [45].

7. Carbohydrates

Carbohydrates are universally present in living beings on our planet. As the first product of photosynthesis, carbohydrates are the starting point for all phytochemicals and also, by extension, for all animal biochemicals. More carbohydrates occur in nature than any other type of natural compound. The most abundant single organic substance on Earth is cellulose, a polymer of glucose, which is the main structural material of plants. Although carbohydrates are primary metabolites, they are incorporated in plenty of secondary metabolites through glycosidation linkages. Polymers of simple sugars and uronic acids produce mucilages and gums [46].

Carbohydrates consist of carbon, hydrogen and oxygen with the last two elements usually present in the same proportions as in water. They are classified into four chemical groups: monosaccharides, disaccharides, oligosaccharides and polysaccharides. Monosaccharides contain from three to nine carbon atoms, although those with five and six carbon atoms (pentoses, $C_5H_{10}O_5$, and hexoses, $C_6H_{12}O_6$) are accumulated in plants in greatest quantity. Condensation of monosaccharides results in the other types according to the number of saccharide units involved. In addition to the important biological and structural function of carbohydrates in plants, some members show medicinal effects such as mucilage. Mucilage, viscous sticky material produced by almost all plants and some microorganisms, plays a protective role in thickening membranes in plants. It also serves in storage of water and food and in seed germination. Chemically it constitutes of a polar glycoprotein and an exopolysaccharide. Mucilage is used medicinally as demulcent. Cactus (and other succulents) and *Linum usitatissimum* (flax seeds) are the major sources of mucilage. The extract of the mucilaginous root of the marshmallow plant (*Althaea officinalis*); used traditionally to make marshmallows, were used as cough suppressant due to its demulcent effect. *Ulmus rubra* (the slippery elm) inner bark, is also used as a demulcent due to its mucilaginous content. Mucilage acts primarily as a local demulcent or emollient when it comes in direct contact with mucous membrane surfaces or skin. Here, they produce a coating of "slime" that soothes and protects exposed or irritated surfaces of the gastrointestinal tract. They are used extensively in the management of inflammatory digestive disorders, especially when there is ulceration. Their relative indigestibility and hydrophilic properties have important influences on bowel behavior [47].

8. Conclusion

According to the abovementioned data, there are several classes of secondary plant metabolites that are responsible for the biological activities of herbal medicines. Eventually, secondary plant metabolites exert their action on molecular targets that differ from one case to the other. These targets may be enzymes, mediators, transcription factors or even nucleic acids. The use of herbal medicines should be based on comprehensive phytochemical studies for the determination of the chemical constituents of the herbs involved. Hence the knowledge of the resultant pharmacological and toxicological effects can be deduced, as well as the possible synergistic or antagonistic effects due to the use of multiple component herbal formulae. For this reason, the isolation and structural elucidation of secondary plant metabolites, though ancient, is still a huge and fast growing approach, and the techniques used for separation and analysis are advancing continuously.

Author details

Rehab A. Hussein* and Amira A. El-Anssary

*Address all correspondence to: rehaba.husein@yahoo.com

Pharmacognosy Department, Pharmaceutical Science Division, National Research Center, Giza, Egypt

References

[1] Seigler DS. Plant Secondary Metabolism. New York: Springer Science: Business Media; 1995. ISBN: 978-1-4613-7228-8; ISBN: 978-1-4615-4913-0 (eBook). DOI: 10.1007/978-1-4615-4913-0

[2] Jones ME, Kossel A. A biographical sketch. Yale Journal of Biology and Medicine. 1953;**26**(1):80-97

[3] Bourgaud F, Gravot A, Milesi S, Gontier E. Production of plant secondary metabolites: A historical perspective. Plant Science. 2001;**161**:839-851

[4] Bennets HW, Underwood EJ, Shier FL. A specific breeding problem of sheep in subterranean clover pastures in Western Australia. Australian Veterinary Journal. 1946;**22**(1):2-12

[5] Goławska S, Sprawka I, Łukasik I, Goławski A. Are naringenin and quercetin useful chemicals in pest-management strategies? Journal of Pest Science. 2014;**87**(1):173-180

[6] Harborne JB, Baxter H. Phytochemical Dictionary: A Handbook of Bioactive Compounds from Plants. London; Washington, DC: Taylor & Francis; 1993

[7] Evans WC. Pharmacognosy. 16th ed. Edinburgh London New York Philadelphia St Louis Sydney Toronto; 2009

[8] Hoffmann D. Medical Herbalism : The Science and Practice of Herbal Medicine. Healing Arts Press One Park Street, Rochester, Vermont; 2003. ISBN: 978-089281749-8

[9] Zbigniew S, Beata Ż, Kamil J, Roman F, Barbara K, Andrzej D. Antimicrobial and anti-radical activity of extracts obtained from leaves of three species of the genus *Pyrus*. Microbial Drug Resistance. 2014;**20**(4):337-343. DOI: 10.1089/mdr.2013.0155

[10] Amann R, Peskar BA. Anti-inflammatory effects of aspirin and sodium salicylate. European Journal of Pharmacology. 2002;**447**(1):1-9

[11] Pelczar MJ, Chan ECS, Krieg NR. Control of microorganisms, the control of microorganisms by physical agents. In: Microbiology. New York: McGraw-Hill International; 1988. pp. 469-509

[12] Eric Y. Botanical medicines for the urinary tract. World Journal of Urology. 2002;**20**(5):285-293

[13] Spiller F, Alves MK, Vieira SM, Carvalho TA, Leite CE, Lunardelli A, Poloni JA, Cunha FQ, de Oliveira JR. Anti-inflammatory effects of red pepper (*Capsicum baccatum*) on carrageenan- and antigen-induced inflammation. The Journal of Pharmacy and Pharmacology. 2008;**60**(4):473-478. DOI: 10.1211/jpp.60.4.0010

[14] Hagerman AE, Butler LG. The specificity of proanthocyanidin-protein interactions. The Journal of Biological Chemistry. 1981;**10**(256):4494-4497

[15] Catarino MD, Silva AMS, Cruz MT, Cardoso SM. Antioxidant and anti-inflammatory activities of *Geranium robertianum* L. decoctions. Food & Function. 2017;**8**(9):3355-3365. DOI: 10.1039/c7fo00881c

[16] Yi Z, Wang Z, Li H, Liu M. Inhibitory effect of tellimagrandin I on chemically induced differentiation of human leukemia K562 cells. Toxicology Letters. 2004;**147**(2):109-119

[17] Puneet G, Aditi S, Vinayak K, Anant GN, Samir D, Nikhil M. *Camellia sinensis* (tea): Implications and role in preventing dental decay. Pharmacognosy Reviews. 2013;**7**(14): 152-156. DOI: 10.4103/0973-7847.120515

[18] Jepson RG, Craig JC. Cranberries for preventing urinary tract infections. Cochrane Database of Systematic Reviews. 2008;**1**:CD001321. DOI: 10.1002/14651858.CD001321. pub4

[19] Avorn J, Monane M, Gurwitz JH, Glynn RJ, Choodnovskiy I, Lipsitz LA. Reduction of bacteriuria and pyuria after ingestion of cranberry juice. Journal of the American Medical Association. 1994;**271**(10):751-754

[20] Xu L, Wu Y, Zhao X, Zhang W. The study on biological and pharmacological activity of coumarins. In: Asia-Pacific Energy Equipment Engineering Research Conference; (AP3ER 2015). pp. 135-138

[21] Montanher AB, Zucolotto SM, Schenkel EP, Fröde TS. Evidence of anti-inflammatory effects of *Passiflora edulis* in an inflammation model. Journal of Ethnopharmacology. 2007;**109**(2):281-288

[22] Serafini M, Peluso I, Raguzzini A. Flavonoids as anti-inflammatory agents. The Proceedings of the Nutrition Society. 2010;**69**(3):273-278. DOI: 10.1017/S002966511000162X

[23] Susana J, Beatriz GM, Fabiana CM, Maria AD, Moacir GP. Antifungal activity of five species of *Polygala*. Brazilian Journal of Microbiology. 2011;**42**(3):1065-1075. DOI: 10.1590/S1517-83822011000300027

[24] Gehm BD, McAndrews JM, Chien P, Jameson JL. Resveratrol, a polyphenolic compound found in grapes and wine, is an agonist for the estrogen receptor. Proceedings of the National Academy of Sciences of the United States of America. 1997;**94**(25):14138-14143

[25] Saeidnia S, Gohari AR, Mokhber-Dezfuli N, Kiuchi F. A review on phytochemistry and medicinal properties of the genus *Achillea*. Daru. 2011;**19**(3):173-186

[26] Sharma PR, Shanmugavel M, Saxena AK, Qazi GN. Induction of apoptosis by a synergistic lignan composition from *Cedrus deodara* in human cancer cells. Phytotherapy Research. 2008;**22**(12):1587-1594. DOI: 10.1002/ptr.2511

[27] Mbaze LM, Lado JA, Wansi JD, Shiao TC, Chiozem DD, Mesaik MA, Choudhary MI, Lacaille-Dubois MA, Wandji J, Roy R, Sewald N. Oxidative burst inhibitory and cytotoxic amides and lignans from the stem bark of *Fagara heitzii* (Rutaceae). Phytochemistry. 2009;**70**(11-12):1442-1447. DOI: 10.1016/j.phytochem.2009.08.007

[28] Tadeusz A. Alkaloids: Chemistry, Biology, Ecology, and Applications. 2nd ed. Amsterdam, Netherlands: Elsevier; 2015. ISBN: 13: 978-0444594334

[29] Benowitz NL. Pharmacology of nicotine: Addiction, smoking-induced disease, and therapeutics. Annual Review of Pharmacology and Toxicology. 2009;**49**:57-71. DOI: 10.1146/annurev.pharmtox.48.113006.094742

[30] Benowitz NL. Clinical pharmacology of caffeine. Annual Review of Medicine. 1990;**41**(1):277-288

[31] Moudi M, Go R, Yong Seok Yien C, Nazre M. Vinca alkaloids. International Journal of Preventive Medicine. 2013;**4**(11):1231-1235

[32] Assa Y, Shany S, Gestetner B, Tencer Y, Birk Y, Bondi A. Interaction of alfalfa saponins with components of the erythrocyte membrane in hemolysis. Biochimica et Biophysica Acta. 1973;**307**(1):83-91

[33] Güçlü-Üstündağ Ö, Mazza G. Saponins: Properties, applications and processing. Critical Reviews in Food Science and Nutrition. 2007;**47**:231-258. ISSN: 1040-8398. DOI: 10.1080/10408390600698197

[34] Hikino H. Recent research on oriental medicinal plants. In: Wanger H, Hiniko H, Farnsworth NR, editors. Economic and Medicinal Plant Research. Vol. 1. London: Academic Press; 1985. pp. 53-85

[35] Bagci E, Yazgın A, Hayta S, Cakılcıoglu U. Composition of the essential oil of *Teucrium chamaedrys* L. (Lamiaceae) from Turkey. Journal of Medicinal Plants Research. 2010;**4**(23): 2587-2589

[36] Akihisa T, Koike K, Kimura Y, Sashida N, Matsumoto T, Ukiya M, Nikaido T. Acyclic and incompletely cyclized triterpene alcohols in the seed oils of theaceae and gramineae. Lipids. 1999;**34**(11):1151-1175

[37] Ishikura H, Mochizuki T, Izumi Y, Usui T, Sawada H, Uchino H. Differentiation of mouse leukemic M1 cells induced by polyprenoids. Leukemia Research. 1984;**8**(5):843-852

[38] Culioli G, Mathe C, Archier P, Vieillescazes C. A lupane triterpene from frankincense (*Boswellia* sp., Burseraceae). Phytochemistry. 2003;**62**:537-541. DOI: 10.1016/S0031-9422(02)00538-1

[39] Fahy E, Subramaniam S, Murphy RC, Nishijima M, Raetz CR, Shimizu T, Spener F, van Meer G, Wakelam MJ, Dennis EA. Update of the LIPID MAPS comprehensive classification system for lipids. Journal of Lipid Research. 2009;**50**(Suppl):S9-S14. DOI: 10.1194/jlr.R 800095-JLR200

[40] Subramaniam S, Fahy E, Gupta S, Sud M, Byrnes RW, Cotter D, Dinasarapu AR, Maurya MR. Bioinformatics and systems biology of the lipidome. Chemical Reviews. 2011;**111**(10):6452-6490. DOI: 10.1021/cr200295k

[41] Richard D, Kefi K, Barbe U, Bausero P, Visioli F. Polyunsaturated fatty acids as antioxidants. Pharmacological Research. 2008;**57**(6):451-455. DOI: 10.1016/j.phrs.2008.05.002 Epub 2008 May 18

[42] Wilhelm R, Hermann M. Bolt "Esters, Organic" Ullmann's Encyclopedia of Industrial Chemistry. Weinheim: Wiley-VCH, Verlag GmbH and Co.KGaA; 2012. DOI: 10.1002/14356007.a09_565.pub2

[43] Pazyar N, Yaghoobi R, Ghassemi MR, Kazerouni A, Rafeie E, Jamshydian N. Jojoba in dermatology: A succinct review. Giornale Italiano di Dermatologia e Venereologia. 2013;**148**(6):687-691

[44] Pichersky E, Noel JP, Dudareva N. Biosynthesis of plant volatiles: Nature's diversity and ingenuity. Science. 2006;**311**(5762):808-811

[45] Masotti V, Juteau F, Bessiere JM, Viano J. Seasonal and phenological variations of the essential oil from the narrow endemic species *Artemisia molinieri* and its biological activities. Journal of Agricultural and Food Chemistry. 2003;**51**:7115-7121. DOI: 10.1021/jf034621y

[46] Asif HM, Akram M, Saeed TM, Khan I, Akhtar N, Ur Rehman R, Ali Shah SM, Ahmed K, Shaheen G. Review paper carbohydrates. International Research Journal of Biochemistry and Bioinformatics. 2011;**1**(1):001-005

[47] Anbalahan N. Pharmacological activity of mucilage isolated from medicinal plants. International Journal of Applied and Pure Science and Agriculture. 2017;**3**(1):98-113. e-ISSN: 2394-5532, p-ISSN: 2394-823X

10

Guidelines for the Development of Herbal-Based Sunscreen

Piergiacomo Buso, Matteo Radice,
Anna Baldisserotto, Stefano Manfredini and
Silvia Vertuani

Abstract

Sun protection is a complex topic, which involves various classes of compounds. The photoprotective effectiveness of a sunscreen involves many biological activities, such as ultraviolet (UV) radiation filter properties and antioxidant, anti-inflammatory, and antimutagenic effects. Formulation strategy is also a key factor. Several studies have examined the role of natural molecules as photoprotective compounds, and a considerable number of commercially available sunscreens contain herbal extracts but not as sunfilters. Indeed, the process of evaluation of UV-filtering and photoprotective activity of herbal compounds presents certain specific difficulties and needs in vitro and in vivo studies. Nowadays, no natural compound or vegetal extract has been approved by any country as official UV filter for sunscreen. With these premises, the aim of this chapter is to define a set of tests, which can help to evaluate the efficacy of an herbal extract in the field of sun protection; in other words, we propose a rational approach to the discovery of natural UV-filtering extract and molecules. The following electronic databases have been used as a source of information: SciFinder, PubMed, Google Scholar, ISI-Web of Science, and Scopus.

Keywords: natural sunscreen, rational development, sustainable resources, SPF (sun protection factor), skin, cosmetic

1. Introduction

The use of herbal extract and natural molecules in the field of solar protection represents a new trend in the cosmetic industry; in fact, over the last few years, a significant increase of the usage of herbal extracts has been registered given the growing interest of the costumer for "green" and "natural" ingredients in the finished product. A large number of studies appearing in scientific literature demonstrate the photoprotective activity of natural products due to UV-filtering activity, antioxidant activity, and DNA-protecting effects [1–3]. Despite these findings, studies regarding photoprotection activity have been developed with a wide range of different methods and different strategies of investigation, thus making difficult to understand both the actual and the claimed potential of the activity. The main cause of this situation is the lack of repeatability of the in vitro SPF tests available nowadays.

In the USA, sunscreen is classified as an OTC (over-the-counter) product. In the European Union (EU) countries, it is listed as cosmetics, and its production must follow the EC Regulation 1223/2009 of the European Parliament on Cosmetic Products. Regarding the SPF determination, the ISO 2444:2010 is nowadays regarded as the reference method; this method involves an in vivo procedure carried out on human volunteers. Due to ethical problems, the in vivo UVAPF determination by the ISO 24442:2011 has been recently substituted by the in vitro ISO 24443:2012 method.

The "gold standard" for the SPF determination nowadays is provided by the ISO 2444:2010 in vivo test. It is not applicable in the initial screening phase of the new filtering compounds due to ethical problems connected to the exposure of healthy subjects to the potentially harmful effects of UV radiation. As far as the UVA Protection Factor (UVAPF) determination is concerned, in 2012, a new in vitro method was established and integrated into the ISO 24443:2012. Also, for in vivo tests, no authority or legislator has released an official statement to support all this. In the sunscreen research field, more effective guidelines for the evaluation of naturally derived actives are required. Despite the numerous scientific reports, there is no officially approved natural commercial sunfilter. Moreover, a consistent number of commercially available solar products (sunscreen) contain herbal derivatives, but an official and a widely approved validation of this method is not available, and so it is indispensable to correct labeling of the final product's UV protection. Hence, the objective of this study is to collect any current data and exhaustive critical overview regarding the use of herbal extract and natural molecules in sunscreens. Finally, the intent of the present chapter is to provide solid types of research methodology approach in order to develop herbal or natural-based sunscreen, useful as a set of guidelines.

1.1. Ultraviolet radiation

Sunlight is composed of about 40% visible light (VIS), 50% infrared light (IR), and 10% ultraviolet light (UV). As far as the biological effects of solar radiation exposure are concerned, ultraviolet radiation is the most important part of the electronic spectrum. Ultraviolet (UV) radiation can be divided into UVC (200–280 nm), UVB (280–315 nm), and UVA (315–400 nm) [2].

UV radiation (sun) is essential to human health; it is necessary for the production of vitamin D3 in the skin. Vitamin D3 is necessary for the intestinal absorption of calcium and phosphorus, and deficiency may cause osteoporosis in adults and growth retardation and skeletal deformities in children. Solar radiation has other therapeutic effects on some skin diseases such as psoriasis and eczema, thus making the outdoors a healthy lifestyle choice [2, 4].

On the other hand, the negative effects of an excessive exposure to UV radiation are well known, and these are harmful to human health; the interaction of the radiation with the most important constituents of human skin (DNA, RNA, proteins, lipids) represents the basis of the UV-mediated negative biological activities [2]. More in particular UVB radiation is responsible for the most known acute negative effect that comes after some hours of UV exposition: the UVB-induced erythema. This radiation also has a potential carcinogenic effect because it can cause direct damage to the DNA and RNA. An over exposition to deeply penetrating radiation, namely, UVA, is responsible for premature skin aging, excessive degradation, and inhibition of the synthesis of collagen fibers [5].

Protection from solar radiation thus represents a complex issue involving various biological activities and factors that influence the efficacy of a sunscreen product, as demonstrated by studies during the last decade. The most important biological activities in the field of sun protection can be summarized in six main categories:

- Filtering activity against UVB/UVA radiation
- Antioxidant and reactive oxygen species scavenging activity
- Antimutagenic activity
- Anticancer properties
- Booster effect
- Safety stability of the active compounds

In our opinion, the research effort should be focused on the discovery of multifunctional compounds or mixtures that present the abovementioned biological activities. Therefore, the reports of in vitro SPF values of herbal extracts and compounds are more valuable if they are accompanied by other types of useful biological activities that are of equal importance in the prevention of skin problems relating to UV exposure [2].

2. Biological activities connected with solar protection

2.1. Antioxidant and reactive oxygen species scavenging activity

Antioxidant effect represents one of the key mechanisms of photoprotective activity of herbal extracts. The UV skin damage depends also on the generation of reactive oxygen species (ROS). ROS are considered as oxidant agents and are responsible for the development of skin disorders like skin aging, lipid peroxidation, and cancer [6]. These species include hydroxyl radicals, peroxyl radicals, superoxide anion, and, mainly, their active precursors: ozone, hydrogen peroxide, and singlet oxygen. ROS react negatively with DNA, proteins, and unsaturated fatty acids that in turn induce carcinogenic processes and inflammatory response from cells. Phenolic/polyphenolic compounds and flavonoids usually represent the main source of natural antioxidant compounds, and several types of research highlight the usefulness of including natural antioxidant extracts in topical products [6–8].

Antioxidant compounds from herbs offer new possibilities and strategies for an effective prevention and treatment of UV-mediated damages and diseases, which are mainly due to the generation of reactive oxygen species suppressing immune reactions. The benefits of natural antioxidants in topical products are nowadays generally accepted in light of the information available [9]. There are several effective in vitro tests for antioxidant activity. Each of them is based on different mechanisms and, thus, evaluates different kinds of oxidative protection. In order to obtain a sufficient evaluation on in vitro antioxidant, it is thus necessary to perform different types of tests to assess the studied compounds on different kinds of oxidative species.

Listed below are some examples of tests that should be carried out to define the whole spectrum of protection. The tests include:

- 1,1-Diphenyl-2-picrylhydrazyl (DPPH) assay
- Luminol photochemiluminescence (PCL) assay
- 2,2′-Azino-bis-3-ethyl-benzothiazoline-6-sulfonic (ABTS) acid assay
- Oxygen radical absorption capacity (ORAC)

2.2. Antimutagenic activity and anticancer properties

UV radiation is capable of damaging DNA and therefore participating in cancer pathogenesis through multiple mechanisms such as immunosuppression, oxidative stress, direct DNA damage, inflammatory response, and p53 tumor suppressor gene mutations. On the other hand, it should be taken into account that immunosuppression might be the desired effect in subjects affected by autoimmune diseases [10].

Several methods are available for a predictive in vitro antimutagenic or anticancer activity evaluation, and it is quite difficult to identify a list of preferred tests [11]. However, a good practice should include at least one of the validated methods in the screening of a new substance or mixture [11].

2.3. Anti-inflammatory activity

UV radiation induces the inflammatory response. UVB-induced cyclooxygenase-2 (COX-2) expression leads to an increase in the production of prostaglandin (PG) metabolites. COX-2 expression in the skin has been linked to the pathophysiology of inflammation and cancer. Exposure to UV radiation is also known to increase the expression of pro-inflammatory cytokines like tumor necrosis factor, interleukin (IL)-1, and interleukin IL-6. These anti-inflammatory properties including various herbal substances and medicines can be evaluated by a number of methods [12, 13].

2.4. Booster effect

This topic is yet quite complex because it is relatively new and not fully explored. There are already known compounds that can boost the SPF of UV filters [10, 14], but the mechanisms that are responsible for booster effects are heterogeneous and often unpredictable; some are linked to the nature of the UV filter(s) that the formulator wants to enhance. It is, in fact, difficult to uniquely define the general characteristics of an ingredient with booster effect, but it is possible to describe the two main aspects of this topic. The three main strategies available to achieve "booster effect" are interaction with the UV filters at the physical-chemical level to improve efficiency (optimize the efficiency of the UV absorber mixture) [10], implement a correct formulation strategy, and improve the film-forming properties (use of emollients and film-forming agents). One of the reasons of the growing importance of the booster effect is the consolidated marketing trend of placing on the market sunscreen products with higher SPF values; as a consequence of this, the formulator has to find all the possible stratagems to use the smallest possible amount of UV filters in the product. Considering the evaluation of herbal materials as "booster ingredients," this activity is, in some cases, identifiable by the in vitro tests that will be described later. Ingredients that improve UV filter distribution and enhance spreadability are also valuable [15].

According to EU regulation [16], Annex VI reports the list of UV filters allowed in cosmetic products.

List of sunscreen ingredients approved in the USA as presented in the sunscreen drug products for over-the-counter human use monograph" (21 CFR 352.10) [17].

3. Guidelines for the determination of SPF in vitro

Currently, several in vitro tests for determination of SPF exist. They are all used for screenings performed in the research and developing phase. The first method proposed is the one by Diffey (1989); it is still the most accredited reference [14]. The fundamental characteristic of all the in vitro methods is that they are based on spectrophotometric measurement of the absorbance (calculated from transmittance) of a thin film of product applied on UV transparent substrates. Substrates should be as close as possible to the physical characteristics of the skin. The amount of product applied varies from 0.7 to 2.0 mg cm^2. There are different types of suitable substrates; they can range from plastic perforated surgical tape such as Transpore™ to standardized plastic plates such as polymethyl methacrylate (PMMA) plates [14]:

- Transpore™ tape: it is a surgical tape (provided by 3M Health Care Company, Maine, USA). It is used according to the Diffey-Robson's method; this tape has a perforated structure, and it allows the distribution of the sunscreen sample in a way similar to the irregular surface of the skin.
- Sand-blasted PMMA plates: this substrate is easy to use and can be supplied with a reproducible roughness. (i.e., Schonberg GmbH, Munich, Germany). The plates have an area of 2 cm^2 and standard roughness of 5 μm. The features of this substrate meet the recommendation of ISO 24443 for in vitro UVA protection assessment.

Our experience in the research of useful compounds in the solar protection field and an accurate bibliographic research indicate that it is possible to point out several factors and variables which are able to affect the accuracy and the repeatability of the in vitro SPF tests. The most important ones are:

- Different compositions of filters
- The formulation of the sunscreens

- The thickness and the homogeneity of the applied sunscreen
- The type of spectrophotometer
- Substrates used and their relative roughness

The main concern, about this type of evaluation, is the lack of data to support correlation to in vivo results [14].

At present, the in vivo method is still the official standard for UVB protection (ISO 2444:2010), and product developers should perform the in vivo test on the final product and the in vitro one during all the phases of the development bringing attention to the ethical issue and on the costs.

In order to provide practical indications, we suggest two methods that have proven, in our experience, to be among the most reliable:

3.1. Method A

This is based on the Diffey-Robson's method [14]. The support used is a Transpore™ surgical perforated tape, cut to have an area of 20 cm^2, in which an amount of 0.0400 $\pm$ 0.002 g (2 mg cm^{-2}) of the product is weighed and laid in small spots through all the area. The tape is then positioned on a scale where the spreading phase is carried out with a finger cot, performing a pattern of six movements in horizontal, vertical, and circular directions and checking the pressure applied in all the movements. As far as the spreading pressure is concern, an internal procedure must be developed by the performing laboratory in order to be repeatable (see the end of this paragraph). At least three tapes have to be prepared for each product, recording five measures each, collecting therefore 15 spectra [14].

3.2. Method B

This method has been recently proposed by us [14], adapting to UVB the ISO 24443:2012 standard for the in vitro UVA protection determination. The support used is a PMMA (polymethyl methacrylate) plastic plate with an area of 25 cm^2 and standardized 5 μm roughness, in which an amount of 0.0320 $\pm$ 0.0005 g (1.3 mg cm^{-2}) of the product is weighed and laid in small spots through all the area. The plate is then positioned on a scale where the spreading phase is carried out performing with pre-saturated finger cot a sequence of six movements in horizontal, vertical, and circular direction and checking the pressure applied throughout the spreading. Before the measurement, the sample lies for a minimum of 15 min in a dark place, allowing the evaporation of volatile components. Three plates have to be prepared for each product, recording five measures each, collecting therefore 15 spectra [14].

In both methods, the spectra were recorded with an appropriate spectrophotometer, wavelength ranging from 290 nm up to 400 nm, with increment step set at 1 nm. The tests carried out for the evaluation of new herbal compounds are usually performed including them, at a known concentration, in a stable formulation suitable for cosmetic use. The obtained SPF data are then compared to those of the same formulation without the studied compounds.

SPF in vitro is defined as follows:

$$\text{In vitro SPF} = \frac{\int_{\lambda=290nm}^{\lambda=400nm} E(\lambda)I(\lambda)d(\lambda)}{\int_{\lambda=290nm}^{\lambda=400nm} E(\lambda)I(\lambda)10^{-A(\lambda)}d(\lambda)} \quad (1)$$

$E(\lambda)$ is the erythema action spectrum (CIE-1987) at the wavelength λ. $I(\lambda)$ is the spectral irradiance received from the UV source at the wavelength λ. $A(\lambda)$ is the monochromatic absorbance of the test product layer at the wavelength λ. $d(\lambda)$ is the wavelength step (1 nm).

Both methods have to be conducted in highly standardized operating conditions with regard to the operator, the environmental conditions, the substrates used, and the instruments. We have worked with spreading pressures of 100 ± 15 g and 200 ± 15 g, and comparing different application pressures on the same substrate, no statistically significant difference subsists in terms of repeatability.

The two fundamental parameters in the in vitro SPF measurement process are in vivo correlation and reproducibility. In our experience, Method B with a spreading pressure of 200 ± 15 g is the most reliable method with respect to reproducibility and accuracy. Nevertheless, Method A can be still considered as a useful in vitro method during the early research phase, especially in laboratories with limited financial resources and limited equipment. In this case, the correlation is not influenced by the choice of operator's pressure (100 ± 15 g or 200 ± 15 g).

The problem of photostability of UV filters should also be considered at this stage. It is necessary, seeking potential human applications, to verify that a new compound or vegetal extract does not present any photostability problems. This evaluation can be performed using solar radiation simulators; this procedure is also indicated in the ISO 24443:2012.

It is very important to assume that, at present, it is possible for a single laboratory to optimize internal methods and protocols to achieve repeatable and predictive in vitro results, whereas it is extremely difficult to develop methods reproducible and equally reliable between different laboratories due to external variables (e.g., the environmental, operator, etc.) [14].

4. Natural compounds in solar radiation protection: current knowledge

In recent years, many plant species have been investigated for their potential uses in the field of solar radiation protection, but much remains to be accomplished. As stated above, this depends on both a large number of under-investigated species and the lack of an official standard in vitro SPF evaluation method, to speed up the screening procedure. Depending on this, and on the many different and incomplete approaches led by different research groups, it is also complex to have a general picture of the existing knowledge. In the aim to achieve a "state of the art," we conducted a detailed bibliographic research on the plants already investigated in biological activities useful for sunscreen products.

In our previous investigation [2], we identified 54 plants, 5 lichens, and 14 pure molecules which have been studied in order to obtain herbal sunscreen products. It is remarkable how many plant extracts showed preliminary natural UV filter activity and, in the same manner, antioxidant properties and/or synergistic photoprotective effects.

Table 1 summarizes a selection of the abovementioned plants, lichens, and pure molecules which have been mentioned at least in two different types of research.

Plant name	Plant part(s) used	Plant extract	Type of compound(s)	Major constituent(s)	Main effect(s)
Calendula officinalis	Flower	Hydroalcoholic extract	Polyphenol, flavonoid	Rutin, narcissin	Prevent UV irradiation-induced oxidative stress
Camellia sinensis	n.r.	n.r.	Polyphenols	EC—(−)epicatechin, ECG—(−)-epicatechin-3-gallate, EGC—(−)-epigallocatechin, EGCG—(−)-epigallocatechin-3-gallate	Anticarcinogenic, anti-inflammatory, photostabilizing capacity
Coffea genus (10 species)	Green dry coffee beans	Chloroform extract	Lipid fraction	Linoleic acid, palmitic acid	UV absorber, emollient
Culcitium reflexum	Leaf	Ethanolic extract	Phenolic compounds, flavonols	Rutin, kaempferol, quercetin, and its glycosylated derivatives and cinnamic acid derivatives	Antioxidant, reduces UVB-induced skin erythema, free-radical-scavenging effect
Fragaria x ananassa	Fruits	n.r.	Anthocyanins and hydrolyzable tannins	Pelargonidin	Antioxidant, reduces UVB-induced skin erythema, anti-inflammatory, diminishing DNA damage on UVA-induced skin damage
Glycine max	Seeds	Soybean cake	Soy isoflavone	Genistein	Antioxidant, reduces skin photo damage and transepidermal water loss (TEWL)
Moringa oleifera	Seeds	Petroleum ether extract	Lipid fraction	n.r.	UV absorber
Pinus pinaster	Bark	Picnogenol	Phenolic compounds, polyphenols, procyanidin derivatives	Catechin, epicatechin, taxifolin, caffeic, ferulic, p-hydroxybenzoic, vanillic, gallic, and protocatechuic acid	Reduces UVB-induced skin erythema, free-radical-scavenging effect
Pimenta pseudocaryophyllus	Leaves	Ethanolic extract	Flavonoids and polyphenolic compounds	n. r.	Inhibits UV-B irradiation-induced inflammation and oxidative stress of the skin Antioxidant, decreases oxidative damages of the skin

Plant name	Plant part(s) used	Plant extract	Type of compound(s)	Major constituent(s)	Main effect(s)
Pongamia glabra	Seeds	n.r.	n.r.	Pongamol, karanjin	UV absorber
Punica granatum	Fruits, peel	methanol extract	Anthocyanidins, hydrolyzable tannins	Delphinidin, cyanidin, and pelargonidin	Decreases in the number of UVB-induced dimers in the human skin, synergic photoprotective activity in nanostrustured lipid carrier
Silybum marianum	Seeds	n.r.	Flavonolignans	Silymarin, Silybin, silydianin, silychristin, isosilybin	Inhibits UVB-induced damage, antioxidant
Vaccinium myrtillus L.	Fruits	n.r., water-soluble extract	Polyphenols, anthocyanins	n.r.	Reduction of UV A-stimulated ROS formation, attenuation of UVA-caused peroxidation of membrane lipids, and depletion of intracellular GSH
Vitis vinifera	Seeds	n.r.	Polyphenols	Flavan-3-ol derivatives, catechin, epicatechin, oligomeric proanthocyanidins	Free-radical-scavenging effect, prevents UVB- and UVC-induced lipid peroxidation, reducing the oxidative stress and apoptosis

n.r.—not reported.

Table 1. Selection of plant extracts useful for sunscreen application.

Lichens are mentioned by several types of research [18–23] as natural sources of photoprotective compounds and phytocomplexes. Some examples of bioactive compounds obtained by lichens are epiphorelic acid I and II, salazinic acid, usnic acid, secalonic acid, and calycine. According to the studies regarding lichens, the main highlighted activities were antioxidant properties and broad-spectrum UV-absorbing capacity. Regarding pure molecules, quercetin and resveratrol have been widely investigated [7, 24–30] for their antioxidant, antiproliferative, and anti-inflammatory properties, including also UVA and UVB filter enhancer activity.

5. Strategies and solutions

UV light is recognized by the US National Institute of Environmental Health Sciences, as the main etiological agent of a large number of skin cancers, sunburns, and oxidative stress (US Tenth Report on Carcinogens). Despite controversial data about photo-irritation, photo-sensitization, and contact dermatitis, synthetic and mineral sunscreens are used to prevent UV-induced skin damage and are very common in several skin care formulations. More often than not, the etiology of a skin disease is multifactorial and includes DNA damages, inflammatory processes, oxidative stress from ROS, lipid peroxidation, etc. All the abovementioned causes need a multi-target approach, which is impossible to obtain with a "magic-bullet" molecule and neither in a blend of UVA/UVB/UVC filters. All synergic photoprotective claims may be integrated with a proven formulation strategy (oleosomes and/or other encapsulation technologies, coatings or stabilizers, film thickness, etc.) in order to stabilize and/or boost the suncare herbal ingredients.

Moreover, in view of the increased demand of natural, herbal ingredients, sunscreens will be the next trend for photoprotective formulations. To this end, it is mandatory to develop natural sunscreen formulations based on a sound scientific investigation to sustain safe and effective products. In these regards, in our laboratory, we have very recently developed a rational approach considering the synergistic properties that a good candidate should possess: proven UVB/UVA absorption capability, antioxidant effects, protection against DNA and other free radical cellular structure-mediated damages, potential synergic protective mechanisms, and, finally, good toxicological profiles and proven formulation efficacy. As a matter of fact, several herbal/natural molecules may provide, in theory, these activities. Herbal extracts are naturally composed of mixtures of synergistic ingredients developed by plants through the evolution process (i.e., polyphenols), to allow the earlier marine organisms to colonize the terrestrial environment inferring resistance to high UV-induced oxidative stress. Taking this into account, as the synthetic strategy goes toward the design of multifunctional molecules inspired by the above natural mechanism [7], herbal sunscreen goes in the same direction but starts from the other side that already is available in the phytocomplex. The weak point of this latter approach is the investigation strategy, often incomplete, that makes literature data not useful. To further complicate the picture, it must be noted that different portions of the plant may be used (leaves, bark, roots, owers, seeds, or fruits), they can be dried either in air or using instruments, and they can be cut or ground into particles and then extracted with either water or organic solvents at different herbs to solvent ratio (i.e., 1:4, w/v). But also fresh herbs are used; in this case, the herb to solvent ratio is usually 1:1. The extraction process might be different in function of the characteristics (physical and chemical) of the ingredients. Thus, the same approach for different compounds cannot be devised. Also, steam distillation is used in the preparation and extraction of essential oils from botanical materials. New technologies, i.e., supercritical carbon dioxide extraction technology, membrane separation technology, enzymatic extraction methods, and so on, are emerging, further complicating the pattern of the relative observed activities.

Taking all this into account, only a few studies on herbal extracts really match the abovementioned strategy. An ideal approach (**Figure 1**) should involve three different steps, typical of drug development:

1. Extraction and characterization of the properties of the extracts (i.e., composition, UV absorption, mutagenicity, cytotoxicity).

2. In vitro evaluation of synergic physiological activity (i.e., lenitive, antiradical, antioxidant, etc.).

3. Formulation strategies, new vehicles development, stabilization, and SPF evaluation in vitro and on volunteers.

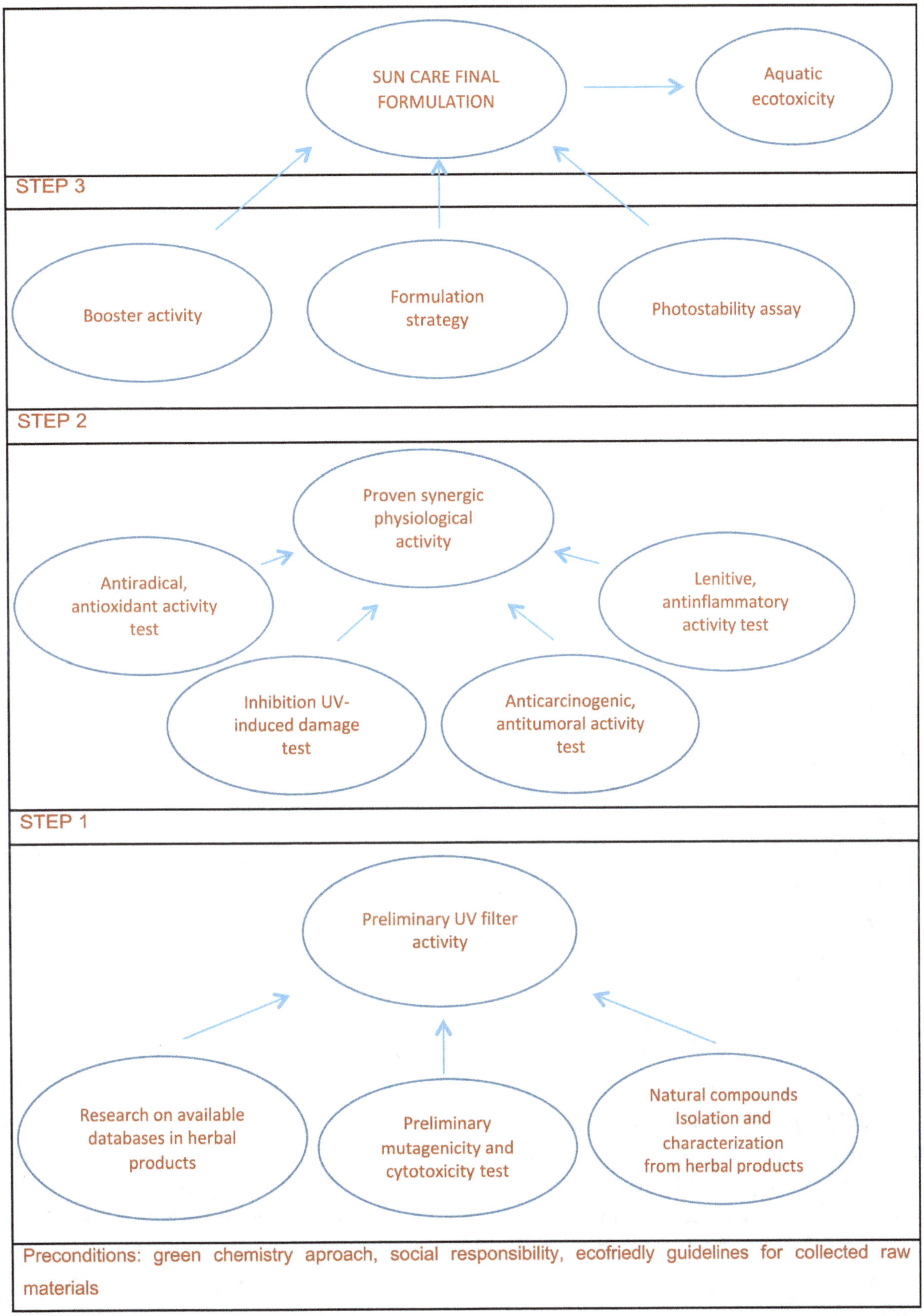

Figure 1. A rational process in suncare active ingredients discovery from herbal extracts.

In our opinion, step 3 represents the main lack of evidence in order to develop a natural sunscreen product. Despite an improving number of recent studies regarding the incorporation of antioxidants into sunscreen [25, 27, 28], none of the researches we reviewed include herbal products and more sophisticated formulations, as nanostructured lipid carrier, elastic niosomes, nanoparticles, microemulsion, etc. We recommend this way as an essential trend for "green" sunscreen research.

6. Natural extracts as a source of active compounds: from ancient to modern times

Scientific reports directed to the discovery of novel natural photoprotective ingredients often describe only the UV-filtering activity (step 1), which is a necessary but not sufficient condition to support the speculation of the effectiveness if inserted into a sunscreen tested on volunteers. The same issue can be referred to the in vitro bioactivity studies (step 2). The hardest challenge is to enhance the already approved findings as models, mentioned in step 3. An extract or natural compound needs to be fully characterized also for its effect in humans in the final product. Without this, it will remain restricted to a scientific investigation, which will be seen as useless to understand the potential of application in substitution of synthetic or mineral filters. Finally, in order to demonstrate real "green" claims, we recommend completing the product development with aquatic ecotoxicity assay. This step is becoming quite relevant [31, 32] and could be a significant benefit for a new sunscreen product.

Natural extracts have often been used as a source of inspiration in the development of new drugs rather than drugs themselves. Thus, while the discovery of synthetic ingredients is based on a rational systematic approach, which takes into account "step-by-step" modifications driven by chemical-physical parameter, the approach to the discovery of herbal ingredients, to be used as extracts, is "experience driven" and mainly based on traditional uses. A step-by-step procedure applied to natural extract would imply (I) the preparation of extracts and eventually phytochemicals from herbs, (II) the phytochemical study of extracts of herbal preparation or compound isolation, (III) the structure/composition elucidation, (IV) the in vitro biological activity evaluation, (V) the compound characterization and principal activity investigation, (VI) and the in vivo proof of the in vitro elucidated activities.

Furthermore, on the one hand, a central government agency of countries with high biodiversity should consider establishing research projects that involve ecological ethics, such as the managing, care, and preservation of the environment. However, on the other hand, the discovery of such ingredients could lead to improving agriculture or farming of these plants which may become an important job opportunity, especially in countries where the land is not favorable for the traditional farming. Finally, biotechnology in fields of plants is already a precious source of ingredients (i.e., secondary metabolites), which can be obtained from cell culture rather than traditional farming, thus saving biodiversity and land to be dedicated to plants for food. This has already been proven possible in the field of medicinal plants (i.e., *Artemisia annua*) [33].

Due to the growing interest in herbal remedies, there is also a significant amount of data available on herbal ingredients (i.e., public databases containing analysis, efficacy tests, extracts preparation) even in relation to their molecular targets [33].

It is already possible, based on existing proofs, to envisage a stage of discovery from herbal ingredients, which includes the preparation of extract (by the same standardized methods) eventual isolation, structure/composition elucidation, and in vitro bioactivity evaluation. In the case of sunscreens, the class of compounds behaving abilities of solar radiation absorption and antioxidant capacities are well known (i.e., polyphenols); what is not known is how much the mixture of other ingredients present in the extract may contribute to the sunscreen activity with complementary mechanisms (i.e., booster activity). This implies that the evaluation of activity in vivo must be conducted for each single extract. As recently reviewed by Si-Yuan Pan et al., the herbal preparation may contain "hundreds" of active compounds, and in addition, the concentrations of some of them might be exceedingly low and thus insufficient for conducting in vivo studies on isolated molecules. They report that from 1960 to 1982 and from over 100,000 crude tested extracts (deriving from more than 30.00 plants) only two compounds, Taxol and camptothecin, were developed into marketable therapeutics [33].

Based on the experience from random trials and observations in animals, ancient people acquired the knowledge of using herbs to treat illnesses. However, herbs used in traditional medicines constitute only a small portion of naturally occurring plants; thus, a large part of work still remains to be developed.

7. Conclusion

In this chapter, we presented a systematic approach based on our experiences and proposed it as a possible standard approach in this field. The steps mentioned in **Figure 1** have to be considered as an initial set of guidelines needed for the development of herbal-based sunscreen. The end result is a complete and rational methodology for the research and development of herbal sunscreen. The authors consider it to be essential to match the initial in vitro studies about UV filter activities with synergic biological activities (antioxidant, anti-inflammatory, inhibitory UV-induced damage effect, etc.) and formulation strategies (boosters, encapsulation, etc.). A solid response in each step may be considered a complete strategy. Finally, regarding natural products and traditional knowledge, an eco-friendly and sustainable approach can complete the investigation process and the management of the industrial supply chains.

We believe that our contribution will be useful to expedite the discovery of sunfilters from herbs. With a solid discovery approach, chances of success will greatly increase.

Acknowledgements

This work was supported by the University of Ferrara (Bando FIR-2016 to Silvia Vertuani) and Ambrosialab srl, Ferrara (Grant 2017). We thank Anna Maria Brincat (Clubclass Residential

Language School, Swieqi, Malta) and Luigi Mastroianni (State Language High School "Giosuè Carducci" Ferrara, Italy) for their careful English revision.

A. Annex VI: List of UV filters allowed in cosmetic products according to EU regulation [11]

List of sunscreen ingredients approved in the USA as presented in the "Sunscreen Drug Products for Over-the-Counter Human Use" monograph (21 CFR 352.10) [12].

Chemical name	**Name of common ingredient glossary**	**Maximum concentration in ready-for-use preparation**
4-Aminobenzoic acid	PABA	5%
N,N,N-Trimethyl-4-(2-oxoborn-3-ylidenemethyl) anilinium methyl sulfate	Camphor benzalkonium methosulfate	6%
Benzoic acid, 2-hydroxy-, 3,3,5-trimethylcyclohexyl ester/ homosalate	Homosalate	10%
2-Hydroxy-4-methoxybenzophenone/oxybenzone	Benzophenone-3	10%
2-Phenylbenzimidazole-5-sulfonic acid and its potassium, sodium, and triethanolamine salts/ensulizole	Phenylbenzimidazole sulfonic acid	8% (as acid)
3,3′-(1,4-Phenylenedimethylene) bis(7, 7-dimethyl-2-oxobicyclo-[2.2.1]hept-1-yl-methanesulfonic acid) and its salts/ecamsule	Terephthalylidene dicamphor sulfonic acid	10% (as acid)
1-(4-tert-Butylphenyl)-3-(4-methoxyphenyl)propane-1,3-dione/ avobenzone	Butyl methoxydibenzoylmethane	5%
alpha-(2-Oxoborn-3-ylidene)-toluene-4-sulphonic acid and its salts	Benzylidene camphor sulfonic acid	6% (as acid)
2-Cyano-3,3-diphenyl acrylic acid, 2-ethylhexyl ester/octocrylene	Octocrylene	10% (as acid)
Polymer of N-{(2 and 4)-[(2-oxoborn-3-ylidene)methyl]benzyl} acrylamide	Polyacrylamidomethyl benzylidene camphor	6%
2-Ethylhexyl 4-methoxycinnamate/octinoxate	Ethylhexyl methoxycinnamate	10%
Ethoxylated ethyl-4-aminobenzoate	PEG-25 PABA	10%
Isopentyl-4-methoxycinnamate/amiloxate	Isoamyl p-methoxycinnamate	10%
2,4,6-Trianilino-(p-carbo-2′-ethylhexyl-1′-oxy)-1,3,5-triazine	Ethylhexyl triazine	5%
Phenol,2-(2H-benzotriazol-2-yl)-4-methyl-6-(2-methyl-3-(1,3,3, 3-tetramethyl-1-(trimethylsilyl)oxy)-disiloxanyl)propyl)	Drometrizole trisiloxane	15%
Benzoic acid, 4,4-((6-((4-(((1,1-dimethylethyl)amino)carbonyl) phenyl)amino)-1,3,5-triazine-2,4-diyl)diimino)bis-, bis (2-ethylhexyl) ester/iscotrizinol (USAN)	Diethylhexyl butamido triazine	10%
3-(4-Methylbenzylidene)-d1 camphor/enzacamene	4-Methylbenzylidene` camphor	4%
3-Benzylidene camphor	3-Benzylidene camphor	2%

Chemical name	Name of common ingredient glossary	Maximum concentration in ready-for-use preparation
2-Ethylhexyl salicylate/octisalate	Ethylhexyl salicylate	5%
2-Ethylhexyl 4-(dimethylamino)benzoate/padimate O (USAN: BAN)	Ethylhexyl dimethyl PABA	8%
2-Hydroxy-4-methoxybenzophenone-5-sulfonic acid and its sodium salt/sulisobenzone	Benzophenone-4, benzophenone-5	5% (as acid)
2,2′-Methylene-bis(6-(2H-benzotriazol-2-yl)-4-(1,1,3,3-tetramethyl-butyl)phenol)/bisoctrizole	Methylene bis-benzotriazolyl tetramethylbutylphenol	10%
Sodium salt of 2,2′-bis(1,4-phenylene)-1H–benzimidazole-4, 6-disulfonic acid)/bisdisulizole disodium (USAN)	Disodium phenyl dibenzimidazole tetrasulfonate	10% (as acid)
2,2′-(6-(4-Methoxyphenyl)-1,3,5-triazine-2,4-diyl)bis(5-((2-ethylhexyl)oxy)phenol)/bemotrizinol	Bis-ethylhexyloxyphenol methoxyphenyl triazine	10%
Dimethicodiethylbenzalmalonate	Polysilicone-15	10%
Titanium dioxide	Titanium dioxide	25%
Benzoic acid, 2-[4-(diethylamino)-2-hydroxybenzoyl]-, hexylester	Diethylamino hydroxybenzoyl hexyl benzoate	10% in sunscreen products

Name of common ingredient glossary	Concentration allowed
Aminobenzoic acid (PABA)	Up to 15%
Avobenzone	Up to 3%
Cinoxate	Up to 3%
Dioxybenzone	Up to 3%
Homosalate	Up to 15%
Menthyl anthranilate	Up to 5%
Octocrylene	Up to 10%
Octyl methoxycinnamate	Up to 7.5%
Octyl salicylate	Up to 5%
Oxybenzone	Up to 6%
Padimate O	Up to 8%
Phenylbenzimidazole sulfonic acid	Up to 4%
Sulisobenzone	Up to 10%
Titanium dioxide	Up to 25%
Trolamine salicylate	Up to 12%
Zinc oxide	Up to 25%
Ensulizole	Up to 4%
Homosalate	Up to 15%

Name of common ingredient glossary	Concentration allowed
Meradimate	Up to 5%
Octinoxate	Up to 7.5%
Octisalate	Up to 5%
Octocrylene	Up to 10%
Oxybenzone	Up to 6%
Padimate O	Up to 8%

Author details

Piergiacomo Buso[2], Matteo Radice[1], Anna Baldisserotto[2], Stefano Manfredini[2,3]* and Silvia Vertuani[2,3]

*Address all correspondence to: mv9@unife.it

1 Department of Earth Sciences, Universidad Estatal Amazónica, Puyo, Pastaza, Ecuador

2 Department of Life Sciences and Biotechnology, Master Course in Cosmetic Science and Technology, University of Ferrara, Ferrara, Italy

3 Ambrosialab Srl, Ferrara, Italy

References

[1] Baker LA, Marchetti B, Karsili TNV, Stavros VG, Ashfold MNR. Photoprotection: Extending lessons learned from studying natural sunscreens to the design of artificial sunscreen constituents. Chemical Society Reviews. 2017;**46**:3770-3791. DOI: 10.1039/c7cs00102a.

[2] Radice M, Manfredini S, Ziosi P, Dissette V, Buso P, Fallacara A, Vertuani S. Herbal extracts, lichens and biomolecules as natural photo-protection alternatives to synthetic UV filters. A systematic review. Fitoterapia. 2016;**114**:144-162. DOI: 10.1016/j.fitote.2016.09.003

[3] Cefali LC, Ataide JA, Moriel P, Foglio MA, Mazzola PG. Plant compounds as active photo protectants in sunscreens. International Journal of Cosmetic Science. 2016;**38**:346-353. DOI: 10.1111/ics.12316

[4] Gonzàlez S, Fernández-Lorente M, Gilaberte-Calzada Y. The latest on skin photoprotection. Clinics in Dermatology. 2008;**26**:614-626. DOI: 10.1016/j.clindermatol.2007.09.010

[5] Valachovic E, Zurbenko I. Skin cancer, irradiation, and sunspots: The solar cycle effect. BioMed Research International. 2014;**11**:734-748. DOI: 10.1155/2014/538574

[6] Thiele JJ, Dreher F, Packer L. Antioxidant defence systems in skin. In: Elsner P, Malbach H, Rougier A, editors. Drugs vs Cosmetics: Cosmeceuticals? New York: Marcel Dekker; 2000. pp. 145-187

[7] Svobodovà A, Psotová J, Walterová D. Natural phenolics in the prevention of UV-induced skin damage. A review. Biomedical Papers. 2003;**147**:137-145. DOI: 10.5507/bp.2003.019

[8] Saewan N, Jimtaisong A. Photoprotection of natural flavonoids. Journal of Applied Pharmaceutical Science. 2013;**3**:129-141. DOI: 10.7324/JAPS.2013.3923

[9] Vayalil PK, Elmets CA, Katiyar SK. Treatment of green tea polyphenols in hydrophilic cream prevents UVB-induced oxidation of lipids and proteins, depletion of antioxidant enzymes and phosphorylation of MAPK proteins in SKH-1 hairless mouse skin. Carcinogenesis. 2003;**24**:927-936. DOI: 10.1093/carcin/bgg025

[10] Bino A, Baldisserotto A, Scalambra E, Dissette V, Vedaldi DE, Salvador A, Durini E, Manfredini S, Vertuani S. Design, synthesis and biological evaluation of novel hydroxy-phenyl-1H-benzimidazoles as radical scavengers and UV-protective agents. Journal of Enzyme Inhibition and Medicinal Chemistry. 2017;**32**(1):527-537. DOI: 10.1080/14756366.2016.1265523

[11] Naranyanan DL, Saladi RN, Fox JL. Ultraviolet radiation and skin cancer. International Journal of Dermatology. 2010;**49**:978-986. DOI: 10.1111/j.1365-4632.2010.04474.x

[12] Clydesdale GJ, Dandie GW, Muller HK. Ultraviolet light induced injury: Immunological and inflammatory effects. Immunology and Cell Biology. 2001;**79**:547-568. DOI: 10.1046/j.1440-1711.2001.01047.x

[13] Nichols JA, Katiyar SK. Skin photoprotection by natural polyphenols: Anti-inflammatory, antioxidant and DNA repair mechanisms. Archives of Dermatological Research. 2010;**302**:71-83. DOI: 10.1007/s00403-009-1001-3

[14] Cvetkovska AD, Manfredini S, Ziosi P, Molesini S, Dissette V, Magri I, Scapoli C, Carrieri A, Durini E, Vertuani S. Factors affecting SPF in vitro measurement and correlation with in vivo results. International Journal of Cosmetic Science. 2017;**39**:310-319. DOI: 10.1111/ics.12377

[15] Perea SE. Solar filters: A strategy of photoprotection. Applied Photochemistry. 2016;**92**:459-478. DOI: 10.1007/978-3-319-31671-0_11

[16] Regulation (EC) N. 1223/2009 of the European Parliament and of the council of 30 November 2009 on cosmetic product [Internet]. 2009. Available from: http://eur-lex.europa.eu/legal-content/EN/TXT/?uri=CELEX:02009R1223-20160812&from=EN [Accessed: 01-08-2017]

[17] Rulemaking history for OTC Sunscreen Drug Products. Available from: https://www.fda.gov/Drugs/DevelopmentApprovalProcess/DevelopmentResources/Over-the-CounterOTCDrugs/StatusofOTCRulemakings/ucm072134.htm#timeandexten [Accessed: 01-08-2017]

[18] Rancan F, Rosan S, Boehm K, Fernàndez E, Hidalgo ME, Quihot W, Rubio C, Boehm F, Piazena H, Oltmanns U. Protection against UVB irradiation by natural filters extracted from lichens. Journal of Photochemistry and Photobiology. B. 2002;**68**:133-139. DOI: 10.1016/S1011-1344(02)00362-7

[19] Kohlhardt-Floehr C, Bohem F, Troppens S, Lademann J, Truscott TG. Prooxidant and antioxidant behaviour of usnic acid from lichens under UVB-light irradiation—Studies in human cells. Journal of Photochemistry and Photobiology. 2010;**B101**:97-102. DOI: 10.1016/j.jphotobiol.2010.06.017

[20] Millot M, Di Meo F, Tomasi S, Boustie J, Trouillas P. Photoprotective capacities of lichen metabolites: A joint theoretical and experimental study. Journal of Photochemistry and Photobiology. 2012;**B111**:17-26. DOI: 10.1016/j.jphotobiol.2012.03.005

[21] Lohézic-Le Dévéhat F, Legouin B, Couteau C, Boustie J, Coiffard L. Lichenic extracts and metabolites as UV filters. Journal of Photochemistry and Photobiology. 2013;**B120**:17-28. DOI: 10.1016/j.jphotobiol.2013.01.009

[22] Boehm F, Clarke K, Edge R, Fernandez E, Navaratnam S, Quilhot W, Rancan F, Truscott TG. Lichens – Photophysical studies of potential new sunscreens. Journal of Photochemistry and Photobiology. 2009;**B95**:40-45. DOI: 10.1016/j.jphotobiol.2008.12.008

[23] Rojas JL, Días-Santos M, Valencia-Islas NA. Metabolites with antioxidant and photoprotective properties from *Usnea roccellina* Motyka, a lichen from Colombian Andes, UK. Journal of Pharmaceutical and BioSciences. 2015;**3**:18-26. DOI: 10.20510/ukjpb/3/i4/89454

[24] Casagrande R, Georgetti SR, Verri WA, Dorta DJ, Dos Santos AC, Fonseca MJV. Protective effect of topical formulations containing quercetin against UVB-induced oxidative stress in hairless mice. Journal of Photochemistry and Photobiology. B. 2006;**84**:21-27. DOI: 10.1016/j.jphotobiol.2006.01.006

[25] Casagrande R, Georgetti SR, Verri WA, Borin MF, Lopez RFV, Fonseca MJV. In vitro evaluation of quercetin cutaneous absorption from topical formulations and its functional stability by antioxidant activity. International Journal of Pharmaceutics. 2007;**328**:183-190. DOI: 10.1016/j.ijpharm.2006.08.006

[26] Freitas JV, Peporine-Lopes N, Gaspar LR. Photostability evaluation of five UV-filters, trans-resveratrol and beta-carotene in sunscreens. European Journal of Pharmaceutical Sciences. 2015;**78**:79-89. DOI: 10.1016/j.ejps.2015.07.004

[27] Freitas JV, Praca FSG, Bentley MVLB, Gaspar LR. Trans-resveratrol and beta carotene from sunscreens penetrate viable skin layers and reduce cutaneous penetration of UV-filters. International Journal of Pharmaceutics. 2015;**484**:131-137. DOI: 10.1016/j.ijpharm.2015.02.062

[28] Souza C, Maia Campos PMBG. Development and photoprotective effect of a sunscreen containing the antioxidants Spirulina and dimethylmethoxy chromanol on sun-induced skin damage. European Journal of Pharmaceutical Sciences. 2017;**104**:52-64. DOI: 10.1016/j.ejps.2017.03.026

[29] Azizoglu GA, Tanriverdi ST, Kose FA, Kirmizibayrak PB, Ozer O. Dual-prevention for UV-induced skin damage: Incorporation of melatonin-loaded elastic Niosomes into Octyl Methoxycinnamate Pickering emulsions. AAPS PharmSciTech. Nov 2017;**18**(8):2987-2998. DOI: 10.1208/s12249-017-0786-1

[30] Bora NS, Pathak MP, Mandal S, Mazumder B, Policegoudra R, Raju PS, Chattopadhyay P. Safety assessment and toxicological profiling of a novel combinational sunprotective dermal formulation containing melatonin and pumpkin seed oil. Regulatory Toxicology and Pharmacology. 2017;**89**:1-12. DOI: 10.1016/j.yrtph.2017.07.004

[31] Molins-Delgado D, Távora J, Díaz-Cruz MS, Barceló D. UV filters and benzotriazoles in urban aquatic ecosystems: The footprint of daily use products. Science of the Total Environment. 2017;**601-602**:975-986. DOI: 10.1016/j.scitotenv.2017.05.176

[32] Campos D, Gravato C, Fedorova G, Burkina V, Soares AMVM, Pestana JLT. Ecotoxicity of two organic UV-filters to the freshwater caddisfly Sericostoma Vittatum. Environmental Pollution. 2017;**228**:370-377. DOI: 10.1016/j.envpol.2017.05.021

[33] Pan SY, Zhou SF, Gao SH, Yu ZL, Zhang SF, Tang MK, Sun JN, Ma DL, Han YF, Fong WF, Ko KM. New perspectives on how to discover drugs from herbal medicines: CAM's outstanding contribution to modern therapeutics. Evidence-based Complementary and Alternative Medicine. 2013;**2013**. Article ID: 627375. DOI: 10.1155/2013/627375

11

Plant-Based Ethnopharmacological Remedies for Hypertension in Suriname

Dennis R.A. Mans, Angela Grant and Nicholaas Pinas

Abstract

Hypertension is the most important modifiable risk factor for cardiovascular, cerebrovascular, and renal diseases which are together among the most frequent causes of morbidity and mortality in the world. Despite the availability of a wide range of effective medicines, many individuals suffering from hypertension use plant-derived preparations for treating their disease. The choice for these alternatives is often associated with the closer relationship of such approaches to specific social, cultural, and religious perceptions about health and disease. However, in most cases, the scientific evidence for clinical efficacy of such medications is scant. The Republic of Suriname is a middle-income country in South America with a relatively high prevalence of hypertension and other cardiovascular diseases. This country harbors descendants of all continents, all of whom have preserved their cultural customs including their ethnopharmacological traditions. As a result, many Surinamese are inclined to treat their diseases including hypertension as they have done for centuries, that is, with plant-based preparations. This chapter has compiled the plants used for treating hypertension in Suriname; extensively evaluates 15 commonly used plants for potential efficacy on the basis of available phytochemical, mechanistic, preclinical, and clinical literature data; and closes with conclusions about their potential usefulness against the disease.

Keywords: hypertension, medicinal plants, Suriname, preclinical studies, clinical studies, phytochemical composition, mechanism of action

1. Introduction

Blood pressure is the force exerted by the heart and the arteries to maintain the flow of blood through the body in order to supply all cells with oxygen and nutrients and remove waste products. This normally occurs at average systolic and diastolic pressures of 120 and 80 mm Hg, respectively [1]. High blood pressure or arterial hypertension (or hypertension for short) is present when these values are persistently above 140 and 90 mm Hg, respectively [1]. This condition initially does not cause symptoms [1]. However, in the long-term, it is one of the most important predisposing factors for potentially fatal coronary artery disease, heart failure, stroke, peripheral vascular disease, vision loss, and chronic kidney disease [1].

Hypertension is classified as primary (or essential) hypertension and secondary hypertension [2]. Primary hypertension accounts for 90–95% of cases, typically begins in the fifth or sixth decade of life, and is associated with nonspecific lifestyle factors such as excess salt intake, obesity and a sedentary lifestyle, cigarette smoking, high alcohol intake, stress, and a family history suggesting the involvement of genetic factors in its etiology [3]. In the remaining 5–10% of cases categorized as secondary hypertension, the elevated blood pressure has an identifiable cause such as renal artery stenosis, chronic kidney disease, sleep apnoea, hyperthyroidism, pheochromocytoma, the use of oral contraceptives, or pregnancy [2].

In both situations, the elevated blood pressure is caused by an increase in the total peripheral resistance, that is, the total resistance to the flow of blood in the systemic circulation. The increased peripheral resistance is most often attributable to abnormalities in the sympathetic nervous system [4] and the renin-angiotensin-aldosterone system [5]. In the former case, the excessive release of adrenaline and noradrenaline leads to overstimulation of β_1- and α_1-adrenoreceptors, contraction of arterial smooth muscles, constriction of the arterioles, and an increased peripheral resistance [4]. In the latter case, excess secretion of renin by juxtaglomerular cells following stimulation of β_1-adrenergic receptors on their surface, along with glomerular underperfusion, leads to the reabsorption of salt and water and the release of renin, enlarging vascular volume and further increasing peripheral resistance [5]. Impairments in the functioning of vasorelaxing factors such as nitric oxide due to endothelial dysfunction as well as that of vasoactive substances such as endothelin, bradykinin, and atrial natriuretic peptide may further contribute to and/or maintain the hypertension [6].

Lifestyle modifications such as dietary changes can lower blood pressure and decrease the risk of health complications. Examples of such alterations are diets low in sodium, high in potassium, rich in vegetables, fruits, and low-fat dairy products (the so-called Dietary Approaches to Stop Hypertension (DASH) diet, as well as vegetarian diets [7]. Lifestyle modifications other than dietary changes shown to reduce hypertension are increased physical exercise, weight loss, and stress reduction [8]. The potential effectiveness of these modifications is similar to, and may even exceed the effects of a single medication [9]. Notably, several randomized controlled trials have demonstrated that even a slight blood pressure decrease of 10 mm Hg reduces the risk of death due to cardiovascular disease by 25% and the risk of stroke-related mortality by 40% [10].

If lifestyle changes are not sufficient to reduce the elevated blood pressure, antihypertensive medications are prescribed. Still, lifestyle changes are recommended in conjunction with medication [6, 11]. Among the commonly used antihypertensives are thiazide-diuretics such as chlorthalidone and hydrochlorothiazide, calcium channel blockers such as nifedipine and amlodipine, β-blockers such as atenolol and metoprolol, angiotensin-converting enzyme (ACE) inhibitors such as captopril and enalapril, and angiotensin receptor blockers such as losartan and candesartan [6, 11]. These medications may be used either alone or at certain combinations [6, 11]. β-blockers are widely used as a first-line treatment for hypertension, but their efficacy may be inferior to those of other antihypertensive drugs [12].

Currently, close to 1 billion adults or over 20% of the world population suffer from hypertension [13]. This leads to enormous medical, economic, and human costs. In the USA alone, the total economic burden of hypertension in terms of healthcare services, medications, and absent workforce was estimated at USD 47 billion to USD 73.4 billion between the years 2009 and 2011 [14]. And management of hypertension accounts for 30% of office visits for individuals of 45–64 years, and for more than 40% of visits in those aged 60–74 years and over 75 years [15].

Hypertension occurs slightly more often in males, individuals of low socioeconomic status, and those of older age [13, 16]. It is correspondingly common in high-, medium-, and low-income countries [13, 17], but prevalence rates vary widely throughout the world, with values as low as 3.4–6.8% in rural India and as high as 68.9–72.5% in Poland [17]. There are also large differences in prevalence rates within certain countries. For instance, African American adults in the USA have among the highest rates in the world at 44% but hypertension is less common in US whites and Mexican Americans [16, 18]. Still, deaths due to non-communicable diseases including those related to hypertension occur more frequently and at earlier stages in low- and middle-income countries when compared to industrialized countries [19]. By 2030, low-income countries are even expected to have eight times more deaths due to these ailments than high-income countries [19].

2. Background on Suriname

2.1. Geography, people, and economy

The Republic of Suriname is located on the north-east coast of South America and borders the Atlantic Ocean to the north, French Guiana to the east, Brazil to the south, and Guyana to the west (**Figure 1**). The country's land area of roughly 165,000 km^2 can be distinguished into a northern narrow low-land coastal area that harbors the capital city Paramaribo as well as other urbanized areas, a broad but sparsely inhabited savannah belt, and a southern forested area that comprises about three-quarters of its surface area and largely consists of dense, pristine, and highly biodiverse tropical rain forest. Roughly 80% of the population of about 570,000 lives in the urbanized northern coastal zone while the remaining 20% populates the rural and interior savannas and hinterlands [20].

Suriname is renowned for its ethnic, religious, and cultural diversity, harboring various Amerindian tribes, the original inhabitants of the country; descendants from runaway enslaved Africans brought in between the sixteenth and the nineteenth century (called Maroons); those from mixed Black and White origin (called Creoles); descendants from contract workers from China, India (called Hindustanis), and Java, Indonesia (called Javanese) who arrived between the second half of the nineteenth century and the first half of the twentieth century; descendants from a number of European countries; and more recently, immigrants from various

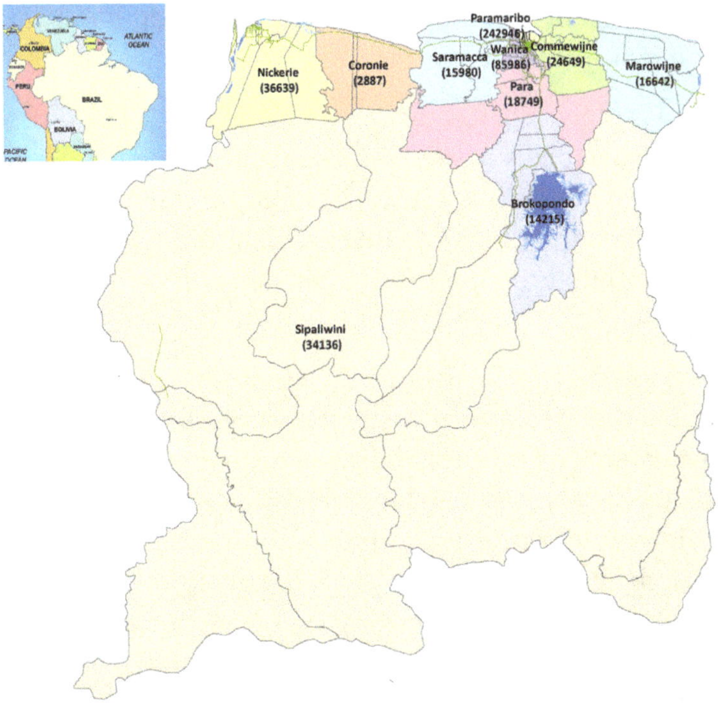

Figure 1. Map of Suriname depicting the administrative districts (from: https://goo.gl/images/gqdxwn). The insert (from: https://goo.gl/images/rWXrAL) indicates the location of Suriname in South America.

Latin American and Caribbean counties including Brazil, Guyana, French Guiana, Haiti, etc. [20]. The largest ethnic groups in the country are the Hindustanis, Maroons, Creoles, and Javanese, accounting for 27.4, 21.7, 17.0, and 15.7%, respectively, of the total population [20]. All ethnic groups have largely preserved their own specific identity [21], making Suriname one of the culturally most diverse countries in the world [22].

Suriname is situated on the Guiana Shield, a Precambrian geological formation estimated to be 1.7 billion years old and one of the regions with the largest expanse of undisturbed tropical rain forest in the world with a very high animal and plant biodiversity [23]. The high mineral density of Suriname's soil contributes to its ranking as the 17th richest country in the world in terms of natural resources and development potential [24]. Suriname's most important economic means of support are crude oil drilling, bauxite and gold mining, agriculture, fisheries, forestry, and ecotourism [24]. These activities contributed substantially to the gross domestic income in 2014 of USD 5.21 billion and the average *per capita* income in that year of USD 9325 [24]. This positions Suriname on the World Bank's list of upper-middle income economies [25].

2.2. Non-communicable diseases

At the same time, as observed in many low- and middle-income countries [19], more and more Surinamese are adapting a Western lifestyle. For instance, only about half of the country's overall population met the levels for physical activity recommended by the World Health Organization (WHO) [26]; almost three-quarters of school children aged 13–15 years had less than 1 hour of physical activity per day and 81% had a high calorie intake [27]; and the average tobacco and alcohol consumption *per capita* in individuals of 15 years and older was unacceptably high [28].

As a result, in 2008, 25.1% of Surinamese was obese [28, 29]; 7.4% had prediabetes and 13.0% diabetes mellitus [30]; the overall estimated prevalence of the metabolic syndrome was 39.2% [31]; and more than 25% of adults had a raised blood pressure [29, 32]. These observations indicate that Suriname, similarly to many other economically developing countries [19], is facing increasing public health threats of lifestyle-related non-communicable diseases including cardiovascular disease.

Indeed, WHO assessments from 2014 attributed 68% of total deaths in Suriname to the four main non-communicable diseases (cardiovascular, neoplastic, diabetic, and chronic respiratory diseases) and estimated that the probability of dying between age 30 and 70 years from these conditions was 14% [29]. Notably, in all approximations and previsions, cardiovascular disease was the most important cause of morbidity and mortality in Suriname. For instance, in 2012, stroke (11%), ischemic heart disease (9.1%), diabetes mellitus (7.3%), and hypertensive heart disease (4.5%) were among the leading causes of mortality, together accounting for about 800 or almost one-third of the total number of deaths in that year [29]. Indeed, with 864 fatalities in 2013 (or more than one-quarter of the total number of 3260 deaths in that year), cardiovascular disease was by far the leading cause of mortality in Suriname, ahead of death due to malignant neoplasms, external causes, perinatal complications, diabetes mellitus, and acute respiratory infections [33].

2.3. Hypertension

The comprehensive, nation-wide Suriname Health Study on non-communicable diseases found an overall prevalence of hypertension of 26.2% [32]. This was in the range of values reported for many other developing countries [34] as well as the relatively large Surinamese diaspora in The Netherlands [35]. Mean values for systolic and diastolic blood pressure were higher in males than in females; increased with older age; and were highest in Creoles Hindustanis, and Javanese, and lowest in Maroons and Amerindians [32]. The prevalence of hypertension in demographic risk factor subgroups differed between ethnic groups, as did the associations of ethnic groups with hypertension [32], implying the need of tailor-made intervention programs to control hypertension in Suriname [32].

The findings from two other Surinamese studies suggest that an urban lifestyle may also contribute to the development of prehypertension and hypertension in Suriname, reporting higher prevalence rates in the urban areas of the country (39 and 41%, respectively [36]), and in an urban middle-income population (31 and 41%, respectively [37]). These studies found neither gender differences nor racial/ethnic differences in the prevalence of hypertension in their participants [36, 37], but prehypertension was more common in urban males than in urban females [36] and after adjusting for age, urban African-Surinamese had significantly higher odds of having hypertension than their Asian counterparts [36].

An apparent ethnic/racial predilection of hypertension was also observed in several Dutch epidemiological studies that included Surinamese migrants. These studies reported a higher incidence of prehypertension, hypertension, malignant hypertension, and related renal complications in participants from Afro-Surinamese and Hindustani descent compared to white individuals [35, 38–40]. These differences were tentatively explained by ethnic disparities in the perception of hypertension (supporting one of the findings of the Suriname Heath Study [32]), as well in drug adherence, blood pressure control, and/or insurance status [38, 40–42].

2.4. Health care system

Suriname's healthcare system is coordinated by the Ministry of Health which is headed by the Minister of Health and the Director of Health (the Chief Medical Officer). The main responsibilities of the ministry are the planning, coordination, inspection, and monitoring and evaluation of, as well as policy development and setting standards to the country's health system [43].

In 2014, the Ministry spent 5.7% of the country's gross domestic product for health expenditures which corresponded to an average *per capita* sum of USD 589. The costs of those who cannot afford these expenses are covered by the Ministry of Social Affairs. Government employees and employees of government-related companies are mandatory insured at the State Health Foundation. Essential pharmaceuticals including those for treating hypertension are imported, stocked, and distributed by the National Pharmaceutical Import and Distribution Company and are in general readily available. These medicines are identified by the Board for Essential Pharmaceuticals that consists of various players in the field of pharmacy and pharmacology in Suriname.

Primary healthcare in Suriname's coastal area and hinterlands is provided by the government-subsidized Regional Health Service and Medical Mission, respectively, each operating about 40 clinics which also dispense medicines. In 2004, Suriname had 0.45 physicians per 1000 population. Secondary care and specialist care including that for patients suffering from complications of hypertension are provided by two private and two government-supported hospitals in Paramaribo and one public hospital in the western district of Nickerie.

The Academic Hospital Paramaribo also functions as training facility for both general practitioners and medical specialists, and has to its disposal a Thorax Center for specialized cardiology care and cardiothoracic surgery. Patients with kidney failure are treated by the government-supported Kidney Dialysis Center. Cases of hypertensive crisis and other medical emergencies can get help around-the-clock from the First-aid Stations of the Academic Hospital Paramaribo and the Sint Vincentius Hospital Suriname.

Patients who need specialized therapy that is not available in Suriname (particularly those suffering from certain malignancies) are sent abroad – in general to the Netherlands or Colombia – for treatment. All expenses are covered by the Ministry of Health that has reserved a special budget for these cases.

2.5. Use of traditional medicines against hypertension in Suriname

Despite the broad availability of affordable and accessible modern health care throughout the entire country, the use of traditional medicines is deeply rooted in all ethnic groups in Suriname [21, 44]. This is probably for an important part attributable to the fact that all ethnic and cultural groups in the country have preserved much of their original cultural and ethnopharmacological practices as a means of strengthening the ethnic identity during the secluded lifestyle the former colonial authorities had forced them into [21, 22]. Furthermore, Suriname's large biodiversity provides ample and readily available raw material that can be processed into traditional medicines [23]. As a result, many disease conditions including hypertension are often treated with traditional plant-based medicines and may be used instead of, or in conjunction with prescription drugs.

The medicinal plants used throughout the country have extensively been discussed in the literature [45], and those used more commonly by Hindustanis, Maroons, and Javanese have also been reviewed [46–48]. Less comprehensive accounts of these plants have been presented as well [49–55]. Together, these publications have compiled 789 Surinamese medicinal plants, 65 of which (roughly 8%) are used for treating hypertension. The latter plants, plant parts, and methods of processing are given in **Table 1**. They belong to 38 different families, the most represented of which are the Fabaceae with 7 species, the Solanaceae with 5 species, the Malvaceae and the Piperaceae with 4 species each, and the Asteraceae and the Cucurbitaceae with 3 species each (**Table 1**). In 31 cases the leaves are used, in 9 cases the whole plant, in 6 cases the fruits, in 5 cases the bark, and in 1–3 cases other plant parts such as roots and flowers (**Table 1**).

Family	Species (Vernacular names in English; Surinamese)	Part(s) used	Mode of preparation
Acanthaceae	*Justicia pectoralis* Jacq. (Freshcut; tonkawiwiri)	Leaves	Infusion
Acanthaceae	*Ruellia tuberosa* L. (Minnieroot; watrakanu)	Roots and leaves	Infusion
Amaranthaceae	*Alternanthera brasiliana* (L.) Kuntze (Brazilian joyweed; weti ede)	Whole plant	Infusion
Anacardiaceae	*Mangifera indica* L. (Mango; manya)	Leaves	Infusion
Anacardiaceae	*Spondias dulcis* L. (Ambarella; pomme cythère)	Fresh fruits; fresh peels	Pressed to obtain juice to drink; infusion
Annonaceae	*Annona muricata* L. (Soursop; zuurzak)	Fresh leaves	Infusion
Apiaceae	*Apium graveolens* L. (Celery; soepgroenten)	Fresh leaves	Infusion
Apocynaceae	*Catharanthus roseus* (L.) G.Don, 1837 (Rosy periwinkle; kotomisi)	Whole plant	Infusion
Apocynaceae	*Geissospermum laeve* (Vell.).Miers (Pao-pereira bark; bergi bita)	Fresh stem bark	Decoction

Family	Species (Vernacular names in English; Surinamese)	Part(s) used	Mode of preparation
Arecaceae	*Cosos nucifera* L. (Coconut tree; kronto)	Dried husk fibers	Infusion
Asteraceae	*Ayapana triplinervis* (Vahl) R.M. King & H. Rob (Water hemp; sekrepatuwiwiri)	Fresh or dried leaves	Infusion
Asteraceae	*Cyanthillium cinereum* (L.) H. Rob (Little ironweed; doifiwiwiri)	Whole plant	Infusion
Asteraceae	*Melampodium camphoratum* (L.F.) Baker (Sand bitters; kanfrubita)	Whole plant	Infusion
Bignoniaceae	*Mansoa alliacea* (Lam.) A.H. Genry (Garlic vine; konofrukutetey)	Leaves and hardwood	Infusion
Boraginaceae	*Cordia schomburgkii* DC. (Canalette; blaka uma)	Fresh leaves	Infusion
Boraginaceae	*Cordia tetrandra* Aubl. (Clammy cherry; tafrabon)	Dried leaves	Infusion
Caricaceae	*Carica papaya* L. (Papaya; papaya)	Fresh fruits	None; fresh fruit eaten
Cecropiaceae	*Cecropia peltata* L. (Trumpet tree; uma busipapaya)	Dried leaves	Infusion
Cecropiaceae	*Cecropia sciadophylla* Mart. (Congo pump; man busipapaya)	Dried leaves	Infusion
Combretaceae	*Terminalia catappa* L. (Tropical almond; zoete amandel)	Leaves	Infusion
Commelinaceae	*Tripogandra serrulata* (Vahl.) Handlos. (Pink trinity; redi gado dede)	Dried leaves	Infusion
Convolvulaceae	*Ipomoea aquatica* Forssk. (Water spinach; dagublad)	Young leaves and stem	Cooked and eaten as a vegetable
Cucurbitaceae	*Cucumis sativus* L. (Cucumber; komkommer)	Fresh fruits	Pressed to obtain juice to drink
Cucurbitaceae	*Cucurbita moschata* Duchesne (Squash; pompoen)	Dried flowers	Infusion
Cucurbitaceae	*Momordica charantia* L. (Bitter melon; sopropo)	Dried whole plant	Infusion
Dilleniaceae	*Davilla nitida* (Vahl.) Kubizki (Sandpaper tree; schuurpapier)	Stem	Pressed to obtain sap to drink

Family	Species (Vernacular names in English; Surinamese)	Part(s) used	Mode of preparation
Euphorbiaceae	*Acalypha hispida* Burm. f. (Red hot cat's tail; pus'pusitere)	Leaves	Infusion
Fabaceae	*Copaifera guyanensis* Desf. (Copaiba; hoepelhout)	Fresh stem bark	Infusion
Fabaceae	*Desmodium adscendens* (Sw.) DC. (Beggar lice; toriman)	Roots	Pressed to obtain sap to drink
Fabaceae	*Hymenaea courbaril* L. (West Indian locust; loksi)	Stem bark	Infusion
Fabaceae	*Machaerium lunatum* (L.f.) Ducke (Manatee bush; brantimaka)	Leaves	Infusion
Fabaceae	*Mimosa pudica* L. (Shy plant; Sing sing tap yu koto)	Whole plant	Infusion
Fabaceae	*Senna alata* (L.) Roxb. (Candle bush; slabriki)	Leaves	Infusion
Fabaceae	*Tamarindus indica* L. (Tamarind; tamarinde)	Leaves	Infusion
Lamiaceae	*Ocimum campechianum* Mill. (Amazonian basil; smeriwiwiri)	Whole plant	Macerated for herbal bath
Lauraceae	*Persea americana* Mill. (Avocado; advocaat)	Dried leaves	Infusion
Malvaceae	*Gossypium barbadense* L. (Sea island cotton; redi katun)	Leaves	Infusion
Malvaceae	*Hibiscus sabdariffa* L. (Roselle; syuru)	Leaves	Infusion
Malvaceae	*Waltheria indica* L. (Sleepy morning; malva)	Leaves	Infusion
Meliaceae	*Azadirachta indica* A. Juss. (Neem; nim)	Leaves	Infusion
Meliaceae	*Carapa guianensis* Aubl. (Crabwood; witte krapa)	Dried stem bark	Decoction
Meliaceae	*Carapa procera* D.C. (African crabwood; rode krapa)	Dried stem bark	Decoction
Musaceae	*Musa sp., Musa x paradisiaca* (Banana; banaan)	Leaves	Infusion
Oxalidaceae	*Averrhoa bilimbi* L. (Bilimbi; birambi)	Fresh fruits	Pressed to obtain juice to drink

Family	Species (Vernacular names in English; Surinamese)	Part(s) used	Mode of preparation
Passifloraceae	*Passiflora cocciea* Aubl. (Scarlet passion flower; sneki markusa)	Leaves and stem	Infusion
Phyllanthaceae	*Phyllanthus amarus* Schumach. & Thonn. (Stonebreaker; finibita)	Whole plant	Infusion
Phytolaccaceae	*Microtea debilis* Sw. (Weak jumby pepper; eiwitblad)	Fresh or dried whole plant or leaves	Infusion
Piperaceae	*Peperomia pellucida* (L.) Kunth. (Pepper elder; konsakawiwiri)	Fresh leaves or whole plant	Pressed to obtain sap to drink
Piperaceae	*Peperomia rotundifolia* (L.) Kunth. (Swan spice; tinsensiwiwiri)	Fresh leaves or whole plant	Pressed to obtain sap to drink
Piperaceae	*Piper betle* L. (Betel; pahnblad)	Leaves	Infusion
Piperaceae	*Piper marginatum* Jacq. (Marigold pepper; aneysiwiwiri)	Leaves	Infusion
Poaceae	*Eleusine indica* L. (Indian goosegrass; mangrasi)	Leaves	Infusion
Poaceae	*Zea mais* L. (Maize; karu)	Ripe ears	Decoction
Rhamnaceae	*Ziziphus jujuba* L. (Jujube; olijf)	Leaves	Infusion
Rubiaceae	*Sipanea pratensis* Aubl. (Water lagaga; wetibaka)	Leaves	Infusion
Sapindaceae	*Paullinia pinnata* L. (Bread and cheese; feyfifingawiwiri)	Leaves	Pressed to obtain sap to drink
Sapotaceae	*Chrysophyllum cainito* L. (Star apple; sterappel)	Dried leaves	Infusion
Scrophulariaceae	*Scoparia dulcis* L. (Licorice weed; sibiwiwiri)	Aerial parts	Infusion
Simarubaceae	*Quassia amara* L. (Bitter wood; kwasibita)	Hard wood	Infusion
Siparunaceae	*Siparuna guianensis* Aubl. (Ant bush; yarakopi)	Aerial parts	Macerated for herbal bath
Solanaceae	*Physalis angulata* L. (Angular winter cherry; batotobita)	Dried leaves	Infusion

Family	Species (Vernacular names in English; Surinamese)	Part(s) used	Mode of preparation
Solanaceae	*Solanum leucocarpon* Dual. (Bitayouli; uma parabita)	Leaves	Macerated for herbal bath
Solanaceae	*Solanum macrocarpum* L. (African eggplant; antruwa)	Fresh fruits	Cooked and eaten as a vegetable
Solanaceae	*Solanum stramoniifolium* Jacq. (Coconilla; makadroyfi)	Fresh fruits	None; fresh fruit eaten
Solanaceae	*Solanum subinerme* Jacq. (Juhuna; droyfimaka)	Leaves	Infusion

Table 1. Plants used for treating hypertension in Suriname.

3. Scientific rationale for using Surinamese plants against hypertension

In this section, 15 plants that are commonly used against hypertension in Suriname, as well as preclinical and clinical indications for their blood pressure-lowering effect and their presumed bioactive constituent(s) and mechanism(s) of action are in detail addressed. The plants are most frequently mentioned as traditional treatments for hypertension in the above-mentioned publications [45–55]. The data are summarized in **Table 2**.

Family	Plant species (Vernacular name in English; Surinamese)	Preclinical evidence	Clinical evidence	Presumed key active constituent(s)	Presumed mechanism of action
Acanthaceae	*Ruellia tuberosa* L. (Minnieroot; watrakanu)	No	No	Unknown	Decreased blood lipid levels
Anacardiaceae	*Mangifera indica* L. (Mango; manya)	Yes	No	Mangiferin	Vasodilation; stimulated diuresis
Annonaceae	*Annona muricata* L. (Soursop; zuurzak)	Yes	No	Alkaloids, essential oils	Vasodilation
Apiaceae	*Apium graveolens* L. (Celery; soepgroente)	Yes	Yes	3-n-butylphthalide	Vasodilation, stimulated diuresis
Arecaceae	*Cocos nucifera* L. (Coconut; kronto)	Yes	Yes	Phenolics, flavonoids	Vasodilation; decreased blood lipid levels; stimulated diuresis

Family	Plant species (Vernacular name in English; Surinamese)	Preclinical evidence	Clinical evidence	Presumed key active constituent(s)	Presumed mechanism of action
Caricaceae	*Carica papaya* L. (Papaya; papaya)	Yes	No	Unknown	Vasodilation; stimulated diuresis
Cucurbitaceae	*Cucumis sativus* L. (Cucumber; komkommer)	Yes	Yes	Unknown	Stimulated diuresis
Fabaceae	*Desmodium adscendens* (Sw.) DC. (Beggar lice; toriman)	No	No	Unknown	Vasodilation
Fabaceae	*Hymenaea courbaril* L. (West Indian locust; loksi)	No	No	Unknown	Unknown
Fabaceae	*Tamarindus indica* L. (Tamarind; tamarinde)	Yes	No	Unknown	Sympatico-inhibition; decreased blood lipid levels
Lauraceae	*Persea americana* Mill. (Avocado; advocaat)	Yes	No	Unknown	Vasodilation; decreased blood lipid levels
Malvaceae	*Gossypium barbadense* L. (Sea island cotton; redi katun)	Yes	No	Unknown	Vasodilation
Malvaceae	*Hibiscus sabdariffa* L. (Roselle; syuru)	Yes	No	Polyphenolics, flavonoids	Vasodilation; stimulated diuresis; decreased blood lipid levels
Meliaceae	*Azadirachta indica* A. Juss. (Neem; nim)	Yes	No	Azadirachtin, nimbinin	Vasodilation
Oxalidaceae	*Averrhoa bilimbi* L. (Bilimbi; birambi)	Yes	No	Unknown	Vasodilation; decreased cardiac output; stimulated diuresis

Table 2. Preclinical and clinical evidence for blood pressure-lowering activity of 15 commonly used plants in Suriname for treating hypertension, the presumed key active constituent(s) in these plants, and their presumed mechanism of action.

3.1. Acanthaceaea – *Ruellia tuberosa* L.

The minnie root *R. tuberosa* (**Figure 2**) is probably native to Central America but has spread to various other tropical regions in South America as well as South and South east Asia. Both the English vernacular name 'cracker plant' and the Surinamese vernacular name *watrakanu* ('water canon') are probably derived from the loud crack emitted when the ripe fruits in a pod with seven to eight seeds burst open on contact with water, hurdling the seeds away. The whole plant, the leaves, and/or the roots are used in various traditional medicinal systems including those in Suriname as an antidiabetic, antipyretic, analgesic, diuretic, antihypertensive, gastroprotective, anthelmintic, antigonorrheal, antioxidant, blood-purifying, and abortifacient agent [46, 48, 49, 55, 56]. Some of these activities were supported by the results from pharmacological studies [57, 58] and could be associated with certain alkaloids, triterpenoids, saponins, sterols, and flavonoids in the plant [59].

So far, no formal experimental evaluations on the presumed antihypertensive activity of *R. tuberosa* have been reported. However, crude extracts from the leaves of the closely related species *R. patula* and *R. brittoniana* as well as n-butanolic extracts and the aqueous layers of both plant extracts displayed cardiotonic effects in isolated rabbit hearts [60]. More importantly, a preparation from *R. patula* elicited a clear blood pressure-lowering effect in pentothal sodium-anesthetized rats [61]. This effect may be attributed, at least partially, to the blood lipid-lowering actions of *Ruellia* preparations [57, 58].

3.2. Anacardiaceae – *Mangifera indica* L.

The mango tree *M. indica* is indigenous to Bangladesh, India, and Pakistan where it is found in the wild. It has been domesticated in India around 2000 BC, and many cultivated varieties have been produced in other tropical countries including Suriname. Both sour, unripe, and sweet, ripe mangoes are widely used in cuisine, among others, in chutneys, curries, pickles, or side dishes, and to prepare juices, smoothies, nectars, jams, and as a flavoring in ice creams, sorbets, fruit bars, and pies.

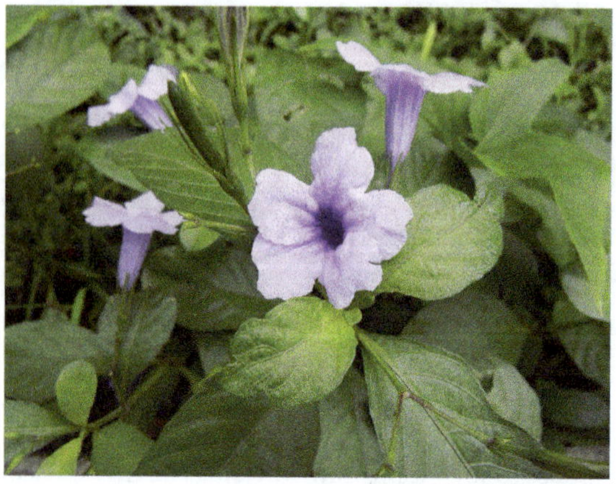

Figure 2. Acanthaceaea – *Ruellia tuberosa* L. (from: https://goo.gl/images/vk862o).

Preparations from flowers, unripe fruits, stone, leaves, stembark, and roots of *M. indica* also have many traditional medicinal uses, among others, to treat certain parasitic infections, uterus disorders, gastrointestinal problems, and syphilis; strengthen the blood vessels; cure varicose veins; and lower an elevated blood pressure [46, 62–64]. Several of these properties have been attributed to a number of bioactive substances in leaves and stem bark of the plant including the polyphenolic compound mangiferin [65]. This compound also displayed notable blood pressure-lowering effects in *in vitro* models and laboratory animals [66].

The apparent antihypertensive effect of *M. indica* preparations and constituents may be attributed to at least two mechanisms, namely the induction of vasodilation and the stimulation of diuresis. Indications for the former possibility are provided by the inhibition of noradrenaline-induced contractions of mesenteric arteries isolated from spontaneously hypertensive rats by a *M. indica* stem bark extract (called 'Vimang' from 'vida del mango' meaning 'life of the mango') [62]. Support for the second possibility comes from the diuretic effect of 'Vimang' in laboratory rats [67].

3.3. Annonaceae – *Annona muricata* L.

The exact origin of the soursop or graviola *A. muricata* (**Figure 3**) is unknown, but it is believed to be native to the Caribbean and the tropical regions of the Americas. It is now widely cultivated for its fruit, the pulp of which contains substantial amounts of vitamin C, vitamin B1, and vitamin B2 and is used to make fruit juice drinks, smoothies, as well as candies, sorbets, and ice cream flavorings. Relatively recently, *A. muricata* fruit and graviola capsules have been promoted as an alternative treatment for cancer. However, there is no medical evidence for such an activity, even though preclinical studies have shown cytotoxic effects of *A. muricata* extracts against cultured cancer cells [68].

Importantly, *Annona* species including *A. muricata* are a rich source of annonaceous acetogenins such as annonacin and annonamine, potent neurotoxins that inhibit mitochondrial

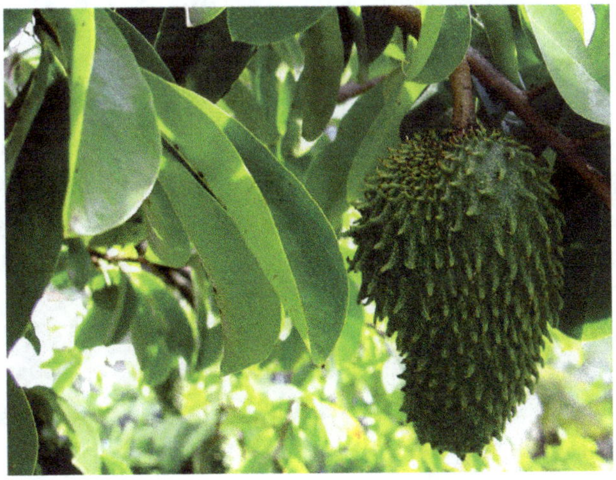

Figure 3. Annonaceae – *Annona muricata* L. (from: https://goo.gl/images/K9WNHr).

complex I, thereby shutting down cellular respiration [69]. These compounds have been associated – although not conclusively – with the unusually high incidence of atypical parkinsonism in the Caribbean island of Guadeloupe where relatively large amounts of *A. muricata* fruits as well as infusions and decoctions from the leaves of the plant are consumed [70].

Nevertheless, all parts of *A. muricata* are extensively used – also in Suriname – as traditional medicines against a wide diversity of conditions, among others, insomnia; nervousness, anxiety, and depression; a hangover; epilepsy; parasitic and helminth infections; diabetes mellitus; cancer; and hypertension [45, 48, 49, 55, 71]. Pharmacological studies with preparations from leaves, bark, and roots of the plant have indeed shown sedative, anxiolytic, smooth muscle-relaxant, antispasmodic, and antihypertensive effects [71–73]. Some of these effects may be attributed to the presence in the plant of bioactive constituents such as alkaloids, flavonol triglycosides, phenolics, and essential oils [71].

Indications for an antihypertensive effect were provided by the decrease in blood pressure in normotensive Sprague-Dawley rats which were intravenously treated with an aqueous leaf extract of *A. muricata* [74]. Furthermore, the extract decreased the phenylephrine-induced contractions of isolated rat and guinea pig aortic rings [74, 75], and relaxed the contractions of isolated rat aortic rings caused by high K^+ while apparently blocking Ca^{2+} channels [74]. These findings suggest that the hypotensive effects of the *A. muricata* leaf extract may involve vasodilation mediated through peripheral mechanisms involving antagonism of Ca^{2+} [74]. This effect has been attributed to alkaloids such as coreximine, anomurine, and reticulin, and some essential oil components such as β-caryophyllene [74].

However, in light of the affinity of both crude extracts and isoquinoline alkaloids isolated from *Annona* species to 5-HT_{1A} receptors *in vitro* [72], and the well-known decreasing effect of 5-HT_{1A} receptor agonists on blood pressure and heart rate [76], it is also possible that the antihypertensive effect of these plants occurs through a central mechanism that causes peripheral vasodilation and stimulates the vagus nerve.

3.4. Apiaceae – *Apium graveolens* L.

The celery *A. graveolens* (**Figure 4**) originates from the Mediterranean region, but many cultivars are now grown throughout the world. This plant has been cultivated since ancient times, initially only for its medicinal qualities, but later also as a vegetable to counter the salt-sickness of winter diets based on salted meats without green vegetables. Today, *A. graveolens* stalks, leaves, and hypocotyl are eaten raw or as an ingredient in salads, cooked as a vegetable, or as a flavoring – either fresh or dried – in soups, stews, and pot roasts.

A. graveolens seeds – which are in fact very small fruits – yield a valuable volatile oil that is used in perfumes and, when ground and mixed with salt, to produce celery salt for enhancing the flavor of, for instance, Bloody Mary cocktails [77]. However, celery seeds contain relatively high levels of the phenylpropene apiole that can cause abortion – sometimes with fatal consequences [78] – as well as liver and kidney damage [79] and severe allergic reactions including potentially fatal anaphylactic shock [80].

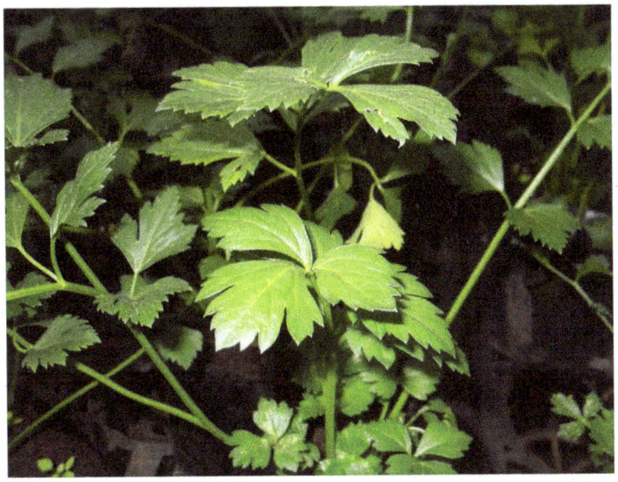

Figure 4. Apiaceae – *Apium graveolens* L. (from: https://goo.gl/images/7RWqQ4).

Nevertheless, *A. graveolens* is extensively used in traditional medicinal systems – including those in Suriname-against numerous diseases ranging from respiratory ailments and liver diseases to menstrual problems and hypertension [45, 81, 82].

Support for an antihypertensive effect of preparations from *A. graveolens* came from the decreased blood pressure and heart rate in salt-induced hypertensive rats, normotensive rats, and normotensive rabbits following intraperitoneal administration of extracts from seeds, stalks, or roots of the plant [83–86]. The results from studies with isolated rat aortic rings suggested that these effects occurred through vasodilation [83] or the stimulation of muscarinic receptors [84]. However, extracts from celery leaves, stalks, and roots have also been reported to stimulate diuresis in several experimental models [87, 88], providing an alternative explanation for their blood pressure-lowering effects.

The antihypertensive effects of *A. graveolens* have been attributed to the presence in the plant of the benzofuran 3-n-butylphthalide [86, 89] that, along with sedanolide, is also primarily responsible for the aroma and taste of celery. Clinical studies indeed showed a reduction in blood pressure of patients who had been given celery juice [90, 91]. These and other clinical data first led to the approval in China of 3-n-butylphthalide for the treatment of cerebral ischemia, and the preparation of clinical studies to assess n-butylphthalide formulated as softgel capsules for its safety in patients with mild to moderate acute ischemic stroke [92].

3.5. Arecaceae – *Cocos nucifera* L.

The coconut tree *C. nucifera* is believed to originate from the South East Asian peninsular region. It has probably spread to many other parts of the world by sea-faring traders and through marine currents, and is now cultivated in many subtropical and tropical countries. Refrigerated coconut water or coconut juice is a much appreciated refreshing drink all over the world; the fleshy coconut 'meat' is used fresh or dried in confections and desserts; coconut milk is frequently added to curries and other spicy dishes; and coconut oil is used for frying and preparing margarine and in various cosmetics [93].

Almost all parts of *C. nucifera* have long been used in traditional medicine for treating many disease conditions, among others, diarrhea, fever and malaria, renal diseases, asthma, diabetes mellitus, hair loss, menstrual disorders, venereal diseases, as an oral contraceptive, and against hypertension [45, 94]. Pharmacological studies with extracts, fractions, and isolated compounds from parts of *C. nucifera* indeed showed a variety of activities ranging from antimicrobial and antiparasitic activities to vasodilatory and antihypertensive effects [95]. Some of these observations may be related to the presence in the plant of polyphenols, tannins, flavonoids, triterpenes, saponins, steroids, alkaloids, and/or fatty acids [94].

Evidence for an antihypertensive activity from *C. nucifera* came from the relaxation of isolated rat aortic rings by an ethanolic extract of *C. nucifera* endocarp and the reduced blood pressure in salt-induced hypertensive rats treated with this preparation [96]; the decreased blood pressure in a rat model of insulin resistance and acquired systolic hypertension following administration of tender coconut water [97]; and the decrease in heart rate of hypertensive Wistar rats which were given coconut water [98]. Notably, in a small clinical study, coconut water given for 2 weeks reportedly lowered the blood pressure in 71% of hypertensive individuals [99], while the fresh vascular sap from the immature, unopened inflorescence given once per day for 5 consecutive weeks led to a decrease in blood pressure as well as a reduction in total serum cholesterol in women with stage one hypertension [100].

The antihypertensive effects have been attributed to vasodilation following the direct activation of the nitric oxide/guanylate cyclase pathway as well as stimulation of muscarinic receptors and/or the cyclooxygenase pathway which would be caused by phenolic compounds and flavonoids [96]; inhibition of lipid peroxidation, upregulation of antioxidant status, and improved insulin sensitivity [97]; a decreased cardiac beating frequency [98]; and/or a (potassium-sparing) diuretic activity [99].

3.6. Caricaceae – *Carica papaya* L.

The papaya plant *C. papaya* probably has its origin in Mexico and the northern parts of South America and has subsequently become naturalized throughout other tropical and subtropical regions. Various cultivars are grown for their edible ripe fruits which are usually consumed raw. The juice from ripe papayas is a popular low-calorie beverage and is also added as a flavoring in candies, jellies, and ice cream; the unripe fruit is incorporated in various dishes; the young leaves and flower buds may be consumed as vegetables; and the ground black seeds are sometimes used as a substitute for black pepper.

The relatively high amount of the protease papain in unripe fruits has been taken advantage of for centuries by the indigenous peoples of the Americans and Caribbean to tenderize meat [101]. Based on this practice, papain is now included as a component in some powdered meat tenderizers [102]. A few other important contemporary uses of papain are its medical use against dyspepsia and other digestive disorders and disturbances of the gastrointestinal tract [103], and its addition to beer as a clarifying agent [104].

Preparations from papaya leaves are traditionally used for treating a wide variety of diseases ranging from dengue fever and malaria to diabetes mellitus, hypercholesterolemia, and hypertension [51, 101, 105]. Some of these claims may be explained, at least partially, by the presence of carotenoids and polyphenols, benzyl isothiocyanates and benzyl glucosinolates, and/or the cyanogenic substance prunasin in papaya skin, pulp, and seeds [101].

Support for the alleged antihypertensive effect of *C. papaya* was provided by the decrease in blood pressure in renal and salt-induced hypertensive Wistar rats treated with a crude ethanol extract from the unripened fruit [106]. This preparation, as well as a pentane extract from papaya seeds and an aqueous extract from papaya leaves relaxed vascular muscle tone of isolated rabbit arterial strips [106], strips of dog carotid artery precontracted with phenylephrine [107], and rat aortic ring preparations [108]. The relaxing effect of the fruit preparation was counteracted by phentolamine, suggesting that *C. papaya* contains (an) antihypertensive substance(s) that mainly exhibits α-adrenoceptor activity [108]. *C. papaya* preparations may also exert a blood pressure-lowering effect by stimulating diuresis, as suggested by the diuretic action of an aqueous root extract in laboratory rats, accomplishing similar effects on electrolyte excretion as hydrochlorothiazide [109].

3.7. Cucurbitaceae – *Cucumis sativus* L.

The cucumber plant *C. sativus* is originally from South Asia, most probably India, where it has been cultivated for more than 3000 years. Nowadays, hundreds of cultivars are grown throughout the world and traded on the global market. The mature fruit contains about 90% water and is relatively low in nutrients, and many enjoy its appetizing flavor and texture, making it a popular ingredient of fresh salads as well as pickles and relishes. Cucumber extracts are also widely used in facial tonics and moisturizers, presumably because their high water and antioxidant content would protect the skin from aging [93].

Preparations from *C. sativus* leaves, seeds, flowers, and fruits are also used in various traditional medicines for treating, among others, bacterial and parasitic infections, kidney and gall stones, as well as thrombosis and hypertension [45, 50, 52, 56, 110]. Preclinical evaluation of the plant parts showed various pharmacological activities including blood pressure-lowering effects [111, 112]. Some of these effects may be associated with the presence in the plant of bioactive compounds such as cucurbitacins, cucumegastigmanes I and II, cucumerin A and B, vitexin, and orientin [111, 112].

Importantly, a Chinese study found a significant reduction in blood pressure and a marked increase in coronary blood flow of patients receiving *C. sativus* vine compound tablets, as well as improved myocardial contraction in laboratory animals while no toxic effects were noted [113]. Furthermore, a relatively recent study conducted in Indonesia reported a reduction in mean blood pressure in elderly patients receiving 100 g of cucumber in juice form for 7 days [114].

The antihypertensive effects of these preparations may be associated with the stimulation of diuresis. Indeed, an ethanolic extract from the leaves of *C. sativus*, either alone or as part of a polyherbal formulation, had a moderately stimulatory effect on diuresis in laboratory rats when compared to furosemide [115]. Also, an ether extract from the seeds of *C. melo* increased diuresis in anesthetized dogs [116], and an aqueous extract from the leaves of *C. trigonus* caused a comparable diuretic effect as hydrochlorothiazide in conscious albino rats [117]. In the former study, urinary chloride excretion was increased suggesting that the extract had decreased tubular reabsorption [116].

3.8. Fabaceae – *Desmodium adscendens* (Sw.) DC.

The glue sticks *D. adscendens* is commonly encountered in forests, grasslands, secondary/disturbed vegetation, old cultivated fields, and roadsidesin tropical areas. The leaves and stems have probably been used for thousands of years by native peoples for a variety of health issues, including liver ailments, respiratory diseases, backache, rheumatism, gonorrhea, ovarian inflammation, and epilepsy [118, 119].

Main compounds in *D. adscendens* are flavonoids, triterpenes, saponins, amines, and alkaloids [120]. Pharmacological studies with *D. adscendens* leaf extracts showed, among others, spasmolytic effects in isolated guineas pig trachea and ilei precontracted with histamine [121, 122].

In Suriname, *D. adscendens* is generally known as '*konkruman*' ('informer') or '*toriman*' ('story teller') because the sticky pods stay clinging to clothing, betraying the unapproved presence of the bearer 'in the field', that is, away from home. Indigenous folklore believes that preparations from the plant attract and hold fortune and prosperity while at the same capturing and removing bad luck and disease [45]. A tea prepared from the macerated roots is also used as an antihypertensive [46]. This effect may be attributable to the above-mentioned relaxing effect of certain constituents of the plant on smooth muscle cells [121, 122] – possibly including those in blood vessel walls – but there are no scientific indications to support this presumption.

3.9. Fabaceae – *Hymenaea courbaril* L.

The courbaril, West Indian locust, or jaṭoba *H. courbaril* (**Figure 5**) is a common tree in the Caribbean, Central America, and South America. The hardwood is very durable and is used for manufacturing furniture, flooring, window frames, staircases, as well as canoes. The seeds are situated in a hard pod and are surrounded by an edible dry pulp that has an unpleasant scent reminiscent of foot odor. For this reason, the tree is also known as 'stinking toe' and 'old man's toe'. However, the pulp has a high content of starches and proteins and a sweet taste. It is often eaten raw; may be dried and powdered for making snacks; and may also be mixed with water to prepare a drink called 'atole'.

The stembark of the tree produces an orange, soft, sticky resin called 'animé', French for 'animated', referring to the large numbers of insects that are entrapped in it [123]. Animé has a pleasant fragrance and is used for the production of incense, perfume, and varnish [123]. Interestingly, the indigenous peoples of the Amazon have used *H. courbaril* resin for centuries to preserve the colors on their pottery [45]. Preparations from this substance, along with those from several other parts of the plant, have traditionally also been used in various South American and African countries for treating a variety of conditions such as anemia, kidney problems, dysfunctions of the respiratory system, and abdominal ailments [45, 123, 124].

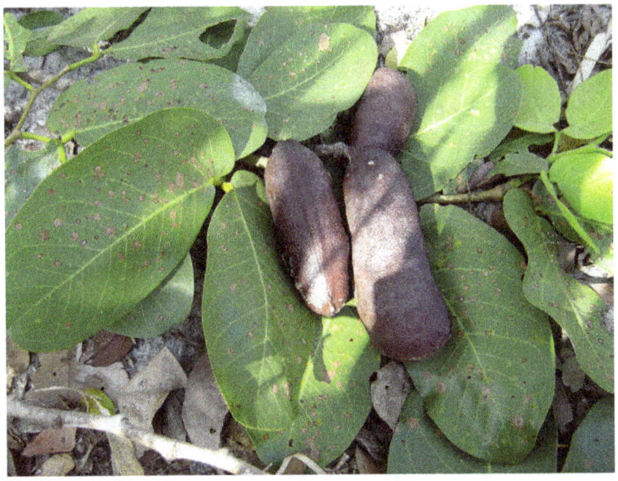

Figure 5. Fabaceae – *Hymenaea courbaril* L. (from: https://goo.gl/images/ePJjyr).

Many bioactive compounds have been identified in leaves, seeds, and trunk resin of *H. courbaril*, including flavonoids, terpenoids, phenolic acids, steroids, and coumarins [124, 125]. Some of these compounds have been related to the myorelaxant, anti-inflammatory, and antimicrobial effects including activity against dengue virus type-2 observed in pharmacological studies with *H. courbaril* preparations [124, 126, 127]. In Suriname, the stembark is used to prepare a tea that would treat a similar variety of ailments as well as hypertension [45]. Whether the latter activity may be associated with vasodilation following relaxation of the smooth muscles [126] including those in the blood vessel walls remains to be determined.

3.10. Fabaceae – *Tamarindus indica* L.

The tamarind *T. indica* is probably indigenous to tropical Africa where it grows in the wild. It has been cultivated for centuries on the Indian subcontinent, and has been introduced in South America including Suriname by Spanish and Portuguese colonists in the sixteenth century. The fruit is a pod with a hard, brown shell that contains up to 12 seeds surrounded by a sweet and sour pulp that is used in cooking, to flavor foods, in refreshing drinks, and as a key ingredient of Worcestershire sauce.

Preparations from *T. indica* leaves, seeds, fruits, and roots are extensively used in folk medicine, among others, for treating abdominal discomfort, microbial and parasitic infestations, as an aphrodisiac, and against hypertension [48, 128, 129]. These parts of the plant contain various phenolic compounds, terpenes, sugars, as well as mucilage and pectin [128, 129]. Some of these constituents have been associated with, among others, antioxidant, anti-hyperlipidemic, and cardioprotective effects of the plant in laboratory models [130].

Furthermore, an aqueous tamarind seed extract produced a decrease in blood pressure, heart rate, as well as serum LDL, cholesterol, and HDL levels in streptozotocin-induced diabetic and hypertensive rats [131]. As well, administration of the dried and pulverized fruit pulp led to a decrease in diastolic blood pressure as well as total cholesterol and LDL-cholesterol levels in human subjects [132]. The blood pressure-lowering effects of the *T. indica* preparations have been suggested to occur through direct sympatho-inhibition [131], protection of the body against oxidative assault that could initiate the development of hypertension [131, 133], and/or lowering of blood lipid levels [133, 134].

3.11. Lauraceae – *Persea americana* Mill.

The avocado tree *P. americana* probably originates from Central America and the western parts of South America and was presumably domesticated as early as 5000 BC. Today, avocados are a successful cash crop with a high commercial value. Avocado is mostly eaten raw; (prolonged) cooking makes it inedible, causing a chemical reaction that confers a bitter taste to it. It is an ingredient of many servings and dishes and is often used in vegetarian cuisine as a substitute for meats because of its relatively high content of monounsaturated fats [135]. The rather expensive oil extracted from avocados is mostly used for salads or dips and in cosmetics and toiletries [136].

The stem bark, fruits, seeds, and leaves of *P. americana* are used in traditional medicine in Africa, the West Indies, as well as South and Central America including Suriname for treating, among others, menstrual problems, gastrointestinal ailments, bronchitis, diabetes mellitus, hypercholesterolemia, and hypertension [45, 46, 49, 52, 55, 137, 138]. Pharmacological evaluations with animal models provided some support for these ethnopharmacological claims [139]. These effects may partially be associated with the aliphatic acetogenins, terpenoid glycosides, furan ring-containing derivatives, flavonoids, and coumarins in various parts of the plant [140].

Evidence for an antihypertensive effect of *P. americana* leaf and seed preparations came from the relaxing effects they produced in isolated guinea pig atrial muscle strips, rat portal veins, and rat thoracic aortic rings precontracted with noradrenaline [141] and the blood pressure-lowering effects they produced in laboratory animals [141–143].

The mechanisms responsible for these effects may involve vasorelaxation by substances that inhibit Ca^{2+} influx and stimulate the synthesis and release of endothelium-derived relaxing factors and vasoactive mediators [144], modulation of ACE activity [145], and/or lowering of total cholesterol, triglycerides, VLDL, and/or LDL [143, 145, 146]. However, a clinical study found no benefit with respect to body weight, BMI, and percentage body fat, and no difference in serum lipids, fibrinogen, blood flow, or blood pressure when avocados were substituted for mixed fats in an energy-restricted diet [147].

3.12. Malvaceae – *Gossypium barbadense* L.

The sea island cotton or Egyptian cotton *G. barbadense* (**Figure 6**) is believed to have emerged in Peru as a cross between *G. herbaceum* L. and *G. raimondii* Ulbrich or *G. gossypioides* (Ulbrich) Standley. It is now widely cultivated in the warmer parts of the world, and is an important industrial and export product of Egypt, the West Indies, Sudan, Peru, and the USA.

Cotton is the soft white fibrous substance that surrounds the seeds of the plant and helps in the dispersal of the seeds [148]. It consists of 88–96% α-cellulose, 3–6% hemicellulose, and 1–2%

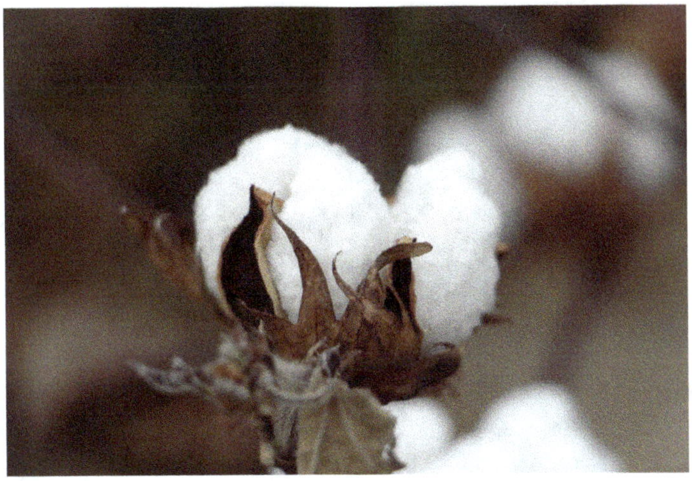

Figure 6. Malvaceae – *Gossypium barbadense* L. (from: https://goo.gl/images/NN46ra).

lignin [148]. Since about 2500 BC, the fibers are used for making sewing thread, yarn, cordage, and fishing nets, and more recently also for making coffee filters, paper, surgical dressings, and nitrocellulose-based explosives [148]. The seed oil can be incorporated in, among others, margarine and mayonnaise, but also in soaps, cosmetics, lubricants, and protective coatings [148]. The oil as well as other parts of *Gossypium* species contains the triterpenoid aldehyde gossypol that causes infertility in males [149]. Other constituents of *G. barbadense* are alkaloids, flavonoids, total phenols, cyanogenic glycosides, and saponins [148, 150].

G. barbadense preparations are widely used in traditional medicine. In many African countries as well as the Guianas including Suriname, preparations from leaves, roots, and seed oil are used for treating a multitude of diseases ranging from eye affections, otitis media, bronchitis, and menstrual problems to malaria, convulsions, gonorrhea, leprosy, and hypertension [45, 51, 52, 55, 151]. Pharmacological studies have supported some of these folk medicinal uses [151, 152].

The presumption of a blood pressure-lowering effect of *G. barbadense* was supported by the dose-dependent hypotensive effect of a fraction of a crude leaf extract in laboratory rats [153]. The results from parallel studies with several agonists and antagonists of acetylcholine receptors suggested that this occurred through an action on the central nervous system comparably to that of the centrally acting α_2-adrenergic agonist clonidine [153]. On the other hand, an aqueous extract from *G. barbadense* leaves decreased the tension of isolated guinea pig aorta rings stimulated with phenylephrine (a selective α_1-adrenergic receptor agonist) by 15–35% [75], suggesting that it may lower an elevated blood pressure by decreasing the peripheral vascular resistance.

3.13. Malvaceae – *Hibiscus sabdariffa* L.

The roselle *H. sabdariffa* (**Figure 7**) probably originates from Africa and is presumably domesticated in Sudan about 6000 years ago. It was initially cultivated for its seed and later for its leaves and bright red colored calyces which are particularly in the USA and Germany

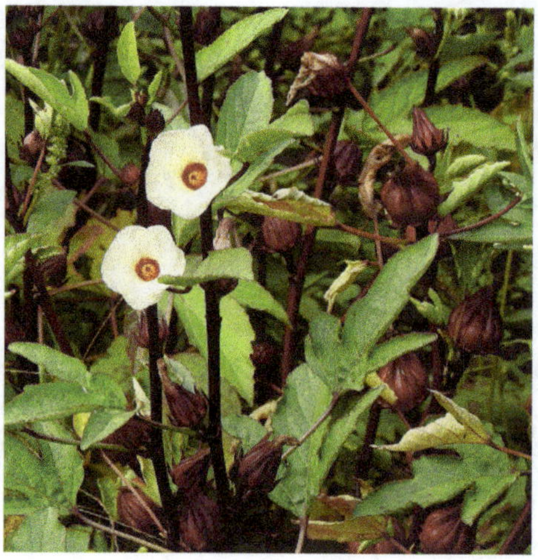

Figure 7. Malvaceae – *Hibiscus sabdariffa* L. (from: https://goo.gl/images/BRZcTZ).

processed to give food colorings. The seed oil can be used for cooking and the seeds are eaten roasted as a snack. However, *H. sabdariffa* seeds probably contain toxic substances and may be better used for manufacturing soaps and shrubs [154]. Young shoots, leaves, and calyces can be included in certain dishes, and fresh or dried calyces are used to prepare flavorful and slightly acidic herbal teas, refreshing beverages that may be carbonated, cocktails with rum, as well as jams.

Preparations from *H. sabdariffa* leaves, calyces, and roots are widely used in traditional medicines because of their presumed antimicrobial, antioxidant, anticancer, hepatoprotective, hypocholesterolemic, antidiabetic, diuretic, and antihypertensive properties [45, 155, 156]. Phytochemical and pharmacological studies supported some of these uses [155, 156].

The results from preclinical studies have associated the potential antihypertensive (and cardioprotective) properties of particularly tea made from roselle calyces with its abundant content of polyphenolic compounds such as chlorogenic acids [157], as well as flavonoid compounds such as kaempferol, quercetin, and anthocyanins [156, 158]. Chlorogenic acids (modestly) reduced an elevated blood pressure [157, 159]. Kaempferol may have a protective effect in heart diseases [160]. Quercetin caused the release of NO from vascular endothelium, increasing renal vasorelaxation and kidney filtration, stimulating diuresis and decreasing blood pressure [161]. And the anthocyanins may exert antioxidant effects which inhibit LDL oxidation, impeding atherosclerosis, an important cardiovascular risk factor [162]. Alternatively, anthocyanins may decrease blood pressure by inhibiting ACE activity [163]. These compounds, along with the flavonoids and the chlorogenic acids, have also been suggested to decrease hypertension by stimulating diuresis following modulation of aldosterone activity [164].

However, comprehensive reviews and a meta-analysis suggest that the evidence for the use of *H. sabdariffa* preparations against hypertension is insufficient and recommend more high-quality animal and human studies to demonstrate benefit from these substances in this condition [162, 165, 166].

3.14. Meliaceae – *Azadirachta indica* A. Juss.

The neem tree *A. indica* is originally from the Asian subcontinent and is now grown in various tropical and semi-tropical regions. The bitter-tasting shoots and flowers are incorporated into various dishes, while preparations from leaves, bark, and fruits are consumed during many Hindu ceremonies, festivals, and commemorations.

A. indica leaves and seeds contain potent antiparasitic, insecticidal, and antimicrobial compounds such as the limonoids azadirachtin and nimbinin [167]. For this reason, dried neem leaves are placed in cupboards and storage facilities for grains to prevent damage from insects and burned to keep away mosquitoes, while the seed oil is used as a key ingredient of non-synthetic ecofriendly pesticides in agriculture, acting as an antifeedant, repellent, and egg-laying deterrent for insects [168]. The seed cake that remains after oil extraction is used as a fertilizer, enriching the soil with organic matter, and at the same time reducing nitrogen loss by inhibiting nitrification and averting damage to crops by termites and nematodes [168]. Neem oil is also a valuable ingredient of a large variety of cosmetics such as soaps, shampoos, balms, creams as well as toothpastes and nail polishes [169].

Parts of *A. indica* have been used for centuries in traditional and alternative medicinal systems in India and Suriname against a wide variety of diseases ranging from microbial infections and malaria to diabetes mellitus and hypertension [45, 170]. Some of these applications are supported by the results from pharmacological studies and may be related to the actions of, among others, azadirachtin and nimbinin [167, 171].

Indications for a potential antihypertensive effect of *A. indica* preparations were provided by the inhibitory effect of *A. indica* yogurt on ACE activity *in vitro* [172], and the blood pressure-lowering effect of leaf extracts in (salt-induced) rat models [173, 174]. Studies with laboratory rabbits suggested that these effects might also be due to vasodilation mediated through a combination of Ca^{2+} channel blockade, NO-inhibitory mechanisms, and cardiac depressant activity [175].

3.15. Oxalidaceae – *Averrhoa bilimbi* L.

The bilimbi *A. bilimbi* (**Figure 8**) presumably originates from Indonesia. It has been introduced in several Southeast Asian countries, and has spread to Australia as well as the Caribbean, Central America, and South America. The fruits can be eaten raw with salt and spice, pickled to obtain sweet and sour side dishes, incorporated in certain dishes as a souring agent, made into jams, or squashed to obtain a cooling beverage. However, *A. bilimbi* fruits (as well as leaves) contain high levels of oxalate [176] which may cause tubular necrosis and acute kidney failure when the concentrated juice is drunk on a daily basis [177].

Parts of *A. bilimbi* have been important sources of medicines since antiquity. Decoctions, infusions, powders, and pastes have been used in several traditional medicinal systems including those in Suriname for preventing and treating many diseases such as skin eruptions, cough, cold, syphilis, diarrhea, obesity, diabetes mellitus, microbial infections, and hypertension [46, 178]. Physicochemical and pharmacological studies supported some of these uses [179].

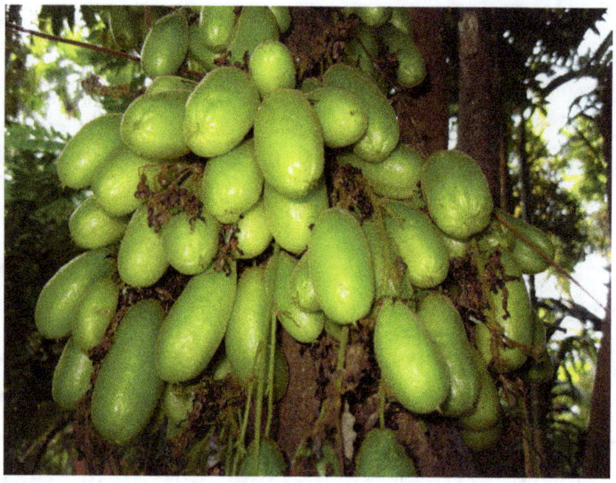

Figure 8. Oxalidaceae – *Averrhoa bilimbi* L. (from: https://goo.gl/images/THfTgV).

Indications for efficacy against hypertension of *A. bilimbi* came from the decreased contractility of isolated guinea pig atria precontracted with norepinephrine upon exposure to an aqueous extract from the leaves [180]. Such an extract also produced a substantial antihypertensive effect in an *in vivo* study with cats [181]. The mechanisms underlying these observations may be associated with a decrease in cardiac output following alterations in intracellular calcium metabolism and/or phenomena involving the muscarinic receptor [180]. It is also possible that the relatively high levels of oxalate in these preparations [176] promote diuresis. A third possible mechanism involves inhibition of ACE activity, as suggested by the *in vitro* ACE-inhibitory effect of an *A. bilimbi* leaf ethanol extract which was comparable to that of captopril [182].

4. Concluding remarks

This chapter has addressed the plants that are used in Suriname for treating hypertension. About 60 of the approximately 800 medicinal plants in Suriname are used against this condition ([45–55]; **Table 1**), indicating both the high need of antihypertensive medications and the high demand for traditional plant-derived for treating this condition in the country. As mentioned above, the prevalence of hypertension and other cardiovascular diseases is relatively high in Suriname [32, 36, 37], while most Surinamese have a long tradition of using ethnopharmacological preparations for treating their diseases [21, 44].

However, an extensive evaluation of 15 plants that are commonly used against hypertension in Suriname indicates that there is little scientific evidence for clinical efficacy against this condition. As shown in **Table 2**, 3 of the 15 plants (*A. graveolens*, *C. nucifera*, and *C. sativus*) had undergone preclinical as well as clinical evaluation against hypertension and turned out positive in at least some of the clinical studies. However, the clinical studies merely comprised a handful, although those with 3-n-butylphthalide in *A. graveolens* were sufficiently encouraging to prepare larger scale clinical evaluations [90–92].

Nine other plants (*M. indica, A. muricata, C. papaya, T. indica, P. americana, G. barbadense, H. sabdariffa, A. indica,* and *A. bilimbi*) have only been tested in preclinical models of hypertension (**Table 2**), relatively few of which involved animal studies. And three of the plants (*R. tuberosa, D. adscendens,* and *H. courbaril*) have never been assessed for potential antihypertensive effects, not even in preclinical models (**Table 2**). On the bright side, with the exception of *H. courbaril,* there were in all cases suggestions about the mechanisms that may be involved in the antihypertensive effects (**Table 2**). Then again, the chemical substances responsible for these effects were only provided for 6 plants (*M. indica, A. muricata, A. graveolens, C. nucifera, H. sabdariffa,* and *A. indica;* **Table 2**).

These data clearly indicate that the scientific evidence accumulated so far to support the use of plant-based traditional medicines in Suriname against hypertension is scant. This raises not only the possibility that patients treat their disease with substances that may be ineffective, but also that they may run the risk of unknown or unforeseen adverse effects. For these reasons, it is necessary to subject these plants to comprehensive phytochemical and pharmacological investigations, elaborate preclinical evaluations, and well-designed and well-executed clinical studies to definitely establish their roles in the treatment of hypertension. Obviously, these enterprises will require considerable efforts from both academia and industry, but may eventually payoff when considering the importance of ancient wisdom and folk medicine to drug discovery and development programs [183].

Author details

Dennis R.A. Mans[1]*, Angela Grant[2] and Nicholaas Pinas[3]

*Address all correspondence to: dennis_mans@yahoo.com

1 Department of Pharmacology, Faculty of Medical Sciences, Anton de Kom University of Suriname, Paramaribo, Suriname

2 National Herbarium of Suriname, Anton de Kom University of Suriname, Paramaribo, Suriname

3 Clinical Laboratory, Diakonessenhuis, Paramaribo, Suriname

References

[1] Beevers G, Lip GY, O'Brien E. ABC of hypertension: The pathophysiology of hypertension. British Medical Journal. 2001;**322**:912-916

[2] Weber MA, Schiffrin EL, White WB, Mann S, Lindholm LH, Kenerson JG, et al. Clinical practice guidelines for the management of hypertension in the community – A statement by the American Society of Hypertension and the International Society of Hypertension. Journal of Clinical Hypertension (Greenwich, Conn.). 2014;**16**:14-26. DOI: 10.1111/jch.12237

[3] Weber MA, Schiffrin EL, White WB, Mann S, Lindholm LH, Kenerson JG, et al. Clinical practice guidelines for the management of hypertension in the community. A statement by the American Society of Hypertension and the International Society of Hypertension. Journal of Hypertension. 2014;**32**:3-15. DOI: 10.1097/HJH.0000000000000065

[4] Esler M, Lambert E, Schlaich M, Schlaich L. Point: Chronic activation of the sympathetic nervous system is the dominant contributor to systemic hypertension. Journal of Applied Physiology (1985). 2010;**109**:1996-1998; discussion 2016. DOI: 10.1152/japplphysiol.00182.2010

[5] Navar LG. Counterpoint: Activation of the intrarenal renin-angiotensin system is the dominant contributor to systemic hypertension. Journal of Applied Physiology (1985). 2010;**109**:1998-2000; discussion 2015. DOI: 10.1152/japplphysiol.00182.2010a

[6] Delacroix S, Chokka RG, Worthley SG. Hypertension: Pathophysiology and treatment. Journal of Neurology & Neurophysiology. 2014;**5**:250. DOI: 10.4172/2155-9562.1000250

[7] Yokoyama Y, Nishimura K, Barnard ND, Takegami M, Watanabe M, Sekikawa A, et al. Vegetarian diets and blood pressure: A meta-analysis. JAMA Internal Medicine. 2014;**174**:577-587. DOI: 10.1001/jamainternmed.2013.14547

[8] Brook RD, Appel LJ, Rubenfire M, Ogedegbe G, Bisognano JD, Elliott WJ, et al. Beyond medications and diet: Alternative approaches to lowering blood pressure: A scientific statement from the American Heart Association. Hypertension. 2013;**61**:1360-1383. DOI: 10.1161/HYP.0b013e318293645f

[9] Mancia G, Fagard R, Narkiewicz K, Redon J, Zanchetti A, Böhm M, et al. 2013 ESH/ESC guidelines for the Management of Arterial Hypertension: The task force for the management of arterial hypertension of the European Society of Hypertension (ESH) and of the European Society of Cardiology (ESC). European Heart Journal. 2013;**34**:2159-2199. DOI: 10.1093/eurheartj/eht151

[10] Law MR, Morris JK, Wald NJ. Use of blood pressure lowering drugs in the prevention of cardiovascular disease: Meta-analysis of 147 randomised trials in the context of expectations from prospective epidemiological studies. British Medical Journal. 2009;**338**:b1665. DOI: 10.1136/bmj.b1665

[11] James PA, Oparil S, Carter BL, Cushman WC, Dennison-Himmelfarb C, Handler J, et al. 2014 evidence-based guideline for the management of high blood pressure in adults: Report from the panel members appointed to the Eighth Joint National Committee (JNC 8). Journal of the American Medical Association. 2014;**311**:507-520. DOI: 10.1001/jama.2013.284427

[12] Wiysonge CS, Bradley HA, Volmink J, Mayosi BM, Opie LH. Beta-blockers for hypertension. Cochrane Database of Systematic Reviews. 2017;**1**:CD002003. DOI: 10.1002/14651858.CD002003.pub5

[13] Mills KT, Bundy JD, Kelly TN, Reed JE, Kearney PM, Reynolds K, et al. Global disparities of hypertension prevalence and control: A systematic analysis of population-based studies

from 90 countries. Circulation. 2016;**134**:441-450. DOI: 10.1161/CIRCULATIONAHA. 115.018912

[14] Cohen JD. Hypertension epidemiology and economic burden: Refining risk assessment to lower costs. Managed Care. 2009;**18**:51-58

[15] Cherry DK, Hing E, Woodwell DA, Rechtsteiner EA. National Ambulatory Medical Care Survey: 2006 summary. National Health Statistics Reports. 2008;**3**:1-39

[16] Kearney PM, Whelton M, Reynolds K, Whelton PK, He J. Worldwide prevalence of hypertension: A systematic review. Journal of Hypertension. 2004;**22**:11-19

[17] Kearney PM, Whelton M, Reynolds K, Muntner P, Whelton PK, He J. Global burden of hypertension: Analysis of worldwide data. Lancet. 2005;**365**:217-223

[18] Roger VL, Go AS, Lloyd-Jones DM, Adams RJ, Berry JD, Brown TM, et al. Heart disease and stroke statistics-2011 update: A report from the American Heart Association. Circulation. 2011;**123**:e18-e209. DOI: 10.1161/CIR.0b013e3182009701

[19] Chan KY, Adeloye D, Grant L, Kolčić I, Marušić A. How big is the 'next big thing'? Estimating the burden of non-communicable diseases in low- and middle-income countries. Journal of Global Health. 2012;**2**:020101. DOI: 10.7189/jogh.02.020101

[20] Algemeen Bureau voor de Statistiek/Censuskantoor. Suriname in cijfers 2013/05. Resultaten achtste (8ste) volks- en woningtelling in Suriname (volume 1) (General Bureau of Statistics/Census office. Suriname in numbers 2013/05. Results of the Eight General Census of Suriname). Demografische en sociale karakteristieken en migratie (Demographic and social characteristics and migration). Paramaribo: Algemeen Bureau voor de Statistiek; 2013

[21] Mans DRA, Ganga D, Kartopawiro J. Meeting of the minds: Traditional herbal medicine in multiethnic Suriname (chapter 6). In: El-Shemy H, editor. Aromatic and Medicinal Plants – Back to Nature. Rijeka: InTech; 2017. pp. 111-132. DOI: 10.5772/66509

[22] Helman A. Cultureel mozaïek Van Suriname. Bijdrage Tot Onderling Begrip (Cultural Mosaic of Suriname. A Contribution to Mutual Understanding). De Walburg Pers: Zutphen; 1977

[23] Hammond DS. Forest conservation and management in the Guiana shield (chapter 1). In: Hammond DS, editor. Tropical Rainforests of the Guiana Shield. Wallingford: CABI Publishing; 2005. pp. 1-14

[24] Algemeen Bureau voor de Statistiek. Suriname in cijfers 303-2014-04 (General Bureau of Statistics. Suriname in numbers 303-2014-04). Basis indicatoren (Basic indicators). Paramaribo: Algemeen Bureau voor de Statistiek; 2014

[25] The World Bank. Suriname overview [Internet]. 2014. Available from: http://www.worldbank.org/en/country/suriname/overview [Accessed: Sep 23, 2017]

[26] Baldew SS, Krishnadath IS, Smits CC, Toelsie JR, Vanhees L, Cornelissen V. Self-reported physical activity behavior of a multi-ethnic adult population within the urban and rural setting in Suriname. BMC Public Health. 2015;**15**:485. DOI: 10.1186/s12889-015-1807-1

[27] Suriname Ministry of Health. Global School-Based Student Health Survey. Paramaribo: Suriname Ministry of Health; 2009

[28] Suriname Ministry of Health Suriname. National Action Plan for the Prevention and Control of Noncommunicable Diseases 2012-2016. Paramaribo: Suriname Ministry of Health; 2009

[29] World Health Organization. Noncommunicable Diseases (NCD) Country Profiles. Suriname. Geneva: World Health Organization; 2014

[30] Krishnadath ISK, Nahar-van Venrooij LM, Jaddoe VWV, Toelsie JR. Ethnic differences in prediabetes and diabetes in the Suriname. Health Study. BMJ Open Diabetes Research & Care. 2016;**4**:e000186. DOI: 10.1136/bmjdrc-2015-000186

[31] Krishnadath ISK, Toelsie JR, Hofman A, Jaddoe VWV. Ethnic disparities in the prevalence of metabolic syndrome and its risk factors in the Suriname Health Study: A cross-sectional population study. BMJ Open. 2016;**6**:e013183. DOI: 10.1136/bmjopen-2016-013183

[32] Krishnadath ISK, Jaddoe VWV, Nahar-van Venrooij LM, Toelsie JR. Ethnic differences in prevalence and risk factors for hypertension in the Suriname Health Study: A cross sectional population study. Population Health Metrics. 2016;**14**:33. eCollection 2016

[33] Punwasi W. Doodsoorzaken in Suriname 2009-2011 (Causes of Daeth in Suriname 2009-2011). Ministerie van Volksgezondheid, Bureau Openbare Gezondheidszorg: Paramaribo; 2012

[34] Ibrahim MM, Damasceno A. Hypertension in developing countries. Lancet. 2012;**380**:611-619. DOI: 10.1016/S0140-6736(12)60861-7

[35] Agyemang C, Bindraban N, Mairuhu G, Montfrans G, Koopmans R, Stronks K, et al. Prevalence, awareness, treatment, and control of hypertension among Black Surinamese, South Asian Surinamese and White Dutch in Amsterdam, The Netherlands: The SUNSET study. Journal of Hypertension. 2005;**23**:1971-1977

[36] Diemer F, Baldew SM, Van Montrans GA, Oehlers GP, Brewster LM. Prehypertension and hypertension in urban Suriname. Journal of Hypertension. 2016;**34**:e358. DOI: 10.1097/01.hjh.0000492391.01413.be

[37] Karamat F, Diemer F, Baldew S, Oehlers G, Van Montfrans G, Brewster L. Prehypertension and hypertension in urban Suriname: The HELISUR study. Journal of Hypertension. 2016;**34**:e551. DOI: 10.1097/01.hjh.0000501508.90665.63

[38] Van den Born BJ, Koopmans RP, Groeneveld JO, van Montfrans GA. Ethnic disparities in the incidence, presentation and complications of malignant hypertension. Journal of Hypertension. 2006;**24**:2299-2304

[39] Agyemang C, van Valkengoed I, van den Born BJ, Stronks K. Prevalence and determinants of prehypertension among African Surinamese, Hindustani Surinamese, and White Dutch in Amsterdam, the Netherlands: The SUNSET study. European Journal of Cardiovascular Prevention and Rehabilitation. 2007;**14**:775-781

[40] Agyemang C, Kunst AE, Bhopal R, Zaninotto P, Unwin N, Nazroo J, et al. Hypertension in Dutch and English ethnic minorities. Blood pressure better controlled in English groups than in Dutch groups. Nederlands Tijdschrift voor Geneeskunde. Dutch. 2011;**155**:A3318

[41] Van Beune EJ, Haafkens JA, Schuster JS, Bindels PJ. 'Under pressure': How Ghanaian, African-Surinamese and Dutch patients explain hypertension. Journal of Human Hypertension. 2006;**20**:946-955

[42] Van Beune EJ, Haafkens JA, Agyemang C, Schuster JS, Willems DL. How Ghanaian, African-Surinamese and Dutch patients perceive and manage antihypertensive drug treatment: A qualitative study. Journal of Hypertension. 2008;**26**:648-656

[43] Ministry of Health. Report of the Director of Health 2005-2007. Paramaribo: Ministry of Health Republic of Suriname; 2008

[44] Mans DRA. "Nature, green in leaf and stem". Research on plants with medicinal properties in Suriname. Clinical and Medical Investigations. 2016;**2**:1-10. DOI: 10.15761/CMI.1000121

[45] Van Andel TR, Ruysschaert S. Medicinale en rituele planten van Suriname (Medicinal and Ritual Plants of Suriname). Amsterdam: KIT Publishers; 2011

[46] Raghoenandan UPD. Etnobotanisch onderzoek bij de Hindoestaanse bevolkingsgroep in Suriname (An Ethnobotanical Investigation among Hindustanis in Suriname). [thesis]. Paramaribo: Anton de Kom Universiteit van Suriname; 1994

[47] Van't Klooster C, van Andel T, Reis R. Patterns in medicinal plant knowledge and use in a Maroon village in Suriname. Journal of Ethnopharmacology 2016;**189**:319-330

[48] Tjong AG. Het gebruik van medicinale planten door de Javaanse bevolkingsgroep in Suriname (The Use of Medicinal Plants by the Javanese in Suriname). Instituut voor de Opleiding van Leraren: Paramaribo; 1989

[49] Stephen HJM. Geneeskruiden van Suriname: hun toepassing in de volksgeneeskunde en in de magie (Herbal Medicines from Suriname: Their Applications in Folk Medicine and Wizardry). Amsterdam: De Driehoek; 1979

[50] May AF. Sranan oso dresi. Surinaams kruidenboek (Surinamese Folk Medicine. A Collection of Surinamese Medicinal Herbs). De Walburg Pers: Paramaribo; 1982

[51] Titjari. Famiri-encyclopedia foe da natoera dresi-fasi. Gezinskruidenboek van de natuurgeneeswijzen. Natuurgeneeswijzen uit het zonnige Suriname (Encyclopedia of Plant-based Forms of Treatment. Folk Medicines from Sunny Suriname). Amsterdam: Sangrafoe; 1985

[52] Heyde H. Surinaamse Medicijnplanten (Surinamese Medicinal Plants). 2nd ed. Westfort: Paramaribo; 1987

[53] Slagveer JL. Surinaams Groot Kruidenboek: Sranan Oso Dresie (Surinamese Herbal Medicines). De West: Paramaribo; 1990

[54] Veth B. Gebruiks- en Medicinale Planten Van de Wayana Indianen in Frans Guyana en Suriname (Useful and Medicinal Plants of the Wayana Indians in French Guiana and Suriname). Utrecht: Nationaal Herbarium Nederland, Universiteit Utrecht; 1990

[55] Sedoc NO. Afrosurinaamse natuurgeneeswijzen: Bevattende meer dan tweehonderd meest gebruikelijke geneeskrachtige kruiden (Afro-Surinamese Natural Remedies: Over two hundred Commonly Used Medicinal Herbs). Paramaribo: Vaco Press; 1992

[56] Chothani DL, Patel MB, Vaghasiya HU, Mishira SH. Review on *Ruellia tuberosa* (cracker plant). Pharmacognosy Journal. 2010;**2**:506-512

[57] Chaitanya BK, Babu SR, Ramesh C, Ravella A, Vardhan J, Atigari DV. Hypolipidemic and anti-oxidant activity of *Ruellia tuberosa* Linn. International Journal of Pharmacy and Biological Sciences. 2012;**2**:63-72

[58] Rajan M, Kumar VK, Kumar PS, Swathi KR, Haritha S. Antidiabetic, antihyperlipidaemic and hepatoprotective activity of methanolic extract of *Ruellia tuberosa* Linn leaves in normal and alloxan induced diabetic rats. Journal of Chemical and Pharmaceutical Research. 2012;**4**:2860-2868

[59] Samy MN, Sugimoto S, Matsunami K, Otsuka H, Kamel MS. Chemical constituents and biological activities of genus *Ruellia*. International Journal of Pharmacognosy. 2015;**2**:270-279. DOI: 10.1007/s10600-013-0549-5

[60] Akhtar MF, Rashid S, Ahmad M, Usmanghani K. Cardiovascular evaluation of *Ruellia patula* and *Ruellia brittoniana*. Journal of Islamic World Academy of Sciences. 1992;**5**:67-71

[61] Ahmad M, Akhtar MF, Miyase T, Rashid S, Ghani KU. Studies on the medicinal herb *Ruellia patula*. International Journal of Pharmacognosy. 1993;**31**:121-129

[62] Beltrán AE, Alvarez Y, Xavier FE, Hernanz R, Rodriguez J, Núñez AJ, et al. Vascular effects of the *Mangifera indica* L. extract (Vimang). European Journal of Pharmacology. 2004;**499**:297-305

[63] Tharanathan RN, Yashoda HM, Prabha TN. Mango (*Mangifera indica* L.), the king of fruits – A review. Food Reviews International. 2006;**22**:95-123. DOI: 10.1080/87559120600574493

[64] Bekoe EO, Kretchy IA, Sarkodie JA, Okraku A, Sasu C, Adjei D, et al. Ethnomedicinal survey of plants used for the management of hypertension sold in the Makola market, Accra, Ghana Emelia Oppong Bekoe. European Journal of Medicinal Plants. 2017;**19**:1-9. DOI: 10.9734/EJMP/2017/32342

[65] Barreto JC, Trevisan MTS, Hull WE, Erben G, De Brito ES, Pfundstein B, et al. Characterization and quantitation of polyphenolic compounds in bark, kernel, leaves, and peel

of mango (*Mangifera indica* L.). Journal of Agricultural and Food Chemistry. 2008;**56**:5599-5610. DOI: 10.1021/jf800738r

[66] Parvez GMM. Pharmacological activities of mango (*Mangifera indica*): A review. Journal of Pharmacognosy and Phytochemistry. 2016;**5**:1-7

[67] Shree Devi MS. Acute toxicity and diuretic activity of *Mangifera indica* L. bark extracts. International Journal of Pharma and Bio Sciences. 2011;**2**:141-146

[68] Tundis R, Xiao J, Loizzo MR. *Annona* species (Annonaceae): A rich source of potential antitumor agents? Annals of the New York Academy of Sciences. 2017;**1398**:30-36. DOI: 10.1111/nyas.13339

[69] Bermejo A, Figadere B, Zafra-Polo MC, Barrachina I, Estornell E, Cortes D. Acetogenins from Annonaceae: Recent progress in isolation, synthesis and mechanisms of action. Natural Product Reports. 2005;**22**:269-303

[70] Lannuzel A, Ruberg M, Michel PP. Atypical parkinsonism in the Caribbean island of Guadeloupe: Etiological role of the mitochondrial complex I inhibitor annonacin. Movement Disorders. 2008;**23**:2122-2128. DOI: 10.1002/mds.22300

[71] Moghadamtousi SZ, Fadaeinasab M, Nikzad S, Mohan G, Ali HM, Kadir HA. *Annona muricata* (Annonaceae): A review of its traditional uses, isolated acetogenins and biological activities. International Journal of Molecular Sciences. 2015;**16**:15625-15658. DOI: 10.3390/ijms160715625

[72] Hasrat JA, De Bruyne T, De Backer JP, Vauquelin G, Vlietinck AJ. Isoquinoline derivatives isolated from the fruit of *Annona muricata* as 5-HTergic 5-HT_{1A} receptor agonists in rats: Unexploited antidepressive (lead) products. The Journal of Pharmacy and Pharmacology. 1997;**49**:1145-1149

[73] Saleem U, Ejaz-ul-Haq M, Chudary Z, Ahmad B. Pharmacological screening of *Annona muricata*: A review. Asian Journal of Agriculture and Biology. 2017;**5**:38-46

[74] Nwokocha CR, Owu DU, Gordon A, Thaxter K, McCalla G, Ozolua RI, et al. Possible mechanisms of action of the hypotensive effect of *Annona muricata* (soursop) in normotensive Sprague-Dawley rats. Pharmaceutical Biology. 2012;**50**:1436-1441. DOI: 10.3109/13880209.2012.684690

[75] Mans DRA, Sallevelt SCEH, Soekhoe R, Bipat R, Toelsie JR. Evaluation of plants with presumed antihypertensive properties for their potential to decrease peripheral resistance using isolated guinea pig aortic rings precontracted with phenylephrine. Academic Journal of Suriname. 2010;**1**:15-19

[76] Dabiré H. Central 5-hydroxytryptamine (5-HT) receptors in blood pressure regulation. Thérapie. 1991;**46**:421-429

[77] Sowbhagya HB. Chemistry, technology, and nutraceutical functions of celery (*Apium graveolens* L.): An overview. Critical Reviews in Food Science and Nutrition. 2014;**54**:389-398. DOI: 10.1080/10408398.2011.586740

[78] Ciganda C, Laborde A. Herbal infusions used for induced abortion. Journal of Toxicology. Clinical Toxicology. 2003;**41**:235-239

[79] Amerio A, de Benedictis G, Leondeff J, Mastrangelo F, Coratelli P. Nephropathy due to apiol. Minerva Nefrologica. 1968;**15**:49-70

[80] Celestin J, Heiner DC. Food-induced anaphylaxis. The Western Journal of Medicine. 1993;**158**:610-611

[81] Gharouni M, Sarkati A. Application of *Apium graveolens* in treatment of hypertension. Journal of Dentistry of Tehran University of Medical Sciences. 2000;**3**:67-69

[82] Al-Asmari AK, Athar MT, Kadasah SG. An updated phytopharmacological review on medicinal plant of Arab region: *Apium graveolens* Linn. Pharmacognosy Reviews. 2017;**11**:13-18. DOI: 10.4103/phrev.phrev_35_16

[83] Tang FF, Guo JX, Zhang J, Li J, Study SM. On hypotensive and vasodilatory effects of celery juice. Food Science. 2007;**28**:322-325

[84] Branković S, Kitić D, Radenković M, Veljković S, Kostić M, Miladinović B, et al. Hypotensive and cardioinhibotory effects of the aqueous and ethanol extracts of celery (*Apium graveolens*, Apiaceae). Acta Medica Medianae. 2010;**49**:13-16

[85] Chai LM, Tian L, Li Y, Liu CS, Wu LY. Antihypertensive effects of roots of *Apium graveolens* extract in renal hypertensive rats. Chinese Journal of Experimental Traditional Medical Formulae. 2010;**16**:101-103

[86] Moghadam MH, Imenshahidi M, Mohajeri SA. Antihypertensive effect of celery seed on rat blood pressure in chronic administration. Journal of Medicinal Food. 2013;**16**:558-563. DOI: 10.1089/jmf.2012.2664

[87] Al Jawad FH, Al Razzuqi RAM, Al Jeboori AA. *Apium graveolens* accentuates urinary Ca^{2+} excretions in experimental model of nephrocalcinosis. International Journal of Green Pharmacy. 2011;**5**:100-102. DOI: 10.4103/0973-8258.85160

[88] Ur Rehman A, Ishaq H, Furqan M, Sheikh D, Raza ML, Naqvi BS, et al. Comparative study of ethanolic and aqueous extracts of *Apium graveolens* L. root with furosemide for its diuretic activity and excretion of urinary metabolites in Wistar rats. Science International (Lahore). 2016;**28**:2503-2507

[89] Zhu J, Zhang Y, Yang C. Protective effect of 3-n-butylphthalide against hypertensive nephropathy in spontaneously hypertensive rats. Molecular Medicine Reports. 2015;**11**:1448-1454. DOI: 10.3892/mmr.2014.2791

[90] Dewi K, Jasaputra DK, Litanto O. The effect of celery ethanol extract (*Apium graveolens* L.) on male adult's blood pressure. Planta Medica Journal. 2010;**1**:27-34

[91] Madhavi D, Kagan D, Rao V, Murray MT. A pilot study to evaluate the antihypertensive effect of a celery extract in mild to moderate hypertensive patients. Natural Medicine Journal. 2013;**5**:1-5

[92] Abdoulaye IA, Guo YJ. A review of recent advances in neuroprotective potential of 3-n-butylphthalide and its derivatives. BioMed Research International. 2016;**2016**: 5012341. DOI: 10.1155/2016/5012341

[93] Mans DRA, Grant A. "A thing of beauty is a joy forever". Plants and plant-based preparations for facial care in Suriname. Clinical and Medical Investigations. 2017;**2**:1-16. DOI: 10.15761/CMI.1000143

[94] Lima EBC, Sousa CNS, Meneses LN, Ximenes NC, Santos Jr MA, Vasconcelos GS, et al. *Cocos nucifera* (L.) (Arecaceae): A phytochemical and pharmacological review. Brazilian Journal of Medical and Biological Research. 2015;**48**:953-964. http://dx.doi.org/10.1590/1414-431X20154773

[95] Aggarwal B, Lamba HS, Sharma PA, Ajeet. Various pharmacological aspects of *Cocos nucifera* – A review. American Journal of Pharmacological Sciences 2017;**5**:25-30. DOI: 10.12691/ajps-5-2-2

[96] Bankar GR, Nayak PG, Bansal P, Paul P, Pai KS, Singla RK, et al. Vasorelaxant and antihypertensive effect of *Cocos nucifera* Linn. Endocarp on isolated rat thoracic aorta and DOCA salt-induced hypertensive rats. Journal of Ethnopharmacology. 2011;**134**:50-54. DOI: 10.1016/j.jep.2010.11.047

[97] Bhagya D, Prema L, Rajamohan T. Therapeutic effects of tender coconut water on oxidative stress in fructose fed insulin resistant hypertensive rats. Asian Pacific Journal of Tropical Medicine. 2012;**5**:270-276. DOI: 10.1016/S1995-7645(12)60038-8

[98] Syafriani R, Sukandar EY, Apriantono T, Sigit JI. The effect of coconut water (*Cocos nucifera* L.) and an isotonic drink on the change of heart rate frequency in the rats induced hypertension. Procedia Chemistry. 2014;**13**:177-180. DOI: 10.1016/j.proche.2014.12.023

[99] Alleyne T, Roache S, Thomas C, Shirley A. The control of hypertension by use coconut water and Mauby; two tropical food drinks. The West Indian Medical Journal. 2005;**54**:3-8

[100] Bhagya D, Gopan S. Effects of coconut neera (*Cocos nucifera* L.) on blood pressure among hypertensive adult women. International Journal of Applied and Pure Science and Agriculture. 2016;**2**:1-7

[101] Ikrama EHK, Stanley R, Netzel M, Fanning K. Phytochemicals of papaya and its traditional health and culinary uses – A review. Journal of Food Composition and Analysis. 2015;**4**:201-211

[102] Khanna N, Panda PC. The effect of papain on tenderization and functional properties of spent hen meat cuts. Indian Journal of Animal Research. 2007;**41**:55-58

[103] Huet J, Looze Y, Bartik K, Raussens V, Wintjens R, Boussard P. Structural characterization of the papaya cysteine proteinases at low pH. Biochemical and Biophysical Research Communications. 2006;**341**:620-626

[104] Fukal L, Kas J. The role of active and inactivated papain in beer chillproofing. Journal of the Institute of Brewing. 1984;**90**:247-249

[105] Sivarajah N. Medicinal uses of *Carica papaya*. Int. Journal of Scientific Research. 2017;**6**:2770-2772

[106] Eno AE, Owo OI, Itam EH, Konya RS. Blood pressure depression by the fruit juice of *Carica papaya* (L.) in renal and DOCA-induced hypertension in the rat. Phytotherapy Research. 2000;**14**:235-239

[107] Wilson RK, Kwan TK, Kwan CY, Sorger GJ. Effects of papaya seed extract and benzyl isothiocyanate on vascular contraction. Life Sciences. 2002;**71**:497-507

[108] Runnie I, Salleh MN, Mohamed S, Head RJ, Abeywardena MY. Vasorelaxation induced by common edible tropical plant extracts in isolated rat aorta and mesenteric vascular bed. Journal of Ethnopharmacology. 2004;**92**:311-316

[109] Sripanidkulchai B, Wongpanich V, Laupattarakasem P, Suwansaksri J, Jirakulsomchok D. Diuretic effects of selected Thai indigenous medicinal plants in rats. Journal of Ethnopharmacology. 2001;**75**:185-190

[110] Saboo SS, Thorat PK, Tapadiya GG, Khadabadi SS. Ancient and recent medicinal uses of Cucurbitaceae family. International Journal of Therapeutic Applications. 2013;**9**:11-19

[111] Mukherjee PK, Nema NK, Maity N, Sarkar BK. Phytochemical and therapeutic potential of cucumber. Fitoterapia. 2013;**84**:227-236. DOI: 10.1016/j.fitote.2012.10.003

[112] Sahu T, Sahu J. *Cucumis sativus* (cucumber): A review on its pharmacological activity. Journal of Applied Pharmaceutical Research. 2015;**3**:4-9

[113] Lu G, Yuan WX, Fan YJ. Clinical and experimental study of tablet cucumber vine compound in treating essential hypertension. Zhong Xi Yi Jie He Za Zhi. 1991;**11**:274-276

[114] Pertami SB. Budiono, Rahayu DYS. Effect of cucumber (*Cucumis sativus*) juice on lowering blood pressure in elderly. Public Health of Indonesia. 2017;**3**:30-36

[115] Palanisamy V, Shanmugam S, Balakrishnan S. Evaluation of diuretic activity of polyherbal formulation. International Journal of Pharmaceutics. 2015;**5**:244-247

[116] Singh RC, Sisodia CS. Pharmacodynamic investigations into the diuretic activity of *Cucumis melo* seed (ether extract). The Indian Journal of Medical Research. 1970; **58**:505-512

[117] Naik VR, Agshikar NV, Abraham GJ. *Cucumis trigonus* Roxb. II. Diuretic activity. Journal of Ethnopharmacology. 1981;**3**:15-19

[118] Adjanohoun E. Contribution to ethnobotanical and floristic studies in the People's Republic of Congo. Traditional Medicine and Pharmacopoeia. 1988;**3**(Suppl):428

[119] Rastogi S, Pandey MM, Rawat AKS. An ethnomedicinal, phytochemical and pharmacological profile of *Desmodium gangeticum* (L.) DC. And *Desmodium adscendens* (Sw.) DC. Journal of Ethnopharmacology. 2011;**136**:283-296. DOI: 10.1016/j.jep.2011.04.031

[120] Muanda FN, Bouayed J, Djilani A, Yao C, Soulimani R, Dicko A. Chemical composition and, cellular evaluation of the antioxidant activity of *Desmodium adscendens* leaves. Evidence-based Complementary and Alternative Medicine. 2011;**2011**:620862. DOI: 10.1155/2011/620862

[121] Addy ME, Burka JF. Effects of *Desmodium adscendens* fractions on antigen-and arachidonic acid-induced contractions of guinea pig airways. Canadian Journal of Physiology and Pharmacology. 1988;**66**:820-825

[122] Addy ME. Several chromatographically distinct fractions of *Desmodium adscendens* inhibit smooth muscle contractions. International Journal of Crude Drug Research. 1989;**27**:81-91

[123] Hussain H, Hussain J, Al Harrasi A, Krohn K. The chemistry and biology of bicoumarins. Tetrahedron. 2012;**68**:2553-2578. DOI: 10.1016/j.tet.2012.01.035

[124] Boniface PK, Baptista Ferreira S, Roland Kaiser C. Current state of knowledge on the traditional uses, phytochemistry, and pharmacology of the genus *Hymenaea*. Journal of Ethnopharmacology. 2017;**206**:193-223. DOI: 10.1016/j.jep.2017.05.024

[125] Nogueira RT, Shepherd GJ, Laverde A, Marsaioli AJ, Imamura PM. Clerodane-type diterpenes from the seed pods of *Hymenaea courbaril* var. *stilbocarpa*. Phytochemistry. 2001;**58**:1153-1157

[126] Bezerra GP, Góis RW, de Brito TS, de Lima FJ, Bandeira MA, Romero NR, et al. Phytochemical study guided by the myorelaxant activity of the crude extract, fractions and constituent from stem bark of *Hymenaea courbaril* L. Journal of Ethnopharmacology. 2013;**149**:62-69. DOI: 10.1016/j.jep.2013.05.052

[127] Zandi K, Teoh B, Sam S, Wong P, Mustafa MR, AbuBakar S. *vitro* antiviral activity of fisetin, rutin and naringenin against dengue virus type-2. Journal of Medicinal Plants Research. 2011;**5**:5534-5539

[128] De Caluw E, Halamov K, van Damme P. *Tamarindus indica* L.: A review of traditional uses, phytochemistry and pharmacology. Afrika Focus. 2010;**23**:53-83

[129] Bagul M, Sonawane SK, Arya SS. Tamarind seeds: Chemistry, technology, applications and health benefits: A review. Indian Food Industry Mag. 2015;**34**:28-35

[130] Bhadoriya SS, Mishra V, Raut S, Ganeshpurkar A, Jain SK. Anti-inflammatory and antinociceptive activities of a hydroethanolic extract of *Tamarindus indica* leaves. Scientia Pharmaceutica. 2012;**80**:685-700

[131] Sole SS, Srinivasan BP. Aqueous extract of tamarind seeds selectively increases glucose transporter-2, glucose transporter-4, and islets' intracellular calcium levels and stimulates β-cell proliferation resulting in improved glucose homeostasis in rats with streptozotocin-induced diabetes mellitus. Nutrition Research. 2012;**32**:626-636. DOI: 10.1016/j.nutres.2012.06.015

[132] Iftekhar AS, Rayhan I, Quadir MA, Akhteruzzaman S, Hasnat A. Effect of *Tamarindus indica* fruits on blood pressure and lipid-profile in human model: An *in vivo* approach. Pakistan Journal of Pharmaceutical Sciences. 2006;**19**:125-129

[133] Lim CY, Junit SM, Abdulla MA, Aziz AA. *In vivo* biochemical and gene expression analyses of the antioxidant activities and hypocholesterolaemic properties of *Tamarindus indica* fruit pulp extract. PLoS One. 2013;**8**:e70058. DOI: 10.1371/journal.pone.0070058

[134] Martinello F, Soares SM, Franco JJ, Santos AC, Sugohara A, Garcia SB, et al. Hypolipemic and antioxidant activities from *Tamarindus indica* L. pulp fruit extract in hypercholesterolemic hamsters. Food and Chemical Toxicology. 2006;**44**:810-818

[135] Dreher ML, Davenport AJ. Hass avocado composition and potential health effects. Critical Reviews in Food Science and Nutrition. 2013;**53**:738-750. DOI: 10.1080/10408398.2011.556759

[136] Swisher HE. Avocado oil: From food use to skin care. J. Amer oil. Chemical Society. 1988;**65**:1704-1706

[137] Karou SD, Tchacondo T, Djikpo Tchibozo MA, Abdoul-Rahaman S, Anani K, Koudouvo K, et al. Ethnobotanical study of medicinal plants used in the management of diabetes mellitus and hypertension in the central region of Togo. Pharmaceutical Biology. 2011;**49**:1286-1297. DOI: 10.3109/13880209.2011.621959

[138] Gbolade A. Ethnobotanical study of plants used in treating hypertension in Edo state of Nigeria. Journal of Ethnopharmacology. 2012;**144**:1-10. DOI: 10.1016/j.jep.2012.07.018

[139] Anita BS, Okokon JE, Okon PA. Hypoglycemic activity of aqueous *Persea americana* mill. Indian Journal of Pharmacology. 2005;**37**:325-326. DOI: 10.4103/0253-7613.16858

[140] Yasir M, Das S, Kharya MD. The phytochemical and pharmacological profile of *Persea americana* mill. Pharmacognosy Reviews. 2010;**4**:77-84. DOI: 10.4103/0973-7847.65332

[141] Ojewole JA, Kamadyaapa DR, Gondwe MM, Moodley K, Musabayane CT. Cardiovascular effects of *Persea americana* mill (Lauraceae) (avocado) aqueous leaf extract in experimental animals. Cardiovascular Journal of Africa. 2007;**18**:69-76

[142] Adeboye JO, Fajonyomi MO, Makinde JM, Taiwo OB. A preliminary study on the hypotensive activity of *Persea americana* leaf extracts in anaesthetized normotensive rats. Fitoterapia. 1999;**70**:15-20. DOI: 10.1016/S0367-326X(98)00015-X

[143] Anaka ON, Ozolua RI, Okpo SO. Effect of the aqueous seed extract of *Persea americana* mill. (Lauraceae) on the blood pressure of Sprague-Dawley rats. African Journal of Pharmacy and Pharmacology. 2009;**3**:485-490

[144] Owolabi MA, Jaja SI, Coker HA. Vasorelaxant action of aqueous extract of the leaves of *Persea americana* on isolated thoracic rat aorta. Fitoterapia. 2005;**76**:567-573

[145] Odubanjo VO, Oboh G, Makinde OA. Inhibitory effect of aqueuos extracts of avocado pear (*Persea americana*) leaf and seed on angiotensin 1-converting enzyme: a

possible means in treating/managing hypertension. Journal of Applied Life Sciences International. 2016;**4**:1-9. DOI: 10.9734/JALSI/2016/21605

[146] Nwaoguikpe RN, Braide W. The effect of aqueous seed extract of *Persea americana* (avocado pear) on serum lipid and cholesterol levels in rabbits. African Journal of Pharmacy and Pharmacological Research. 2011;**1**:23-29

[147] Pieterse Z, Jerling JC, Oosthuizen W, Kruger HS, Hanekom SM, Smuts CM, et al. Substitution of high monounsaturated fatty acid avocado for mixed dietary fats during an energy-restricted diet: Effects on weight loss, serum lipids, fibrinogen, and vascular function. Nutrition. 2005;**21**:67-75

[148] Riello G. Cotton: The Fabric that Made the Modern World. Cambridge: Cambridge University Press; 2013

[149] Coutinho EM. Gossypol: A contraceptive for men. Contraception. 2002;**65**:259-263

[150] Muhammad Z, Masanawa AA, Pyeng AK. Phytochemical and mineral analysis of methanolic extract of *Gossypium barbadense* L. (cotton leaves). Annals of Experimental Biology. 2014;**2**:11-15

[151] Cecilia EO, Olalekan EO, Oluwafemi B, Tolulope OM. Possible *in vitro* antioxidant potential of *Gossypium barbadense* leaf aqueous extract and its effect on lipid profile and liver enzymes of albino rats. Research Journal of Pharmaceutical, Biological and Chemical Sciences. 2014;**5**:129-136

[152] Chaturvedi A, Nag TN. Medicinal value of cotton. International Journal of MediPharm Research. 2015;**1**:147-149

[153] Hasrat JA, Pieters L, Vlietinck AJ. Medicinal plants in Suriname: Hypotensive effect of *Gossypium barbadense*. The Journal of Pharmacy and Pharmacology. 2004;**56**:381-387

[154] Ismail A, Ikram EHK, Nazri HSM. Roselle (*Hibiscus sabdariffa* L.) seeds – nutritional composition protein quality and health benefits. Food. 2008;**2**:1-16

[155] Da-Costa-Rocha I, Bonnlaender B, Sievers H, Pischel I, Heinrich M. *Hibiscus sabdariffa* L. – A phytochemical and pharmacological review. Food Chemistry 2014;**165**:424-443. DOI: 10.1016/j.foodchem.2014.05.002

[156] Okereke CN, Iroka FC, Chukwuma MO. Phytochemical analysis and medicinal uses of *Hibiscus sabdariffa*. International Journal of Herbal Medicine. 2015;**2**:16-19

[157] Zhao Y, Wang J, Ballevre O, Luo H, Zhang W. Antihypertensive effects and mechanisms of chlorogenic acids. Hypertension Research. 2011;**35**:370-374. DOI: 10.1038/hr.2011.195

[158] Grajeda-Iglesias C, Figueroa-Espinoza MC, Barouh N, Baréa B, Fernandes A, de Freitas V, et al. Isolation and characterization of anthocyanins from *Hibiscus sabdariffa* flowers. Journal of Natural Products. 2016;**79**:1709-1718. DOI: 10.1021/acs.jnatprod.5b00958

[159] Onakpoya IJ, Spencer EA, Thompson MJ, Heneghan CJ. The effect of chlorogenic acid on blood pressure: A systematic review and meta-analysis of randomized clinical trials. Journal of Human Hypertension. 2014;**29**:77-81. DOI: 10.1038/jhh.2014.46

[160] Calderon-Montaño JM, Burgos-Moron E, Perez-Guerrero C, Lopez-Lazaro M. A review on the dietary flavonoid kaempferol. Mini Reviews in Medicinal Chemistry. 2011;**11**:298-344

[161] Alarcón-Alonso J, Zamilpa A, Aguilar FA, Herrera-Ruiz M, Tortoriello J, Jimenez-Ferrer E. Pharmacological characterization of the diuretic effect of *Hibiscus sabdariffa* Linn (Malvaceae) extract. Journal of Ethnopharmacology. 2012;**139**:751-756. DOI: 10.1016/j.jep.2011.12.005

[162] Hopkins AL, Lamm MG, Funk JL, Ritenbaugh C. *Hibiscus sabdariffa* L. in the treatment of hypertension and hyperlipidemia: A comprehensive review of animal and human studies. Fitoterapia. 2013;**85**:84-94. DOI: 10.1016/j.fitote.2013.01.003

[163] Ojeda D, Jiménez-Ferrer E, Zamilpa A, Herrera-Arellano A, Tortoriello J, Alvarez L. Inhibition of angiotensin convertin enzyme (ACE) activity by the anthocyanins delphinidin- and cyanidin-3-O-sambubiosides from *Hibiscus sabdariffa*. Journal of Ethnopharmacology. 2010;**127**:7-10. DOI: 10.1016/j.jep.2009.09.059

[164] Jiménez-Ferrer E, Alarcón-Alonso J, Aguilar-Rojas A, Zamilpa A, Jiménez-Ferrer CI, Tortoriello J, et al. Diuretic effect of compounds from *Hibiscus sabdariffa* by modulation of the aldosterone activity. Planta Medica. 2012;**78**:1893-1898. DOI: 10.1055/s-0032-1327864

[165] Ngamjarus C, Pattanittum P, Somboonporn C. Roselle for hypertension in adults. Cochrane Database of Systematic Reviews. 2010;**1**:CD007894. DOI: 10.1002/14651858.CD007894.pub2

[166] Wahabi HA, Alansary LA, Al-Sabban AH, Glasziuo P. The effectiveness of *Hibiscus sabdariffa* in the treatment of hypertension: A systematic review. Phytomedicine. 2010;**17**:83-86. DOI: 10.1016/j.phymed.2009.09.002

[167] Djibril D, Mamadou F, Gérard V, Geuye MDC, Oumar S, Rigal L. Physical characteristics, chemical composition and distribution of constituents of the neem seeds (*Azadirachta indica* A. Juss) collected in Senegal. Research Journal of Chemical Sciences. 2015;**5**:52-58

[168] Lokanadhan S, Muthukrishnan P, Jeyaraman S. Neem products and their agricultural applications. Journal of Biopesticides. 2012;**5**(Suppl):72-76

[169] Mak-Mensah EE, Firempong CK. Chemical characteristics of toilet soap prepared from neem (*Azadirachta indica* A. Juss) seed oil. Asian Journal of Plant Science & Research. 2011;**1**:1-7

[170] Kumar VS, Navaratnam V. Neem (*Azadirachta indica*): Prehistory to contemporary medicinal uses to humankind. Asian Pacific Journal of Tropical Biomedicine. 2013;**3**:505-514. DOI: 10.1016/S2221-1691(13)60105-7

[171] Alzohairy MA. Therapeutics role of *Azadirachta indica* (neem) and their active constituents in diseases prevention and treatment. Evidence-based Complementary and Alternative Medicine. 2016;**2016**:7382506. DOI: 10.1155/2016/7382506

[172] Shori AB, Baba AS. Antioxidant activity and inhibition of key enzymes linked to type-2 diabetes and hypertension by *Azadirachta indica*-yogurt. Journal of Saudi Chemical Society. 2013;**17**:295-301

[173] Koley KM, Lal J. Pharmacological effects of *Azadirachta indica* (neem) leaf extract on the ECG and blood pressure of rat. Indian Journal of Physiology and Pharmacology. 1994;**38**:223-225

[174] Obiefuna I, Young R. Concurrent administration of aqueous *Azadirachta indica* (neem) leaf extract with DOCA-salt prevents the development of hypertension and accompanying electrocardiogram changes in the rat. Phytotherapy Research. 2005;**19**:792-795

[175] Shah AJ, Gilani AH, Hanif HM, Ahmad S, Khalid S, Bukhari IA. Neem (*Azadirachta indica*) lowers blood pressure through a combination of Ca^{++} channel blocking and endothelium-dependent muscarinic receptors activation. International Journal of Pharmacology. 2014;**10**:418-428

[176] De Lima G, de Almeida ME, Dos Santos LL. Physicochemical characteristics of bilimbi (*Averrhoa bilimbi*). Revista Brasileira de Fruticultura 2011;**23**:421-423

[177] Bakul G, Unni VN, Seethaleksmy NV, Mathew A, Rajesh R, Kurien G, et al. Acute oxalate nephropathy due to '*Averrhoa bilimbi*' fruit juice ingestion. Indian Journal of Nephrology. 2013;**23**:297-300. DOI: 10.4103/0971-4065.114481

[178] Alsarhan AN, Sultana N, Kadir MR, Aburjai T. Ethnopharmacological survey of medicinal plants in Malaysia, the Kangkar Pulai region. International Journal of Pharmacology. 2012;**8**:679-686. DOI: 10.3923/ijp.2012.679.686

[179] Alhassan AM, Ahmed QU. *Averrhoa bilimbi*Linn.: A review of its ethnomedicinal uses, phytochemistry, and pharmacology. Journal of Pharmacy & Bioallied Sciences. 2016;**8**:265-271. DOI: 10.4103/0975-7406.199342

[180] Bipat R, Toelsie JR, Joemmanbaks RF, Gummels JM, Klaverweide J, Jhanjan N, et al. Effects of plants popularly used against hypertension on norepinephrine-stimulated guinea pig atria. Pharmacognosy Magazine. 2008;**4**:12-19

[181] Winarti C, Marwati T. Effect of bilimbi leaf extracts on decrease blood pressure. Jurnal Pascapanen Pertanian. 2009;**6**:54-61

[182] Muthia R, Suganda AG, Sukandar EY. Angiotensin-1-converting enzyme (ACE) inhibitory activity of several Indonesian medicinal plants. Research Journal of Pharmaceutical, Biological and Chemical Sciences. 2017;**8**(Suppl.):192-199

[183] Mans DRA. From forest to pharmacy: Plant-based traditional medicines as sources for novel therapeutic compounds Academia Journal of Medicinal Plants 2013;**1**:101-110. DOI: http://dx.doi.org/10.15413/ajmp.2013.0117

Permissions

All chapters in this book were first published in HM, by InTech Open; hereby published with permission under the Creative Commons Attribution License or equivalent. Every chapter published in this book has been scrutinized by our experts. Their significance has been extensively debated. The topics covered herein carry significant findings which will fuel the growth of the discipline. They may even be implemented as practical applications or may be referred to as a beginning point for another development.

The contributors of this book come from diverse backgrounds, making this book a truly international effort. This book will bring forth new frontiers with its revolutionizing research information and detailed analysis of the nascent developments around the world.

We would like to thank all the contributing authors for lending their expertise to make the book truly unique. They have played a crucial role in the development of this book. Without their invaluable contributions this book wouldn't have been possible. They have made vital efforts to compile up to date information on the varied aspects of this subject to make this book a valuable addition to the collection of many professionals and students.

This book was conceptualized with the vision of imparting up-to-date information and advanced data in this field. To ensure the same, a matchless editorial board was set up. Every individual on the board went through rigorous rounds of assessment to prove their worth. After which they invested a large part of their time researching and compiling the most relevant data for our readers.

The editorial board has been involved in producing this book since its inception. They have spent rigorous hours researching and exploring the diverse topics which have resulted in the successful publishing of this book. They have passed on their knowledge of decades through this book. To expedite this challenging task, the publisher supported the team at every step. A small team of assistant editors was also appointed to further simplify the editing procedure and attain best results for the readers.

Apart from the editorial board, the designing team has also invested a significant amount of their time in understanding the subject and creating the most relevant covers. They scrutinized every image to scout for the most suitable representation of the subject and create an appropriate cover for the book.

The publishing team has been an ardent support to the editorial, designing and production team. Their endless efforts to recruit the best for this project, has resulted in the accomplishment of this book. They are a veteran in the field of academics and their pool of knowledge is as vast as their experience in printing. Their expertise and guidance has proved useful at every step. Their uncompromising quality standards have made this book an exceptional effort. Their encouragement from time to time has been an inspiration for everyone.

The publisher and the editorial board hope that this book will prove to be a valuable piece of knowledge for researchers, students, practitioners and scholars across the globe.

List of Contributors

Elisabetta Carata and Bernardetta Anna Tenuzzo
Department of Biological and Environmental Science and Technology, Lecce, Italy

Luciana Dini
Department of Biological and Environmental Science and Technology, Lecce, Italy
CNR-Nanotech Centro Ecotekne, Lecce, Italy

Ezekwesili-Ofili Josephine Ozioma and Okaka Antoinette Nwamaka Chinwe
Department of Applied Biochemistry, Nnamdi Azikiwe University, Awka, Nigeria

Merlin L.K. Mensah
Department of Herbal Medicine, Faculty of Pharmacy and Pharmaceutical Sciences, Kwame Nkrumah University of Science and Technology, Kumasi, Ghana

Gustav Komlaga and Rita A. Dickson
Department of Pharmacognosy, Faculty of Pharmacy and Pharmaceutical Sciences, Kwame Nkrumah University of Science and Technology, Kumasi, Ghana

Arnold D. Forkuo
Department of Pharmacology, Faculty of Pharmacy and Pharmaceutical Sciences, Kwame Nkrumah University of Science and Technology, Kumasi, Ghana

Caleb Firempong
Departments of Biochemistry and Biotechnology, Faculty of Science, Kwame Nkrumah University of Science and Technology, Kumasi, Ghana

Alexander K. Anning
Department of Theoretical and Applied Biology, Faculty of Science, Kwame Nkrumah University of Science and Technology, Kumasi, Ghana

María Eugenia Martínez Valenzuela and Rolando Chamy Maggi
Escuela de Ingeniería Bioquímica, Facultad de Ingeniería, Pontificia Universidad Católica de Valparaíso, Valparaíso, Chile

Katy Díaz Peralta
Departamento de Química, Universidad Técnico Federico Santa María, Valparaíso, Chile

Lorena Jorquera Martínez
Escuela de Ingeniería en Construcción, Facultad de Ingeniería, Pontificia Universidad Católica de Valparaíso, Valparaíso, Chile

Preethi Vidya Udagama and Vindya Udalamaththa
Department of Zoology and Environment Sciences, Faculty of Science, University of Colombo, Colombo, Sri Lanka

Tariku Laelago
Hossana College of Health Sciences, Hossana, Ethiopia

Nontokozo Z. Msomi and Mthokozisi B.C. Simelane
Department of Biochemistry, School of Life Science, University of KwaZulu-Natal, Pietermaritzburg, South Africa

Tina Maver
Faculty of Mechanical Engineering, Laboratory for Characterisation and Processing of Polymers, University of Maribor, Maribor, Slovenia

Manja Kurečič and Karin Stana Kleinschek
Faculty of Mechanical Engineering, Laboratory for Characterisation and Processing of Polymers, University of Maribor, Maribor, Slovenia
Institute for Chemistry and Technology of Materials, Graz University of Technology, Graz, Austria

Dragica Maja Smrke
University Medical Centre Ljubljana, Ljubljana, Slovenia

Uroš Maver
Faculty of Medicine, Institute of Biomedical Sciences and Institute for Palliative Medicine and Care, University of Maribor, Maribor, Slovenia
Faculty of Medicine, Department of Pharmacology, University of Maribor, Maribor, Slovenia

Rehab A. Hussein and Amira A. El-Anssary
Pharmacognosy Department, Pharmaceutical Science Division, National Research Center, Giza, Egypt

Matteo Radice
Department of Earth Sciences, Universidad Estatal Amazónica, Puyo, Pastaza, Ecuador

Piergiacomo Buso and Anna Baldisserotto
Department of Life Sciences and Biotechnology, Master Course in Cosmetic Science and Technology, University of Ferrara, Ferrara, Italy

Stefano Manfredini and Silvia Vertuani
Department of Life Sciences and Biotechnology, Master Course in Cosmetic Science and Technology, University of Ferrara, Ferrara, Italy
Ambrosialab Srl, Ferrara, Italy

Dennis R.A. Mans
Department of Pharmacology, Faculty of Medical Sciences, Anton de Kom University of Suriname, Paramaribo, Suriname

Angela Grant
National Herbarium of Suriname, Anton de Kom University of Suriname, Paramaribo, Suriname

Nicholaas Pinas
Clinical Laboratory, Diakonessenhuis, Paramaribo, Suriname

Index

www.ingramcontent.com/pod-product-compliance
Lightning Source LLC
LaVergne TN
LVHW080946210926
848485LV00004B/788